Nutrition to Improve Pregnancy and Childbirth

Nutrition to Improve Pregnancy and Childbirth

Editor: Jena Lin

AMERICAN
MEDICAL PUBLISHERS
www.americanmedicalpublishers.com

AMERICAN
MEDICAL PUBLISHERS
www.americanmedicalpublishers.com

Cataloging-in-Publication Data

Nutrition to improve pregnancy and childbirth / edited by Jena Lin.
p. cm.
Includes bibliographical references and index.
ISBN 978-1-63927-763-6
1. Pregnancy--Nutritional aspects. 2. Prenatal care. 3. Pregnancy. 4. Nutrition--Requirements.
5. Childbirth--Nutritional aspects. I. Lin, Jena.
RG559 .N883 2023
618.24--dc23

American Medical Publishers,
41 Flatbush Avenue,
1st Floor, New York,
NY 11217, USA

ISBN 978-1-63927-763-6 (Hardback)

Contents

Preface

I am honored to present to you this unique book which encompasses the most up-to-date data in the field. I was extremely pleased to get this opportunity of editing the work of experts from across the globe. I have also written papers in this field and researched the various aspects revolving around the progress of the discipline. I have tried to unify my knowledge along with that of stalwarts from every corner of the world, to produce a text which not only benefits the readers but also facilitates the growth of the field.

Nutrition is the physiological and biochemical process used by an organism in order to sustain life. It involves absorption, ingestion, assimilation, catabolism, biosynthesis and excretion. Nutrition in pregnancy is significant for the healthy growth of the fetus. The nutrition required during pregnancy differs from non-pregnant condition. During pregnancy, energy requirements are high and there is also requirement of particular micronutrients. Folic acid, folate and DHA omega 3 are important substances which a woman should consume in adequate amounts during pregnancy. These are also important while nursing to support the health and well-being of the infant. Various micronutrients such as iron, vitamin D, calcium and vitamin E are recommended during this period. Certain foods such as deli meats and unpasteurized dairy should be avoided as they might contain parasites and bacteria, which can result in illness. The topics covered in this extensive book deal with the core aspects of nutrition and its importance in pregnancy and childbirth. It is appropriate for students seeking detailed information in this area as well as for experts.

Finally, I would like to thank all the contributing authors for their valuable time and contributions. This book would not have been possible without their efforts. I would also like to thank my friends and family for their constant support.

Editor

1

Dietary Patterns in Pregnancy and Effects on Nutrient Intake in the Mid-South: The Conditions Affecting Neurocognitive Development and Learning in Early Childhood (CANDLE) Study

Eszter Völgyi [1], Kecia N. Carroll [2], Marion E. Hare [1,3], Karen Ringwald-Smith [4], Chandrika Piyathilake [5], Wonsuk Yoo [1] and Frances A. Tylavsky [1,*]

1 Department of Preventive Medicine, University of Tennessee Health Science Center, 66 N. Pauline, Memphis, TN 38163, USA; E-Mails: evoelgyi@uthsc.edu (E.V.); mhare@uthsc.edu (M.E.H.); wyoo1@uthsc.edu (W.Y.)

2 Department of Pediatrics, Vanderbilt University Medical Center, 2200 Children's Way, Nashville, TN 37232, USA; E-Mail: kecia.carroll@vanderbilt.edu

3 Department of Pediatrics, University of Tennessee Health Science Center, 50 N. Dunlap, Memphis, TN 38103, USA

4 St. Jude Children's Research Hospital, 262 Danny Thomas Place, Memphis, TN 38105, USA; E-Mail: karen.smith@stjude.org

5 Department of Nutrition Sciences, University of Alabama at Birmingham, 326 Webb Nutrition Sciences Building, 1675 University Blvd., AL 35294, USA; E-Mail: piyathic@uab.edu

* Author to whom correspondence should be addressed; E-Mail: ftylavsk@uthsc.edu

---

Abstract: Dietary patterns are sensitive to differences across socio-economic strata or cultural habits and may impact programing of diseases in later life. The purpose of this study was to identify distinct dietary patterns during pregnancy in the Mid-South using factor analysis. Furthermore, we aimed to analyze the differences in the food groups and in macro- and micronutrients among the different food patterns. The study was a cross-sectional analysis of 1155 pregnant women (mean age 26.5 ± 5.4 years; 62% African American, 35% Caucasian, 3% Other; and pre-pregnancy BMI 27.6 ± 7.5 kg/m^2). Using food frequency questionnaire data collected from participants in the Conditions Affecting Neurocognitive Development and Learning in Early Childhood (CANDLE) study between 16 and 28 weeks of gestation, dietary patterns were identified using factor analysis. Three major dietary patterns, namely, Healthy, Processed, and US Southern were identified among pregnant women from the Mid-South. Further analysis of the three main patterns revealed four mixed dietary patterns, *i.e.*, Healthy-Processed, Healthy-US Southern, Processed-US Southern, and overall Mixed. These dietary patterns were different ($p < 0.001$) from each other in almost all the food items, macro- and micro nutrients and aligned across socioeconomic and racial groups. Our study describes unique dietary patterns in the Mid-South, consumed by a cohort of women enrolled in a prospective study examining the association of maternal nutritional factors during pregnancy that are known to affect brain and cognitive development by age 3.

Keywords: nutrient intake; pregnancy; mixed dietary patterns; food frequency questionnaire

---

1. Introduction

Pregnancy is a time when *in utero* exposures may impact the long term programming for onset of diseases in offspring [1–3]. Dietary intake during pregnancy has the potential to influence birth outcomes [4,5] and cognitive development via gene expression [6]. As dietary habits are often cultural and influenced by the food available for consumption, understanding the characteristics of diet within a study population may provide a basis for future interventions to improve lifelong health.

Multivariate statistical methods such as factor analysis has become a well-accepted and popular method [7] to describe dietary patterns in nutritional research. Much of the work has investigated the effects of diet on the risk of adverse outcomes such as colorectal cancer [8–10], diabetes and obesity [11,12], and stroke [13]. More recently this approach has been used to characterize diet during pregnancy and relate patterns to nutrient intake, lifestyle and socio-demographic characteristics [14–16]. These efforts have provided evidence that dietary patterns may reflect differences in nutrient intake and are sensitive to differences across socio-economic strata or cultural habits.

The Conditions Affecting Neurocognitive Development and Learning in Early childhood (CANDLE) study is a prospective study that includes a cohort of mother-child dyads. Enrollment for this cohort occurs during the second trimester of pregnancy. The study's primary aim is to identify factors from *in utero* through early childhood that contribute to cognitive development by age 3. Consistent with life course theory [17] capturing dietary exposure during gestation may be critical in untangling the role of nutrition in the trajectory of early childhood cognitive development. The objectives of this study are to describe a unique process to determine dietary patterns from a food frequency questionnaire (FFQ) that are region specific for the Mid-South, and to examine how these patterns relate to socio-demographic status of the study population, and nutrients (omega 3 fatty acids, folate, pyridoxine, iron, zinc, cobalamin, choline) [18] plausibly linked to neurocognitive development.

2. Experimental Section

2.1. Study Population

Data from pregnant women who enrolled in the CANDLE study between December 2006 and July 2011 were included in this study. Inclusion criteria included being: a resident of Shelby County

Tennessee, able to speak and understand English, aged between 16 and 40 years old, and 16–28 weeks of gestation with a singleton pregnancy.

Exclusion criteria included: an existing chronic disease requiring medication (hypertension, insulin dependent or Type II diabetes mellitus, sickle cell disease or trait, renal disease, hepatitis, lupus erythematous, scleroderma, pulmonary disease, heart disease, human immunodeficiency virus); pregnancy complications including maternal red cell alloimmunization (Rh factor incompatibility permitted); prolapsed or ruptured membranes; oligohydraminios; complete placenta previa; and not intending to deliver at one of four participating hospitals. The study was conducted in accordance with the Helsinki Declaration and was approved and reviewed by the Institutional Review Board of the University of Tennessee Health Science Center. Informed consent was given by all subjects 18 years or older and assent was given by those aged 16–17.9 years with consent provided by their legally authorized representative prior to the assessments.

2.2. Demographic, Lifestyle and Socioeconomic Assessment

Research assistants collected information on family income, participant race, ethnicity, marital status, and parity and household composition through self-administered questionnaires. Pre-pregnancy body height and weight were recorded based on self report of the women. We calculated pre-pregnancy body mass index (BMI) as weight (kg) per height (m^2).

2.3. Dietary Assessment

The Block (2005) food frequency questionnaire (FFQ) was administered during the second trimester by trained research assistants to elicit usual intake of 111 food and beverage groups from the previous three months. Interviewers were trained by registered dietitians and re-certified by a registered dietician based on a taped interview every six months to obtain the frequency of intake and quantity consumed with the aid of standardized food pictures. The FFQ was processed by Nutrition Quest (Berkley, CA, USA) to yield macro and micronutrients, serving size and frequency of intake of the food items. The full Block FFQ has been shown to be a valid and reliable method to describe nutrient intake from diet for groups and rank individuals according to nutrients [19–23].

Of 1503 women who completed the enrollment visit, we excluded respondents who reported implausibly low (<1000) or high (>5000) kcal/day of total energy intake ($n = 152$). Willett [24] reports using an allowable energy range of 500–3500 for non-pregnant, non-lactating women which we adapted for the increased energy needs of pregnancy. Due to technical issues, 196 participants' FFQ data was unable to be retrieved for determining nutrient intake. The final sample size for this study was 1155.

2.4. Food Pattern Determination

Exploratory factor analysis with principal component extraction and varimax rotation method was performed on the frequency of the 111 food and beverage groups to extract the factors that make up distinct dietary patterns. To decide the number of factors to retain, we used the scree plot and the eigenvalues of the principal components, and subjective criteria. We tested solutions for number of models with two to five factors in order to evaluate the interpretability of the dietary patterns. Food groups with a factor loading above 0.30 were considered as the most important contributors to each factor, and were used to identify the dietary patterns. Three factors were identified in our population. These single dietary patterns were termed "Healthy", "Processed", and "US-Southern" based on the food groups that loaded for each of the three factors. For each participant, a factor score in the respective single dietary pattern was estimated as a sum of the daily frequency of intake of each food group multiplied by the loading score for the food group. Theoretically the food groups with high daily intake and high factor loading contributed most to the individual's score in the respective single dietary pattern.

Because the total explained variance of the three single dietary patterns was 15.4%, we explored the use of rank percentiles in order to combine the three major dietary factors, as done elsewhere [16]. After carefully evaluating the factor scores, combined food patterns were created based on the individuals' rank order in each single factor. Five quintiles were created in each factor based on the individual's factor scores. (1) Single food patterns (Healthy, Processed, and US Southern dietary patterns) were created if the woman was at least two quintiles higher in one factor than in the other two single dietary factors. (2) A combined dietary pattern was assigned if the individual was at least two quintiles higher in two single dietary patterns than in the third factor. In this way, combined dietary patterns were created as Healthy-Processed (H-P), Healthy-US Southern (H-S), and Processed-US Southern (P-S). (3) If the study participant had less than two quintiles difference between all three single dietary patterns, she was classified with the overall Mixed dietary pattern. As a result, women were grouped into seven mutually exclusive dietary patterns (Healthy, Processed, US Southern, H-P, H-S, P-S, and Mixed), reflecting their primary food choices. Initially, we separated dairy products, salad dressing, and some meat products into low fat and high fat groups. Differential consumption of these foods did not seem to have effect on factor loadings; therefore, we kept low and high fat items in one group.

2.5. Statistical Analysis

All continuous data were checked for normality by Shapiro-Wilk's W test and for homogeneity by Levene's test before each analysis. Descriptive results are reported as mean ± SE. Body mass index for adults was classified as underweight (<18.5 kg/m^2), normal (18.5–24.9 kg/m^2), overweight (25–29.9 kg/m^2), and obese (≥30.0 kg/m^2). Median test and Kruskal-Wallis ANOVA were used to describe the differences in the demographics and food items among the dietary patterns. Analysis of covariance (ANCOVA) with daily energy intake (kcal/day) as a covariate was used to describe the differences in the macro- and micronutrients among the dietary patterns. The *post-hoc* group differences were evaluated using a Tukey adjustment for multiple comparisons. Multiple regression analysis was performed to describe the explained variance in the macro- and micronutrients by the energy adjusted dietary patterns. All analyses were performed using Statistica v10 (StatSoft Inc., Tulsa, OK, USA) and JMP v9.0 (SAS Institute, Cary, NC, USA). A *p*-value of less than 0.05 was considered statistically significant.

3. Results

3.1. Description of the Study Participants

Overall, the mean age of the study population was 26.5 ± 5.4 years (range 16 to 40 years). One third of the women in the study population were obese (30%) and one quarter were overweight (24%) before their pregnancies. The women were predominantly African-American (AA) (62%) and 54% of the total sample had a high school degree or less. The number of individuals living in the household ranged from 2 to 11 with the average household size of 4.3 persons, and 37% were single (data not shown).

3.2. Dietary Patterns

Factor loadings of the food items for each of the single dietary patterns that had a minimum of 0.30 factor loading are presented in Table 1. The Healthy dietary pattern was characterized by high factor loadings of vegetables, fruits, non-fried fish and chicken, and water. The Processed dietary pattern represents those who consume primarily processed meat, fast food items (items typically obtained from Western-style fast food restaurants), snacks, sweets, and soft drinks. The US Southern pattern was characterized by the typical US Southern foods such as eggs, cooked cereals, peaches, corn, fried fish, beans, greens, cabbage, sweet potatoes, liver, pig's feet, neck bones oxtails, and tongue, pork, and real fruit juices.

Our statistical approach resulted in 135 (12%) women categorized as Healthy; 98 (8%) as Processed; 120 (10%) as US Southern; 136 (12%) as P-S; 123 (11%) as H-P; 98 (8%) as H-S; and 445 (39%) as Mixed (Table 2). The seven dietary patterns reflect differences in the daily frequency of intakes for the 62 food and beverage groups that loaded from factor analyses from ($p < 0.001$). There were no differences in foods that were commonly consumed by all participants such as cold cereal and milk on cereal and for foods consumed relatively infrequently by only a few participants (menudo, oysters and diet shakes). Overall the daily frequency of the food and beverage items/groups reflects the influence of the respective single pattern when combining the single diet pattern scores. The overall Mixed dietary pattern obtained from the Healthy, Processed and US Southern reflect foods from all of the single, *i.e.*, H-P pattern represents primarily healthy foods but contains some pertinent processed foods. The largest group of mixed patterns contained pertinent food items from all single diet patterns. There were no food items that distinguished it from the three single and three combined dietary patterns. The contribution of the food items from the single diet patterns' (Healthy, US Southern, Processed) to the mixed groups (H-S, H-P, S-P) could be considered as positive influences (fruits, nuts, seeds, vegetables) or negative influences (salty snacks, higher fat items) on the nutrient density of the diets. For example, in the H-S group there was a slightly higher intake of yogurt than those who reported a "pure US Southern diet", which has positive influences on calcium and the B complex nutrients. On the other hand, in the H-S group, there was a mildly negative influence of salty snacks that could increase a lower nutrient dense diet. Of the 62 food groups that loaded on the three main groups, there were increases in daily frequency for 39 "healthy" foods that would boost the nutrient density of the diet (62%) and a negative influence on nutrient density from 6 (10%) "less healthy foods" for those in the H-S pattern (Table 2). In contrast the mixed groups that had combined with the Processed group, showed a 25% increase in "negative nutrient dense foods" and 32% increase in nutrient dense foods for the H-P pattern and only a 20% increase in positive nutrient dense foods for those consuming a P-S pattern. From regression analyses the energy adjusted dietary patterns explained 90% of the variance in total fat intake, 84% for protein, 89% for carbohydrate. Regression analyses also showed the energy adjusted dietary patterns explained 62% of the variance for omega3, 65% for sugar, 62% for fiber, 75% for iron, 76% for zinc, 65% for B_6, 51% for B_{12}, 59% for folate, 78% for thiamine, 76% for niacin, 74% for riboflavin, 73% for total choline and 78% for free choline. The explained variances are based on the R^2 of the regression model.

Table 1. Factor loadings of food and beverage items/groups in the three main factors.

Food Item (Variance Explained)	**Healthy (5.8%)**	**Processed (5.1%)**	**US Southern (4.4%)**
BREAKFAST ITEMS			
Eggs			**0.344**
Breakfast sausage including in sandwiches/biscuits		**0.301**	**0.311**
Bacon			**0.367**
Cooked cereals (oatmeal, grits, cream of wheat)			**0.320**
Breakfast or cereal bars	**0.308**		
DAIRY			
Yogurt, including frozen	**0.434**		
Cheese, sliced or spreads		**0.332**	
Milk as a beverage	**0.303**		
FRUITS			
Banana	**0.334**		
Apples or pears	**0.355**		
Peaches or nectarines, fresh			**0.352**
Canned fruit			**0.374**
Strawberries or other berries in season	**0.383**		
VEGETABLES			
Broccoli	**0.331**		**0.312**
Carrots or mixed vegetables with carrots	**0.471**		
Corn			**0.316**
Green beans or green peas			**0.407**
Spinach, cooked	**0.370**		
Greens (collards, turnip, or mustard)			**0.517**
Sweet potatoes, yams			**0.360**
Fried potatoes (French fries, home fries, hash browns)		**0.563**	

Table 1. *Cont.*

Cole slaw, cabbage, Chinese cabbage			**0.444**
Green salad, lettuce salad	**0.600**		
Tomatoes, raw	**0.524**		
Other vegetables (squash, cauliflower, okra, peppers)	**0.547**		
Pinto, black or baked beans, chili with beans	**0.304**		
Vegetable, vegetable-beef or tomato soup	**0.337**		
BREADS			
Sandwich buns		**0.469**	
Bagels, English muffins, dinner rolls	**0.339**		
Cornbread, corn muffins, hush puppies			**0.380**
Sliced bread (white, dark, whole wheat)		**0.310**	
CONDIMENTS			
Salad dressing, regular or low fat	**0.541**		
Mayonnaise, sandwich breads		**0.372**	
Ketchup, salsa or chili peppers		**0.450**	
Mustard, barbecue sauce, soy sauce, gravy *etc.*		**0.322**	
SWEETS AND SNACKS			
Donuts		**0.304**	
Cake, snack cakes, cupcakes, Ho-Hos, pastries		**0.437**	
Cookies		**0.407**	
Chocolate candy		**0.392**	
Candy, hard, skittles, starburst *etc.*		**0.358**	
Snack chips like potato chips, tortilla chips, Fritos, Doritos, popcorn		**0.552**	
MEAT, FISH, POULTRY, MEAT SUBSTITUTES			
Pizza		**0.328**	
Meat substitutes (veggie burgers, chicken, hot dogs or lunch meats)	**0.346**		
Hamburgers or cheese burgers		**0.504**	

Table 1. *Cont.*

Hot dogs or sausage (Polish, Italian or chorizo)		**0.342**	
Lunch meats (turkey or regular)		**0.393**	
Tacos, burritos, enchiladas, tamales with meat or chicken		**0.306**	
Ribs, spareribs			**0.373**
Liver (chicken livers or liverwurst)			**0.319**
Pigs feet, neck bones, oxtails, tongue			**0.419**
Beef or pork dishes (beef stew, pot pie, hamburger helper)			**0.319**
Fried chicken (nuggets, wings or patties)		**0.497**	
Roasted or broiled chicken or turkey	**0.354**		
Fried fish or fish sandwich			**0.378**
Fish not fried	**0.435**		
Peanut Butter	**0.378**		
Peanuts, sunflower seeds, or other nuts and seeds	**0.348**		
BEVERAGES			
100% orange or grapefruit juice			**0.310**
Hi-C, Cranberry Juice Cocktail, Hawaiian Punch, Tang		**0.309**	
Kool-aid, lemonade, sports drinks, or fruit flavored drinks		**0.356**	
Soft drinks (Coke, Sprite, Orange) regular or diet		**0.377**	
Water tap or bottled	**0.320**		

Only those food items are presented that had a minimum of 0.30 factor loading.

In a supplementary table, all food and beverage items' factor loadings are available for each main factor (Supplementary Table S1).

Table 2. Average monthly frequency of intake of food groups in the seven dietary patterns [1].

Food Groups	Healthy (n = 135)	Processed (n = 98)	Southern (n = 120)	H-P (n = 123)	H-S (n = 98)	P-S (n = 136)	Mixed (n = 445)
BREAKFAST ITEMS							
Eggs	4.4 ± 0.6	4.6 ± 0.7	7.2 ± 0.6	4.3 ± 0.6	10 ± 0.7	7.9 ± 0.6	5.7 ± 0.3
Breakfast sausage including in sandwiches/biscuits	0.8 ± 0.5	4.9 ± 0.6	5.8 ± 0.5	3.0 ± 0.5	3.3 ± 0.6	9.7 ± 0.5	4.0 ± 0.3
Bacon	1.7 ± 0.6	5.5 ± 0.6	7.4 ± 0.6	2.9 ± 0.6	5.2 ± 0.6	8.5 ± 0.5	4.5 ± 0.3
Cooked cereals (oatmeal, grits, cream of wheat)	5.2 ± 0.7	2.8 ± 0.8	7.5 ± 0.7	3.1 ± 0.7	11.0 ± 0.8	5.2 ± 0.7	5.1 ± 0.4
Breakfast or cereal bars	6.6 ± 0.6	2.4 ± 0.7	2.8 ± 0.6	7.0 ± 0.6	4.9 ± 0.7	1.8 ± 0.6	4.6 ± 0.3
DAIRY							
Yogurt, including frozen	11.1 ± 0.7	2.0 ± 0.8	3.5 ± 0.7	7.2 ± 0.7	9.6 ± 0.8	2.8 ± 0.7	5.6 ± 0.4
Cheese, sliced or spreads	16.3 ± 0.8	18.9 ± 1.0	10.7 ± 0.9	21.2 ± 0.9	13.9 ± 1.0	15.5 ± 0.8	15.5 ± 0.5
Milk as a beverage	16.7 ± 1.0	6.9 ± 1.2	8.7 ± 1.1	14.7 ± 1.1	14.7 ± 1.2	7.2 ± 1.0	12.0 ± 0.6
FRUITS							
Banana	9.7 ± 0.7	3.7 ± 0.8	6.2 ± 0.8	6.8 ± 0.7	11.2 ± 0.8	5.4 ± 0.7	6.6 ± 0.4
Apples or pears	11.1 ± 0.7	3.2 ± 0.8	7.4 ± 0.8	6.2 ± 0.7	13.7 ± 0.8	7.2 ± 0.7	7.3 ± 0.4
Canned fruit	2.5 ± 0.3	5.0 ± 0.8	7.9 ± 0.8	4.3 ± 0.6	8.8 ± 1.0	7.7 ± 0.8	6.1 ± 0.4
Peaches or nectarines, fresh	2.3 ± 0.5	1.3 ± 0.6	5.0 ± 0.5	1.9 ± 0.5	7.4 ± 0.6	3.5 ± 0.5	3.2 ± 0.3
Strawberries or other berries in season	9.2 ± 0.6	2.8 ± 0.7	4.7 ± 0.7	6.3 ± 0.7	9.8 ± 0.7	3.9 ± 0.6	5.9 ± 0.3
VEGETABLES							
Broccoli	4.3 ± 0.5	1.9 ± 0.6	4.2 ± 0.5	3.8 ± 0.5	8.6 ± 0.6	3.7 ± 0.5	4.1 ± 0.3
Carrots or mixed vegetables with carrots	6.6 ± 0.5	1.3 ± 0.6	2.4 ± 0.5	4.5 ± 0.5	7.5 ± 0.6	2.0 ± 0.5	3.7 ± 0.3
Corn	3.4 ± 0.5	3.2 ± 0.5	4.9 ± 0.5	5.0 ± 0.5	6.8 ± 0.5	4.9 ± 0.5	5.0 ± 0.3
Green beans or green peas	5.1 ± 0.5	3.6 ± 0.6	6.5 ± 0.5	5.5 ± 0.5	10.2 ± 0.6	5.6 ± 0.5	6.3 ± 0.3
Spinach, cooked	2.6 ± 0.3	0.6 ± 0.4	1.3 ± 0.3	1.9 ± 0.3	4.5 ± 0.4	0.6 ± 0.3	1.2 ± 0.2
Greens (collards, turnip, or mustard)	0.6 ± 0.3	1.0 ± 0.4	3.3 ± 0.4	0.9 ± 0.3	4.8 ± 0.4	3.1 ± 0.3	2.3 ± 0.2
Sweet potatoes, yams	1.4 ± 0.2	0.8 ± 0.3	1.8 ± 0.2	0.8 ± 0.2	3.3 ± 0.3	1.4 ± 0.2	1.3 ± 0.1
Fried potatoes (French fries, home fries, hash browns)	3.0 ± 0.6	13.1 ± 0.7	4.6 ± 0.6	8.9 ± 0.6	4.0 ± 0.7	11.7 ± 0.6	7.6 ± 0.3
Cole slaw, cabbage, Chinese cabbage	1.00 ± 0.2	0.7 ± 0.3	2.0 ± 0.3	0.8 ± 0.3	4.1 ± 0.3	1.7 ± 0.2	1.6 ± 0.1
Green salad, lettuce salad	13.20 ± 0.6	3.9 ± 0.7	5.0 ± 0.6	10.4 ± 0.6	12.1 ± 0.7	3.5 ± 0.6	7.6 ± 0.3

Table 2. *Cont.*

Tomatoes, raw	10.40 ± 0.6	2.6 ± 0.7	2.2 ± 0.6	9.7 ± 0.6	7.5 ± 0.7	2.2 ± 0.6	5.3 ± 0.3
Other vegetables (squash, cauliflower, okra, peppers)	7.00 ± 0.4	0.7 ± 0.5	1.4 ± 0.5	5.1 ± 0.5	8.4 ± 0.5	1.0 ± 0.4	2.7 ± 0.2
Pinto, black or baked beans, chili with beans	3.30 ± 0.3	1.6 ± 0.3	1.3 ± 0.3	2.9 ± 0.3	2.3 ± 0.3	1.6 ± 0.3	2.2 ± 0.1
Vegetable, vegetable-beef or tomato soup	2.1 ± 0.2	0.6 ± 0.3	1.2 ± 0.2	1.2 ± 0.2	2.3 ± 0.3	0.7 ± 0.2	1.5 ± 0.1
BREADS							
Sandwich buns	3.0 ± 0.5	9.4 ± 0.5	3.1 ± 0.5	7.1 ± 0.5	2.5 ± 0.5	6.6 ± 0.5	5.5 ± 0.3
Bagels, English muffins, dinner rolls	4.8 ± 0.4	2.2 ± 0.5	1.6 ± 0.5	6.1 ± 0.5	3.6 ± 0.5	1.9 ± 0.4	3.7 ± 0.2
Cornbread, corn muffins, hush puppies	0.6 ± 0.3	2.0 ± 0.4	2.1 ± 0.3	1.1 ± 0.3	2.3 ± 0.4	3.8 ± 0.3	2.5 ± 0.2
Sliced bread (white, dark, whole wheat)	12.6 ± 0.8	15.8 ± 1.0	8.3 ± 0.9	16.2 ± 0.9	11.1 ± 1	11.2 ± 0.8	12.2 ± 0.5
CONDIMENTS							
Salad dressing, regular or low fat	12.1 ± 0.6	4.9 ± 0.7	5.2 ± 0.7	10.7 ± 0.7	11.9 ± 0.7	4.4 ± 0.6	8.5 ± 0.3
Mayonnaise, sandwich breads	3.3 ± 0.6	9.8 ± 0.7	3.5 ± 0.7	6.9 ± 0.6	4 ± 0.7	8.7 ± 0.6	6.1 ± 0.3
Ketchup, salsa or chili peppers	6.3 ± 0.6	11.9 ± 0.7	3.4 ± 0.7	11 ± 0.6	3.7 ± 0.7	9 ± 0.6	6.7 ± 0.3
Mustard, barbecue sauce, soy sauce, gravy, *etc.*	6.3 ± 0.6	8.5 ± 0.7	3.3 ± 0.6	9.3 ± 0.6	5.5 ± 0.7	6.4 ± 0.6	6.0 ± 0.3
SWEETS AND SNACKS							
Donuts	0.7 ± 0.2	1.2 ± 0.2	0.4 ± 0.2	1.6 ± 0.2	0.4 ± 0.2	1.5 ± 0.2	1.1 ± 0.1
Cake, snack cakes, cupcakes, Ho-Hos, pastries	1.8 ± 0.5	8.2 ± 0.5	1.5 ± 0.5	4.6 ± 0.5	1.3 ± 0.5	5.3 ± 0.5	2.9 ± 0.3
Cookies	3.6 ± 0.5	5.5 ± 0.5	1.5 ± 0.5	7.1 ± 0.5	1.7 ± 0.5	4.0 ± 0.5	3.7 ± 0.3
Chocolate candy	4.2 ± 0.6	9.6 ± 0.7	1.3 ± 0.6	8.2 ± 0.6	1.9 ± 0.7	5.5 ± 0.6	4.3 ± 0.3
Candy, hard, skittles, starburst, *etc.*	2.3 ± 0.6	6.6 ± 0.6	2.4 ± 0.6	4.8 ± 0.6	2.4 ± 0.6	6.1 ± 0.6	4.3 ± 0.3
Snack chips like potato chips, tortilla chips, Fritos, Doritos, popcorn	6.3 ± 0.7	17.9 ± 0.8	4.5 ± 0.7	12.1 ± 0.7	5.2 ± 0.8	14.6 ± 0.7	8.7 ± 0.4
MEAT, FISH, POULTRY, MEAT SUSTITUTES							
Pizza	2.7 ± 0.4	5.2 ± 0.4	2.7 ± 0.4	4.6 ± 0.4	2.4 ± 0.4	5.5 ± 0.4	3.7 ± 0.2
Meat substitutes (veggie burgers, chicken, hot dogs or lunch meats)	1.7 ± 0.2	0.0 ± 0.2	0 ± 0.2	0.8 ± 0.2	0.5 ± 0.2	0.0 ± 0.2	0.2 ± 0.1
Hamburgers or cheese burgers	1.7 ± 0.4	9.0 ± 0.5	3.2 ± 0.4	4.6 ± 0.4	2 ± 0.5	7.9 ± 0.4	4.2 ± 0.2
Hot dogs or sausage (Polish, Italian or chorizo)	0.8 ± 0.3	3.9 ± 0.4	2.6 ± 0.4	2.0 ± 0.4	1.9 ± 0.4	5.8 ± 0.3	2.6 ± 0.2
Lunch meats (turkey or regular)	4.8 ± 0.6	9.5 ± 0.7	4.1 ± 0.6	7.8 ± 0.6	4.6 ± 0.7	9.0 ± 0.6	6.2 ± 0.3
Tacos, burritos, enchiladas, tamales with meat or chicken	2.2 ± 0.3	3.8 ± 0.3	1.8 ± 0.3	3.8 ± 0.3	1.8 ± 0.3	3.4 ± 0.3	2.7 ± 0.2
Ribs, spareribs	0.2 ± 0.1	0.5 ± 0.1	0.6 ± 0.1	0.2 ± 0.1	0.5 ± 0.1	1.2 ± 0.1	0.6 ± 0.1

Table 2. *Cont.*

Liver (chicken livers or liverwurst)	0.1 ± 0.1	0.1 ± 0.1	0.2 ± 0.1	0.0 ± 0.1	0.7 ± 0.1	0.3 ± 0.1	0.2 ± 0.1
Pig's feet, neck bones, oxtails, tongue	0.0 ± 0.1	0.2 ± 0.1	0.4 ± 0.1	0.0 ± 0.1	0.2 ± 0.1	0.8 ± 0.1	0.2 ± 0.1
Beef or pork dishes (beef stew, pot pie, hamburger helper)	0.6 ± 0.1	1.5 ± 0.2	1.8 ± 0.2	0.8 ± 0.2	1 ± 0.2	2.7 ± 0.2	1.3 ± 0.1
Fried chicken (nuggets, wings or patties)	1.2 ± 0.5	8.2 ± 0.6	4.4 ± 0.5	3.9 ± 0.5	3.0 ± 0.6	9.5 ± 0.5	5.1 ± 0.3
Roasted or broiled chicken or turkey	5.2 ± 0.4	2.6 ± 0.5	2.1 ± 0.4	4.5 ± 0.4	5.9 ± 0.5	2.4 ± 0.4	3.9 ± 0.2
Fried fish or fish sandwich	0.3 ± 0.2	1.1 ± 0.2	1.6 ± 0.2	0.6 ± 0.2	1.2 ± 0.2	2.4 ± 0.2	1.4 ± 0.1
Fish not fried	2.5 ± 0.2	0.3 ± 0.2	0.4 ± 0.2	1.6 ± 0.2	1.7 ± 0.2	0.3 ± 0.2	0.8 ± 0.1
Peanut Butter	6.7 ± 0.5	2.4 ± 0.6	1.9 ± 0.6	8.6 ± 0.6	4.8 ± 0.6	2.0 ± 0.5	4.1 ± 0.3
Peanuts, sunflower seeds, or other nuts and seeds	5.5 ± 0.4	0.9 ± 0.5	1.5 ± 0.5	3.7 ± 0.4	4.3 ± 0.5	1.3 ± 0.4	2.3 ± 0.2
BEVERAGES							
100% orange or grapefruit juice	5.4 ± 0.8	8.3 ± 0.9	9.4 ± 0.8	8.3 ± 0.8	12.5 ± 0.9	10.5 ± 0.8	9.4 ± 0.4
Hi-C, Cranberry Juice Cocktail, Hawaiian Punch, Tang	0.8 ± 0.6	6.6 ± 0.8	5.5 ± 0.7	2.6 ± 0.7	3.3 ± 0.8	9.2 ± 0.6	4.7 ± 0.4
Kool-aid, lemonade, sports drinks, or fruit flavored drinks	3.4 ± 0.7	10.9 ± 0.9	5.8 ± 0.8	5.6 ± 0.8	3.5 ± 0.9	12.8 ± 0.7	6.7 ± 0.4
Soft drinks (Coke, Sprite, Orange) regular or diet	5.9 ± 0.8	17.4 ± 0.9	2.7 ± 0.8	12.6 ± 0.8	2.5 ± 0.9	11.0 ± 0.8	7.5 ± 0.4
Water tap or bottled	29.9 ± 0.6	23 ± 0.7	25.3 ± 0.7	28.8 ± 0.7	29 ± 0.7	21.6 ± 0.6	26.9 ± 0.3
Coffee, regular or decaffeinated	9.7 ± 0.6	1.7 ± 0.7	0.4 ± 0.7	7.4 ± 0.7	1.2 ± 0.7	0.7 ± 0.6	2.0 ± 0.3

H-P, Healthy-Processed pattern; H-S, Healthy-US Southern pattern; P-S, Processed-US Southern pattern.

[1] All values represent means ± SE; ANOVA conducted to examine differences across the seven dietary patterns for each food item showed differences at $p < 0.001$.

3.3. Characteristics of Participants

The characteristics of the study participants according by dietary patterns appear in Table 3. Compared to the US Southern, Processed or Mixed dietary patterns women with the Healthy dietary pattern were more likely to be older ($p < 0.0001$), have a higher level of education ($p < 0.0001$), less likely to be single mothers ($p < 0.0001$), and less likely to be obese prior to pregnancy ($p = 0.0044$). The diet patterns aligned across race categories (Figure 1). Healthy and H-P patterns were consumed more by Caucasians and women in the "other" race category (Asians, American Indians, Alaska Native, Native Hawaiian, other Pacific Islander). In contrast, African Americans disproportionately were the highest consumers of the Processed, US Southern, P-S, and H-S dietary patterns. There were no significant differences in ethnicity, household size, and parity among the dietary patterns.

The differences in mean daily macronutrient and energy adjusted mean daily micronutrient intakes among the dietary patterns appear in Table 4. Energy intake and all macro- and micronutrient intake differed among the dietary patterns ($p < 0.001$). The lowest consumption of energy adjusted nutrients was mirrored by low consumption of fruits and vegetables. The Processed and the P-S patterns had the highest energy intakes, and the Healthy and the US Southern had the lowest. The Healthy, US Southern and H-S patterns had the lowest fat and total sugar intake and highest protein intake while Processed and P-S the highest fat and sugar intake and the lowest protein intake. Regarding carbohydrate intake, there was little difference between patterns, with a significant difference found only between the Healthy and the P-S patterns ($p = 0.011$), where the Healthy group had the highest, and P-S had the lowest intake. The Healthy, H-P and H-S diets were the highest in fiber, while the Processed and P-S were the lowest. Cholesterol intake was high in the US Southern patterns and low in the Healthy and Processed patterns. The vitamin, mineral, and trace element intake was the highest in the US Southern and H-S and lowest in the Processed dietary patterns.

Table 3. Basic characteristics of the study participants by dietary patterns.

Variable	Healthy	Processed	US Southern	H-P	H-S	P-S	Mixed	p [1]
N	135	98	120	123	98	136	445	
Age, y (mean ± SE)	30.3 ± 0.38	24.1 ± 0.49	25.2 ± 0.52	28.5 ± 4.95	27.7 ± 0.74	23.4 ± 0.40	26.2 ± 0.24	<0.0001
Height, cm (mean ± SE)	166 ± 0.64	163 ± 0.79	163 ± 0.65	164 ± 0.67	166 ± 0.74	163 ± 0.59	164 ± 0.24	0.0009
Pre-pregnancy weight, kg (mean ± SE)	68.3 ± 1.40	75.1 ± 2.35	78.1 ± 2.45	72.4 ± 1.69	77.5 ± 2.10	71.9 ± 1.82	76.2 ± 0.99	0.0005
Race, *n* (%)								
Caucasian	121 (90)	19 (19)	8 (7)	97 (79)	13 (13)	3 (2)	140 (32)	<0.001
African American	7 (5)	79 (81)	110 (92)	24 (20)	74 (76)	131 (98)	294 (66)	
Other	7 (5)	0 (0)	2 (2)	2 (2)	11 (11)	0 (0)	9 (2)	
Ethnicity, *n* (%)								
Hispanic	3 (2)	0 (0)	1 (1)	4 (3)	2 (2)	1 (1)	15 (3)	0.2424
Non-Hispanic	132 (98)	97 (100)	119 (99)	117 (97)	95 (98)	133 (99)	425 (97)	
Pre-pregnancy BMI [2], *n* (%)								
Underweight	7 (5)	3 (3)	5 (4)	1 (1)	3 (3)	9 (7)	19 (4)	0.0044
Normal	83 (61)	38 (39)	48 (40)	64 (52)	37 (38)	55 (40)	146 (33)	
Overweight	19 (14)	25 (25)	17 (14)	28 (23)	23 (23)	36 (26)	134 (30)	
Obese	26 (19)	32 (33)	47 (39)	30 (24)	35 (36)	36 (26)	145 (33)	
Parity, *n* (%)								
Primipara	66 (49)	44 (45)	57 (48)	49 (40)	37 (38)	47 (65)	189 (42)	0.2051
Multipara	69 (51)	54 (55)	63 (53)	74 (60)	61 (62)	89 (35)	256 (58)	
Education, *n* (%)								
Less than high school	0 (0)	16 (16)	16 (13)	3 (2)	7 (7)	29 (21)	37 (8)	<0.0001
High school or GED	23 (17)	55 (56)	62 (52)	37 (30)	41 (42)	80 (59)	216 (49)	
Technical school	8 (6)	10 (10)	12 (10)	9 (7)	11 (11)	17 (13)	49 (11)	
College or professional	102 (77)	17 (17)	30 (25)	74 (60)	39 (40)	9 (7)	143 (32)	

Table 3. *Cont.*

Marital Status, *n* (%)								
Single	5 (4)	53 (54)	71 (59)	12 (10)	39 (40)	84 (62)	160 (36)	<0.0001
Co-habitation	127 (95)	43 (44)	45 (38)	110 (90)	54 (54)	48 (35)	272 (61)	
Do not know	2 (1)	2 (2)	4 (3)	0 (0)	4 (4)	4 (3)	12 (3)	
Household size, (mean ± SE)	3.9 ± 0.1	4.7 ± 0.2	4.4 ± 1.2	4.1 ± 0.1	4.2 ± 0.2	4.6 ± 0.2	4.3 ± 0.1	0.0188
Insurance, *n* (%)								
Medicaid (Tenncare)	17 (13)	69 (70)	78 (65)	31 (25)	50 (51)	118 (87)	246 (55)	<0.0001
Other	117 (87)	28 (29)	39 (33)	92 (75)	44 (45)	17 (13)	188 (42)	
Missing	1 (0)	1 (1)	3 (2)	0 (0)	4 (4)	1 (0)	11 (3)	

H-P, Healthy-Processed pattern; H-S, Healthy-US Southern pattern; P-S, Processed-US Southern pattern. The numbers do not always add up because of rounding errors.

[1] To test the significant differences, Kruskal-Wallis ANOVA and median test were performed.

[2] Based on the categories established by the Institute of Medicine [25] for adults and based on age specific cut offs between age 16 and 18 years [26,27].

Figure 1. Distribution of dietary patterns during pregnancy in the Conditions Affecting Neurocognitive Development and Learning in Early Childhood (CANDLE) Cohort by race. (**a**) African American; (**b**) Caucasian; (**c**) Other.

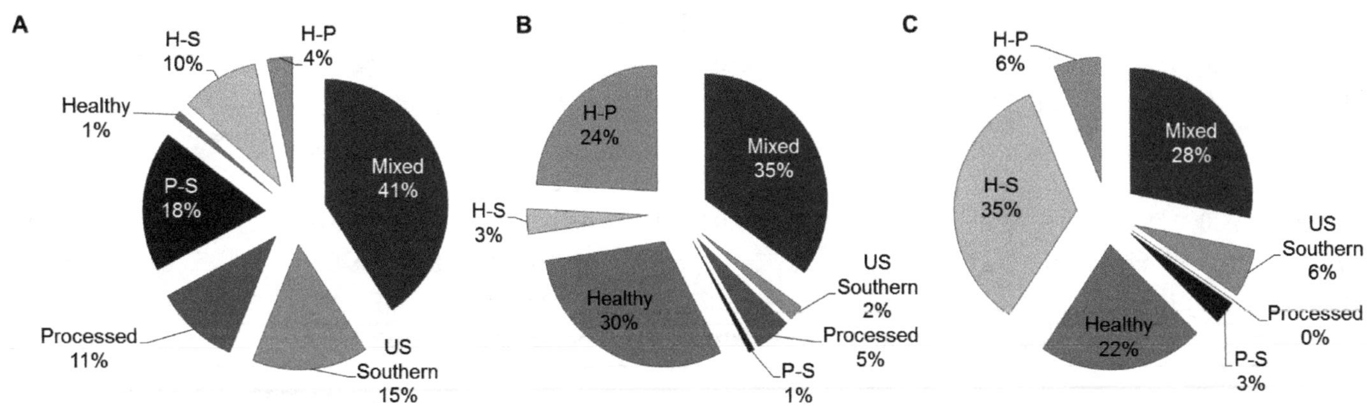

Table 4. Daily intake of total energy, macro- and energy adjusted micronutrients in the seven dietary patterns.

Nutrient	Healthy (n = 135)	Processed (n = 98)	Southern (n = 120)	H-P (n = 123)	H-S (n = 98)	P-S (n = 136)	Mixed (n = 445)	ANCOVA [1] p
Energy (kcal/day)	1801 ± 73.4 ^{a}	2958 ± 86.2 ^{b}	1887 ± 77.9 ^{a}	2579 ± 76.9 ^{c}	2347 ± 86.2 ^{c}	3081 ± 73.2 ^{b}	2360 ± 40.5 ^{c}	<0.0001
Fat (% of E)	34.3 ± 0.43	37.6 ± 0.50	36.3 ± 0.46	36.6 ± 0.45	35.8 ± 0.50	37.9 ± 0.43	36.3 ± 0.24	<0.0001
Protein (% of E)	16.5 ± 0.20	13.5 ± 0.24	14.8 ± 0.21	14.9 ± 0.21	15.9 ± 0.24	14.2 ± 0.20	14.9 ± 0.11	<0.0001
Carbohydrate (% of E)	52.0 ± 0.56	50.4 ± 0.66	50.9 ± 0.59	50.5 ± 0.59	50.7 ± 0.66	49.2 ± 0.56	50.7 ± 0.31	0.0351
Saturated fat (g)	30.1 ± 0.50	33.6 ± 0.59	32.5 ± 0.53	32.2 ± 0.51	29.9 ± 0.58	34.0 ± 0.51	32.0 ± 0.27	<0.0001
Omega 3 fatty acids (g)	2.17 ± 0.05 ^{b}	1.75 ± 0.06 ^{c}	2.09 ± 0.06 ^{b}	2.08 ± 0.05 ^{b}	2.44 ± 0.06 ^{a}	1.82 ± 0.05 ^{c}	2.10 ± 0.03 ^{b}	<0.0001
Total Sugar (g)	10.6 ± 0.64	21.7 ± 0.75	13.2 ± 0.68	16.5 ± 0.67	8.60 ± 0.75	19.4 ± 0.64	15.2 ± 0.35	<0.0001
Fiber (g)	27.4 ± 0.48	15.4 ± 0.55	20.8 ± 0.50	22.3 ± 0.49	26.0 ± 0.54	15.2 ± 0.48	20.5 ± 0.26	<0.0001
Fe (mg)	19.2 ± 0.32 ^{a,b}	15.6 ± 0.37 ^{d}	17.6 ± 0.34 ^{c}	17.9 ± 0.33 ^{b,c}	19.5 ± 0.37 ^{a}	16.1 ± 0.32 ^{d}	17.7 ± 0.17 ^{c}	<0.0001
Zn (mg)	14.3 ± 0.23	12.2 ± 0.26	12.9 ± 0.24	13.3 ± 0.23	13.5 ± 0.26	12.5 ± 0.23	13.2 ± 0.12	<0.0001
Vit B6 (mg)	2.69 ± 0.05 ^{a}	1.93 ± 0.06 ^{c}	2.37 ± 0.05 ^{b}	2.40 ± 0.05 ^{b}	2.72 ± 0.06 ^{a}	2.03 ± 0.05 ^{c}	2.33 ± 0.03 ^{b}	<0.0001
Vit B12 (µg)	6.54 ± 0.20 ^{ah}	5.00 ± 0.23 ^{d}	6.01 ± 0.20 ^{a,b,c}	5.64 ± 0.20 ^{c,d}	6.69 ± 0.22 ^{a}	5.76 ± 0.20 ^{b,c,d}	6.03 ± 0.10 ^{a,b,c}	<0.0001
Folate (µg)	777 ± 17.0	544 ± 19.7	656 ± 17.9	715 ± 17.4	775 ± 19.4	559 ± 17.1	671 ± 9.11	<0.0001
Thiamine (mg)	2.09 ± 0.03 ^{a}	1.62 ± 0.04 ^{d}	1.95 ± 0.03 ^{b}	1.89 ± 0.03 ^{b,c}	2.10 ± 0.04 ^{a}	1.76 ± 0.03 ^{c,d}	1.91 ± 0.02 ^{b}	<0.0001
Niacin (mg)	27.4 ± 0.45 ^{a}	23.0 ± 0.53 ^{d}	24.7 ± 0.48 ^{c,d}	25.8 ± 0.46 ^{a,b,c}	27.1 ± 0.52 ^{a,b}	24.0 ± 0.46 ^{c,d}	25.5 ± 0.24 ^{b,c}	<0.0001
Riboflavin (mg)	2.77 ± 0.04 ^{a}	2.00 ± 0.05 ^{d}	2.40 ± 0.05 ^{c}	2.46 ± 0.04 ^{b,c}	2.65 ± 0.05 ^{a,b}	2.11 ± 0.04 ^{d}	2.42 ± 0.02 ^{c}	<0.0001
Total Choline (mg)	386 ± 7.08 ^{b}	272 ± 8.22 ^{f}	377 ± 7.44 ^{b,c}	334 ± 7.23 ^{d,e}	435 ± 8.08 ^{a}	328 ± 7.11 ^{e}	354 ± 3.79 ^{c,d}	<0.0001
Free Choline (mg)	98.3 ± 1.33 ^{a}	63.8 ± 1.54 ^{d}	79.5 ± 1.39 ^{c}	88.2 ± 1.35 ^{b}	94.0 ± 1.51 ^{a,b}	65.9 ± 1.33 ^{d}	81.9 ± 0.71 ^{c}	<0.0001

H-P, Healthy-Processed pattern; H-S, Healthy-US Southern pattern; P-S, Processed-US Southern pattern. Results are given as mean ± SE.

[1] Covariate: Energy intake (kcal/day).

[a,b,c,d,e,f] Means that do not share the same superscript are significantly different from each other.

4. Discussion

Three major dietary patterns, namely Healthy, Processed and US Southern were identified among pregnant women from the Mid-South using factor analysis. Combining the factor scores with quintile rankings of the factors we developed seven distinct mutually exclusive dietary patterns. This is the first study that examined dietary patterns within a geographical region that includes a diverse socioeconomic sample from the US. These dietary patterns were different ($p < 0.001$) from each other in almost all the food items, macro- and micro nutrients and aligned across socioeconomic and racial groups.

Dietary patterns are known to vary with age, gender, economics, and cultural habits [28]. Residents of Shelby County Tennessee reflect a diverse population that includes a preponderance of African-Americans across a wide range of incomes. The CANDLE study has enrolled participants reflective of the birth mothers of Shelby County Tennessee, thus diet characterization must be sensitive to the different segments of the population. Our approach to identifying dietary patterns appears to have been successful in identifying various segments of our study population based on race, income, and education. While this report is not unique with regard to dietary patterns [15] as they relate to segments of the population, it did identify types and combinations of foods that have distinct differences in nutrient composition with regard to nutrients linked to neurocognitive development [18,29].

Our findings that healthy eating patterns are reflective of older and more educated individuals are in concert with other reports [14]. Our Southern diet pattern is reflective of foods traditionally ascribed to the southeastern US [30]. The identified patterns in this paper are comparable and representative of the Southern US regions that differ from the national patterns [31–33]. Substantial segments of our sample retained core southern foods while also incorporating items from the healthy and from the processed foods patterns, reflecting a wider variety of food selection that translated into different nutrient intakes. Those with the H-S dietary pattern had higher levels of omega-3 fatty acids, iron, vitamin B_6, folate, thiamine, niacin, riboflavin, total choline, and free choline than those with the pure Southern diet pattern, implying that individuals in this category capitalized on the foods with the highest nutrient density of both eating patterns. The Processed dietary pattern was characterized by a lower nutrient density and high energy content, yielding a decreased energy adjusted nutrient intake when combined with other dietary patterns. This is consistent with diets associated with food globalization, urbanization, and lower economic status [34]. The diversity of food selection among the African-American and Caucasian participants in our study underscores cultural sensitivity at the local level is important when collecting dietary information [30].

One limitation of our study was the significant amount of missing data due to technical problems and too low or high energy intake. The excluded sample consisted mainly of African American women due to the study design at recruitment. Therefore the missing sample is not representative of the overall study population presented in this paper, but after stratification, it is representative of the African American study population. Since our results show racial difference in the distribution of study participants across the dietary patterns, we think that this limitation has no significant effect on our analysis.

Statistical approaches have been well documented in establishing dietary patterns. Depicting dietary patterns using factor analyses can account for 15%–32% of the variance in dietary intake [7,15,35,36]. Explained variance in factor analysis is influenced by the amount of variables that are used in the analysis. Our result of the 15.4% is comparable with previously published literature in Mexican Americans [37], however they used 63 food items to identify dietary patterns which means potentially less variance, as the 111 items in our analysis. Most approaches are based on a 1 or 2 step process that may or may not allow for accurate calculation of total variance. However, the dietary patterns in our study accounted for 89%–90% of the variance in energy adjusted macronutrients and 50%–78% of the variance in the energy adjusted micronutrients. Thus, our patterns may be more robust in examining associations with cognitive development than single nutrients alone.

The complexity of a two-step process in assigning dietary patterns allowed us to capture mixed patterns. An individual with a high score on one factor may have another high score on another factor; therefore, the person's dietary pattern is a mixed pattern and not a pure dietary pattern of the highest score. The interpretation of these cases is analytically challenging because there are no cutoffs for these cases. Investigators using factor analysis should be cautious about this problem. To overcome this problem, we created mixed dietary patterns based on the individuals' rank orders in each factor. In this way H-P, H-S, P-S, and overall Mixed patterns were identified. The analysis of the individual food items and energy, macronutrient, and micronutrient intake of these patterns confirm that they are significantly distinct from the other main food patterns. Knudsen and colleagues [16] have used this method of analysis where they identified two factors, *i.e.*, healthy and unhealthy patterns, and then created a third, mixed dietary pattern based on quintiles of the factor scores. Two thirds of their study population belonged to this intermediate group, which is consistent with our results. We found that 70% of the participants in our study ate foods consistent with the mixed dietary pattern.

Our statistical approach was to use all 111 food groups compared to condensing the food items into smaller groups. While decreasing the number of groups may increase the variance explained by the factor analysis, it decreases the ability to identify unique dietary patterns within sub groups of the population perspective [38]. For example condensing food items to 46 groups may yield two-three factors and thus limits the description of the dietary patterns. We also examined if incorporating the fat content of food item yielded additional information pertinent to dietary patterns. In our sample, this did not yield any additional information.

The goal of determining diet patterns is often to identify combinations of foods and beverages that reflect a specific type of diet that may be beneficial or harmful to a health outcome. The strengths and limitations of classifying individuals into specific patterns are that they may reflect an overall pattern of intake that may be targeted for community interventions; however, this may not be useful in examining a specific nutrient/disease relationship. Use of the seven patterns may not be readily translated into individual diet counseling, but it does identify key foods that could be targeted for community-based interventions to improve nutrient intake. Selectively over or under reporting by individuals of various socio-demographic groups, may bias the results of a study using nutrients as the exposure [39]. Diet patterns appear to be unaffected by under reporting or the report of consuming a food item [40]. Our approach in classifying diets, clearly links consumption of more processed foods (low nutrient density) with a higher percentages of overweight and obesity, thereby suggesting that under reporting may not be a large factor in this study.

5. Conclusions

Our study is the first to provide unique dietary patterns consumed by a cohort of women living in the mid-southern US. The diet patterns reflect a gamut of food stuffs that describe the traditional southern diet in the US, a highly processed diet, a primarily healthy food and dietary pattern combinations that reflect nutrition transition. The goal of creating diet patterns for this prospective study is to use examine the association of maternal nutritional factors during pregnancy to brain and cognitive development by age 3. How the dietary patterns during pregnancy relate to the child's cognitive development or help explain epigenetic expression of disease or health condition remains to be determined. In our longitudinal study, we will investigate whether maternal nutrient intake and diet patterns during pregnancy are somewhat stable and examine the influence on early childhood development as part of the life course history.

Acknowledgments

This project was supported by The Urban Child Institute. The funding source had no role in the design, implementation or interpretation of this work or in the manuscript preparation. We gratefully acknowledge the participant recruitment and sample collection by CANDLE staff, and particularly the mothers and children who consented to participate.

References

1. Barker, D.J. The fetal origins of adult hypertension. *J. Hypertens.* **1992**, *10*, S39–S44.
2. Barker, D.J. The fetal origins of diseases of old age. *Eur. J. Clin. Nutr.* **1992**, *46*, S3–S9.
3. Barker, D.J.; Martyn, C.N. The maternal and fetal origins of cardiovascular disease. *J. Epidemiol. Community Health* **1992**, *46*, 8–11.
4. Christian, P. Micronutrients, birth weight, and survival. *Annu. Rev. Nutr.* **2010**, *30*, 83–104.
5. Haider, B.A.; Yakoob, M.Y.; Bhutta, Z.A. Effect of multiple micronutrient supplementation during pregnancy on maternal and birth outcomes. *BMC Public Health* **2011**, *11*, doi:10.1186/1471-2458-11-S3-S19.
6. Gecz, J.; Mulley, J. Genes for cognitive function: Developments on the X. *Genome Res.* **2000**, *10*, 157–163.
7. Newby, P.K.; Tucker, K.L. Empirically derived eating patterns using factor or cluster analysis: A review. *Nutr. Rev.* **2004**, *62*, 177–203.
8. Dixon, L.B.; Balder, H.F.; Virtanen, M.J.; Rashidkhani, B.; Mannisto, S.; Krogh, V.; van Den Brandt, P.A.; Hartman, A.M.; Pietinen, P.; Tan, F.; *et al.* Dietary patterns associated with colon and rectal cancer: Results from the Dietary Patterns and Cancer (DIETSCAN) Project. *Am. J. Clin. Nutr.* **2004**, *80*, 1003–1011.
9. Fung, T.; Hu, F.B.; Fuchs, C.; Giovannucci, E.; Hunter, D.J.; Stampfer, M.J.; Colditz, G.A.; Willett, W.C. Major dietary patterns and the risk of colorectal cancer in women. *Arch. Intern. Med.* **2003**, *163*, 309–314.
10. Slattery, M.L.; Boucher, K.M.; Caan, B.J.; Potter, J.D.; Ma, K.N. Eating patterns and risk of colon cancer. *Am. J. Epidemiol.* **1998**, *148*, 4–16.

11. Gittelsohn, J.; Wolever, T.M.; Harris, S.B.; Harris-Giraldo, R.; Hanley, A.J.; Zinman, B. Specific patterns of food consumption and preparation are associated with diabetes and obesity in a Native Canadian community. *J. Nutr.* **1998**, *128*, 541–547.
12. Van Dam, R.M.; Rimm, E.B.; Willett, W.C.; Stampfer, M.J.; Hu, F.B. Dietary patterns and risk for type 2 diabetes mellitus in U.S. men. *Ann. Intern. Med.* **2002**, *136*, 201–209.
13. Fung, T.T.; Stampfer, M.J.; Manson, J.E.; Rexrode, K.M.; Willett, W.C.; Hu, F.B. Prospective study of major dietary patterns and stroke risk in women. *Stroke* **2004**, *35*, 2014–2019.
14. Northstone, K.; Emmett, P.; Rogers, I. Dietary patterns in pregnancy and associations with socio-demographic and lifestyle factors. *Eur. J. Clin. Nutr.* **2008**, *62*, 471–479.
15. Northstone, K.; Emmett, P.M.; Rogers, I. Dietary patterns in pregnancy and associations with nutrient intakes. *Br. J. Nutr.* **2008**, *99*, 406–415.
16. Knudsen, V.K.; Orozova-Bekkevold, I.M.; Mikkelsen, T.B.; Wolff, S.; Olsen, S.F. Major dietary patterns in pregnancy and fetal growth. *Eur. J. Clin. Nutr.* **2008**, *62*, 463–470.
17. Elder, G.H., Jr. The life course as developmental theory. *Child Dev.* **1998**, *69*, 1–12.
18. Bourre, J.M. Effects of nutrients (in food) on the structure and function of the nervous system: Update on dietary requirements for brain. Part 1: Micronutrients. *J. Nutr. Health Aging* **2006**, *10*, 377–385.
19. Block, G.; Coyle, L.M.; Hartman, A.M.; Scoppa, S.M. Revision of dietary analysis software for the Health Habits and History Questionnaire. *Am. J. Epidemiol.* **1994**, *139*, 1190–1196.
20. Mares-Perlman, J.A.; Klein, B.E.; Klein, R.; Ritter, L.L.; Fisher, M.R.; Freudenheim, J.L. A diet history questionnaire ranks nutrient intakes in middle-aged and older men and women similarly to multiple food records. *J. Nutr.* **1993**, *123*, 489–501.
21. Johnson, B.A.; Herring, A.H.; Ibrahim, J.G.; Siega-Riz, A.M. Structured measurement error in nutritional epidemiology: Applications in the Pregnancy, Infection, and Nutrition (PIN) Study. *J. Am. Stat. Assoc.* **2007**, *102*, 856–866.
22. Subar, A.F.; Thompson, F.E.; Kipnis, V.; Midthune, D.; Hurwitz, P.; McNutt, S.; McIntosh, A.; Rosenfeld, S. Comparative validation of the Block, Willett, and National Cancer Institute food frequency questionnaires: The Eating at America's Table Study. *Am. J. Epidemiol.* **2001**, *154*, 1089–1099.
23. Block, G.; Hartman, A.M.; Dresser, C.M.; Carroll, M.D.; Gannon, J.; Gardner, L. A data-based approach to diet questionnaire design and testing. *Am. J. Epidemiol.* **1986**, *124*, 453–469.
24. Willet, W. *Nutritional Epidemiology*, 2nd ed.; Oxford University Press: New York, NY, USA, 1998.
25. IOM. *Weight Gain During Pregnancy: Reexamining the Guidelines*; The National Academies Press: Washington, DC, USA, 2009.
26. Cole, T.J.; Bellizzi, M.C.; Flegal, K.M.; Dietz, W.H. Establishing a standard definition for child overweight and obesity worldwide: International survey. *BMJ* **2000**, *320*, 1240–1243.
27. Cole, T.J.; Flegal, K.M.; Nicholls, D.; Jackson, A.A. Body mass index cut offs to define thinness in children and adolescents: International survey. *BMJ* **2007**, *335*, doi:10.1136/bmj.39238.399444.55.
28. Satia, J.A. Dietary acculturation and the nutrition transition: An overview. *Appl. Physiol. Nutr. Metab.* **2010**, *35*, 219–223.

29. Bourre, J.M. Effects of nutrients (in food) on the structure and function of the nervous system: Update on dietary requirements for brain. Part 2: Macronutrients. *J. Nutr. Health Aging* **2006**, *10*, 386–399.
30. Bovell-Benjamin, A.C.; Dawkin, N.; Pace, R.D.; Shikany, J.M. Use of focus groups to understand African-Americans' dietary practices: Implications for modifying a food frequency questionnaire. *Prev. Med.* **2009**, *48*, 549–554.
31. Smith, S.L.; Quandt, S.A.; Arcury, T.A.; Wetmore, L.K.; Bell, R.A.; Vitolins, M.Z. Aging and eating in the rural, southern United States: Beliefs about salt and its effect on health. *Soc. Sci. Med.* **2006**, *62*, 189–198.
32. Tucker, K.L.; Maras, J.; Champagne, C.; Connell, C.; Goolsby, S.; Weber, J.; Zaghloul, S.; Carithers, T.; Bogle, M.L. A regional food-frequency questionnaire for the US Mississippi Delta. *Public Health Nutr.* **2005**, *8*, 87–96.
33. Jefferson, W.K.; Zunker, C.; Feucht, J.C.; Fitzpatrick, S.L.; Greene, L.F.; Shewchuk, R.M.; Baskin, M.L.; Walton, N.W.; Phillips, B.; Ard, J.D. Use of the Nominal Group Technique (NGT) to understand the perceptions of the healthiness of foods associated with African Americans. *Eval. Program Plann.* **2010**, *33*, 343–348.
34. Popkin, B.M. Global nutrition dynamics: the world is shifting rapidly toward a diet linked with noncommunicable diseases. *Am. J. Clin. Nutr.* **2006**, *84*, 289–298.
35. Smith, A.D.; Emmett, P.M.; Newby, P.K.; Northstone, K. A comparison of dietary patterns derived by cluster and principal components analysis in a UK cohort of children. *Eur. J. Clin. Nutr.* **2011**, *65*, 1102–1109.
36. Sotres-Alvarez, D.; Herring, A.H.; Siega-Riz, A.M. Latent class analysis is useful to classify pregnant women into dietary patterns. *J. Nutr.* **2010**, *140*, 2253–2259.
37. Tseng, M.; DeVellis, R.F.; Maurer, K.R.; Khare, M.; Kohlmeier, L.; Everhart, J.E.; Sandler, R.S. Food intake patterns and gallbladder disease in Mexican Americans. *Public Health Nutr.* **2000**, *3*, 233–243.
38. Tucker, K.L. Dietary patterns, approaches, and multicultural perspective. *Appl. Physiol. Nutr. Metab.* **2010**, *35*, 211–218.
39. Bailey, R.L.; Mitchell, D.C.; Miller, C.; Smiciklas-Wright, H. Assessing the effect of underreporting energy intake on dietary patterns and weight status. *J. Am. Diet. Assoc.* **2007**, *107*, 64–71.
40. Millen, A.E.; Tooze, J.A.; Subar, A.F.; Kahle, L.L.; Schatzkin, A.; Krebs-Smith, S.M. Differences between food group reports of low-energy reporters and non-low-energy reporters on a food frequency questionnaire. *J. Am. Diet. Assoc.* **2009**, *109*, 1194–1203.

2

The Association between the Macronutrient Content of Maternal Diet and the Adequacy of Micronutrients during Pregnancy in the Women and Their Children's Health (WATCH) Study

Michelle Blumfield [1,2], Alexis Hure [3], Lesley MacDonald-Wicks [1], Roger Smith [2,3], Stephen Simpson [4], David Raubenheimer [5] and Clare Collins [1,2,*]

[1] School of Health Sciences, University of Newcastle, Callaghan, New South Wales 2308, Australia; E-Mails: Michelle.Blumfield@newcastle.edu.au (M.B.); Lesley.Wicks@newcastle.edu.au (L.M.-W.)

[2] Mothers and Babies Research Centre, Hunter Medical Research Institute, John Hunter Hospital, Level 3, Endocrinology, Locked Bag 1, Hunter Region Mail Centre, New South Wales 2310, Australia; E-Mail: Roger.Smith@newcastle.edu.au

[3] School of Medicine and Public Health, Faculty of Health, University of Newcastle, Callaghan, New South Wales 2308, Australia; E-Mail: Alexis.Hure@newcastle.edu.au

[4] School of Biological Sciences, University of Sydney, Sydney, New South Wales 2006, Australia; E-Mail: Stephen.Simpson@sydney.edu.au

[5] Institute of Natural Sciences, Massey University, Albany 0632, New Zealand; E-Mail: D.Raubenheimer@massey.ac.nz

* Author to whom correspondence should be addressed; E-Mail: Clare.Collins@newcastle.edu.au

---

Abstract: Nutrition during pregnancy can induce alterations in offspring phenotype. Maternal ratio of protein to non-protein (P:NP) energy has been linked to variations in offspring body composition and adult risk of metabolic disease. This study describes the dietary patterns of pregnant women by tertiles of the P:NP ratio and compares diet to Australian recommendations. Data are from 179 Australian women enrolled in the Women and Their Children's Health Study. Diet was assessed using a validated 74-item food frequency questionnaire. Food group servings and nutrient intakes were compared to the Australian Guide to Healthy Eating and Australian Nutrient Reference Values. Higher maternal P:NP tertile was positively associated with calcium (P = 0.003), zinc (P = 0.001) and servings of dairy ($P = 0.001$) and meat ($P = 0.001$) food groups, and inversely associated with the energy dense, nutrient poor non-core ($P = 0.003$) food group. Micronutrient intakes were optimized with intermediate protein (18%E–20%E), intermediate fat (28%E–30%E) and intermediate carbohydrate (50%E–54%E) intakes, as indicated in tertile two. Results suggest a moderate protein intake may support pregnant women to consume the largest variety of nutrients across all food groups.

Keywords: maternal; pregnancy; dietary intake; nutrition; nutrient requirements; protein

---

1. Introduction

Maternal nutrition during pregnancy can induce permanent alterations in offspring phenotype [1] and subsequently influence the risk of non-communicable diseases, such as obesity in adult life [2]. Variations in maternal macronutrient proportions have been shown to independently affect offspring outcomes, such as growth and body composition [3–7], insulin sensitivity [8], appetite [9], nutrient metabolism [9] and overall energy homeostasis [8] in both pre- and post-natal environments [10]. Effects are predicted to continue into adulthood and may have long-term consequences for the risk of metabolic disease [11].

However, the nutrient intakes required to optimize the short-term or long-term health of the offspring is undefined. Recent evidence has indicated that the ratio of protein to non-protein (P:NP) energy in the diet may play an important role in the development of obesity and subsequent non-communicable diseases [12]. This is due to regulatory mechanisms prioritizing the maintenance of an adequate protein intake level at the partial expense of carbohydrate and fat intake [12]. This phenomenon is explained by the protein leverage hypothesis [12], which may lead to overconsumption of carbohydrate coupled with increased energy intake, potentially leading to an increase in adiposity and an increased risk of obesity and metabolic disorders.

During pregnancy, protein availability is a key determinant of fetal growth [13]. Amino acids regulate pancreatic β cell differentiation, replication and insulin secretion [14]. There is currently insufficient evidence to provide a prescription for dietary protein content in pregnant women. However, studies suggest both maternal low protein [4,15–17] and high protein [3,17–19] intakes have poor outcomes for fetal body composition and metabolic health, such as restricted growth [3,17], increased adiposity [18], elevated cholesterol [4,16], elevated triglyceride [4,16] and leptin concentrations [4], impaired glucose tolerance [4,16] and insulin resistance [4,15].

We have recently shown in human pregnancy that the maternal macronutrient profile is associated with fetal adiposity and fat distribution [7]. Specifically, fetal abdominal subcutaneous fat was inversely associated with %E protein in the maternal diet, irrespective of whether fat or carbohydrate were the dilutents of protein [7]. This raises questions as to what these women were eating during pregnancy to provide these varying intakes of macronutrients.

While it is evident that macronutrients play an important function in the development of offspring adiposity, micronutrients also influence the regulation of body fat [20] and the aetiology of other health outcomes (e.g., folate and neural tube defects) [21]. However, the dietary patterns that pregnant women adopt to achieve different proportions of dietary protein and whether these eating patterns provide the essential micronutrients required for pregnancy is unclear. Therefore, the aim of this study was to: (i) describe the dietary patterns of pregnant women by tertiles of the P:NP ratio, and (ii) appraise the nutritional adequacy of eating patterns compared to Australian food group and micronutrient recommendations in order to provide evidence that may guide the development of an optimal P:NP ratio during pregnancy.

2. Experimental Section

2.1. Sample

Details of the sample have been previously described [7,22,23]. Briefly, the Women and Their Children's Health (WATCH) Study is a prospective, longitudinal cohort that was initiated in July 2006 in Newcastle, Australia [22,24]. Of the 179 women recruited, 156 women who reported usual diet during pregnancy in the WATCH Study were included in the analysis. Ethics approval for the study was obtained from the Hunter New England Human Research Ethics Committee.

Demographic and social characteristics for the WATCH Study cohort and the sub-sample of pregnant participants with dietary data have been reported elsewhere [7,23]. Compared to the Australian population, the WATCH sample used in this analysis contained a higher proportion of women with post-year 12 higher school certificate qualifications (72.9% *vs.* 52.5%), a relative advantage based on postcode using the Index of Relative Socio-economic Advantage and Disadvantage (IRSAD) scale ≥5 (70.4% *vs.* 50.0%), but a similar proportion of overweight/obesity (46.2% *vs.* 44.0%) and indigenous ethnicity (3.1% *vs.* 2.5%) [7].

2.2. Data Collection

Dietary data were collected between 18 and 24 weeks and again at 36 to 40 weeks gestation using a validated 74-item food frequency questionnaire (FFQ), the Dietary Questionnaire for Epidemiological Studies. The tool was previously validated against weighed-food records in young women [25]. The FFQ includes food and beverage data, but does not ask about vitamin and mineral supplement use. The dietary intake reference period was the previous three months. Therefore, dietary data collected between 18 to 24 weeks and 36 to 40 weeks gestation referred to a reference period of 6 to 24 weeks gestation (early pregnancy) and 24 to 40 weeks gestation (late pregnancy), respectively. Positive moderate to strong pairwise correlations have been previously reported in this sub-sample between all dietary variables in early and late pregnancy ($0.46 < r < 0.78$; $P < 0.001$) [7]. Therefore, dietary intake during pregnancy was determined by averaging the reported early and late pregnancy intake data.

Food servings per day were calculated using portion sizes described in the Australian Guide to Healthy Eating (AGHE) [26], or standard portions derived from NUTTAB 2006, a national food composition database of Australian foods [27].

Questions on maternal demographic and social data were modeled on those in the Women's Health Australia survey [28].

2.3. Australian Food and Nutrient Recommendations

Australia's national food selection guide, the AGHE [26], was designed to encourage daily consumption from each of the five core food groups of breads/cereals (grains), lean meat and substitutes (including eggs, nuts and legumes), vegetables, fruit and dairy, in proportions that are consistent with the Dietary Guidelines for Australians [29]. A non-core food group contains energy dense, nutrient poor foods that do not belong to the core groups and are recommended to be consumed in limited amounts due to their high energy density and/or minimal nutrient contribution. Recommended servings for each food group have been developed for pregnant women [26].

Specific daily nutrient intake targets to optimize health and/or avoid nutritional deficiency have been recommended in the National Health and Medical Research Council of Australia nutrient reference values (NRVs) [30]. The most appropriate NRVs for comparison with population group intakes are estimated average requirements (EAR) and adequate intake (AI) [30]. The EAR is the daily nutrient level estimated to meet the requirements of half the healthy individuals in a particular life stage and gender group, with the proportion below the EAR providing a suitable approximation of the prevalence of inadequacy [30]. When an EAR is not able to be set, an AI is used instead, this being the average daily nutrient intake level that is assumed to be adequate [30].

2.4. Statistical Analysis

To improve the validity of the dietary analyses, the energy cut-off values recommended by Meltzer *et al.* (2008) were applied by excluding those who reported daily energy intakes <4.5 or >20.0 MJ/day (n = 7) [31]. Participants that remained (n = 149) were considered to have plausible dietary data.

Participants with plausible dietary data were divided into tertiles based on their reported P:NP ratio during pregnancy. The proportion of protein to carbohydrate and fat, each expressed as a percentage of total energy, was used to create P:NP tertiles.

Main outcome measures included maternal intake of vitamins, minerals and daily servings of food group intake. Dietary intake was also analyzed to determine those meeting AGHE and NRV dietary recommendations. Data were tested for normality. Normally distributed data are reported as mean (SD) and not normally distributed data as median (IQR). Multiple comparisons for the non-parametric dietary data were performed using the Kruskal-Wallis test.

Parametric response surfaces for the median daily intake of each micronutrient were fitted over macronutrient intake arrays and then visualized by using nonparametric thin-plate splines [32]. This approach allowed the complex relationship between the response variable (each individual micronutrient) and the two major axes of % protein and % fat in the maternal diet to be visualized.

All data manipulation and statistical analyses were performed using Intercooled Stata 11.0 (Stata, College Station, TX, USA) [33]. Graphics were performed using *R* software [34]. *P*-values <0.05 were considered statistically significant.

3. Results

Maternal characteristics and pregnancy outcomes for the sub-group of women with plausible dietary data are presented in Table 1. Differences between women in the WATCH cohort with available dietary data (n = 156) and women without dietary data (n = 23) have been previously reported [7]. Briefly, women who reported dietary data were more likely to be married or in a *de facto* relationship (P = 0.03) and less likely to be at socio-economic disadvantage (P = 0.04) [7]. No significant differences were found between women with plausible (n = 149) and implausible dietary data (n = 7).

Table 2 reports the dietary composition during pregnancy for participants in the WATCH Study by tertile of the P:NP ratio. Pregnant women in the high P:NP ratio group achieved a higher P:NP ratio compared to women in the low P:NP ratio group by consuming a reduced total amount of carbohydrate and increased quantity of protein, as opposed to any changes in total fat intake (Table 2). Micronutrient intakes of calcium (P < 0.01) and zinc (P < 0.01) were positively associated with P:NP tertile, while for vitamin C (P = 0.008) and vitamin E (P = 0.003), there was a negative association with P:NP tertile (Table 2).

Table 3 reports the daily food group servings of women during pregnancy, by tertile of the P:NP ratio. Pregnant women in high P:NP ratio group reported greater median daily servings of dairy (2.1 *vs.* 1.8; P < 0.001) and meat (2.0 *vs.* 1.4; P < 0.001) and lower servings of fruit (1.7 *vs.* 2.6; P = 0.014) and extras (3.6 *vs.* 4.6; P = 0.003) compared to women in the low P:NP ratio group. While significantly lower intakes of sweet non-core foods were reported by women in the high P:NP ratio group (1.2 *vs.* 1.5; P = 0.003), lower servings of savory non-core foods (2.1 *vs.* 2.6) also contributed to the decrease in extra servings. Pregnant women in medium P:NP ratio group reported the highest intake of fruit (2.7 servings) and vegetables (2.4 servings).

Table 1. Maternal characteristics and pregnancy outcomes for the participants in the WATCH study with plausible dietary data, by tertile of the protein to non-protein ratio (n = 149) [1,2].

Characteristic	Low P:NP ratio 0.21 (0.19, 0.22) [3] n = 50	Medium P:NP ratio 0.24 (0.23, 0.25) n = 50	High P:NP ratio 0.28 (0.27, 0.30) n = 49	All women 0.24 (0.21, 0.27) n = 149
Age (year)	27.8 ± 5.2 [4]	29.6 ± 5.7	29.5 ± 5.5	29.0 ± 5.5
Height (cm)	165.0 ± 6.4	166.1 ± 6.3	163.3 ± 6.8	164.8 ± 5.6
Born in Australia [*n* (%)] [5]	49 (98.0)	45 (90.0)	45 (91.8)	139 (93.3)
Aboriginal, not Torres Strait Islander [*n* (%)]	2 (4.0)	0 (0)	3 (6.1)	5 (3.4)
Married or in *de facto* relationship [*n* (%)]	41 (82.0)	45 (90.0)	43 (87.8)	129 (86.6)
Education [*n* (%)] [6]	28 (56.0)	43 (86.0)	40 (81.6)	111 (74.5)
Socioeconomic status, IRSAD [7] decile ≤5 [*n* (%)] [8]	15 (30.0)	12 (24.0)	17 (34.7)	57 (38.3)
Smoked during pregnancy [*n* (%)]	7 (14.0)	3 (6.0)	5 (10.2)	15 (10.2)
Prepregnancy weight (kg)	64.5 (57.0, 79.0)	67.3 (56.0, 78.5)	65.0 (60.0, 80.0)	69.7 ± 17.0
Weight gain during pregnancy (kg)	12.9 ± 6.2	14.2 ± 7.8	12.6 ± 6.0	13.2 ± 6.7
Nulliparous [*n* (%)]	15 (30.0)	25 (50.0)	23 (46.9)	63 (42.3)
Preterm delivery before 37 weeks of gestation	0 (0)	7 (14.0)	6 (12.2)	13 (8.7)
Infant birthweight (g)	3608 (3185, 3910)	3575 (3100, 3980)	3420 (3049, 3718)	3500 (3100, 3820)

P:NP: protein to non-protein; [1] Plausible data is defined as energy intakes ≥4.5 and ≤20.0 MJ/d; [2] The proportion of protein to carbohydrate and fat, each expressed as a percentage of total energy, was used to create P:NP tertiles;. [3] Median: 25th and 75th percentiles in parentheses (all such values); [4] Mean ± standard deviation (all such values); [5] Other countries include England (n = 4), Belgium (n = 1), Canada (n = 1), Malaysia (n = 1), New Zealand (n = 1), Papua New Guinea (n = 1) and the United States (n = 1); [6] Maternal education level ≥ Australian year 12 high school certificate. Pregnant women in the low P:NP ratio group reported lower education compared to women in the medium P:NP ratio group (Kruskal-Wallis P = 0.005); [7] IRSAD, index of relative socioeconomic advantage and disadvantage; [8] Relative disadvantage and lack of advantage based on postcode (IRSAD decile ≤5).

Table 2. Dietary composition during pregnancy for participants in the WATCH Study with plausible dietary data, by tertile of the protein to non-protein ratio (n = 149) [1,2].

Dietary composition	Low P:NP ratio [3] 0.21 (0.19, 0.22) [4] n = 50		Medium P:NP ratio 0.24 (0.23, 0.25) n = 50		High P:NP ratio 0.28 (0.27, 0.30) n = 49		P [4]
	Median	IQR	Median	IQR	Median	IQR	
Macronutrients							
Energy (kJ)	7316.6	5994.7–9527.9	8158.6	6483.2–9624.9	7294.7	5943.9–8872.4	
Protein (%E)	16.8 [a,b]	15.9–17.2	18.8 [a,c]	18.2–19.4	21.4 [b,c]	20.7–22.5	<0.001 [a,b,c]
Total fat (%E)	37.8	35.1–40.5	37.7	35.8–40.7	37.7	35.3–40.4	
Saturated fat (%E)	16.3	14.1–18.9	16.2	13.9–17.5	15.8	13.7–18.7	
Monounsaturated fat (%E)	12.5	11.7–13.5	13.1	12.2–14.1	13.3	12.3–14.6	
Polyunsaturated fat (%E)	5.0	4.1–6.7	5.2	4.1–6.7	5.0	4.0–5.8	
Total carbohydrate (%E)	43.5 [a,b]	41.2–46.0	41.2 [a,c]	38.7–43.4	39.0 [b,c]	36.1–41.3	<0.001 [a,b], <0.01 [c]
Sugars (%E)	20.1 [a]	18.1–23.4	19.6	17.7–21.2	18.2 [a]	15.7–21.0	<0.01 [a]
Starch (%E)	23.0 [a]	20.8–25.0	21.5	20.4–23.3	20.3 [a]	18.4–21.7	<0.001 [a]
Fiber (%E)	3.7	3.2–4.5	4.3	3.7–4.9	4.0	3.4–4.4	
Cholesterol (mg)	223.0 [a]	170.9–319.8	300.5	210.3–350.2	273.1 [a]	224.0–372.2	<0.01 [a]
Vitamins							
Vitamin A (RE µg)	793.1	600.6–1025.1	860.8	707.8–1119.7	741.0	585.2–971.9	
Retinol (µg)	415.1	315.0–541.1	451.6	348.3–520.2	378.7	295.9–501.7	
β-carotene (µg)	2004.2	1454.1–2980.2	2322.1	1663.3–3254.4	2198.0	1460.1–2642.4	
Thiamin (mg)	1.6	1.3–2.0	1.7	1.3–2.2	1.5	1.2–1.9	
Riboflavin (mg)	2.4	1.9–3.1	2.6	2.1–3.6	2.5	2.1–3.2	
Niacin Equivalents (mg)	33.9	26.5–44.2	41.8	32.4–48.0	37.9	32.2–49.4	
Niacin (mg)	19.6	15.0–26.2	23.1	18.1–28.0	21.0	16.7–27.4	
Folate (µg)	279.7	205.2–356.0	298.1	243.2–355.4	244.4	205.3–350.0	
Vitamin C (mg)	161.9	90.9–207.2	153.2 [a]	116.5–190.3	105.0 [a]	81.4–166.9	<0.01 [a]
Vitamin E (mg)	6.5	4.6–8.3	6.7 [a]	5.5–8.2	5.3 [a]	4.3–7.2	<0.01 [a]

Table 2. *Cont.*

Minerals							
Calcium (mg)	867.2 [a,b]	715.9–1006.9	965.6 [a]	811.5–1305.6	1067.8 [b]	826.0–1279.6	<0.01 [a,b]
Iron (mg)	11.9	8.9–15.2	12.9	10.1–16.3	11.7	9.6–15.4	
Magnesium (mg)	259.6	202.2–322.0	291.5	240.9–361.0	272.2	218.2–356.0	
Phosphorus (mg)	1299.5	1093.0–1626.9	1588.8	1277.0–1911.0	1548.5	1254.4–1905.2	
Potassium (mg)	2586.	2026.8–3200.1	3010.9	2612.6–3505.5	2848.8	2204.8–3491.2	
Sodium (mg)	2255.9	1805.1–2868.3	2566.9	2091.6–3184.1	2404.6	2072.6–2941.5	
Zinc (mg)	9.2 [a,b]	7.6–12.7	12.2 [a]	9.3–14.3	11.1 [b]	9.9–14.8	<0.01 [a,b]

P:NP: protein to non-protein; IQR: interquartile range; %E: percentage of total energy; RE: retinol equivalents; [1] Plausible data is defined as energy intakes ≥4.5 and ≤20.0 MJ/day; [2] The proportion of protein (%E) to carbohydrate (%E) and fat (%E), was used to create P:NP tertiles; [3] Median: 25th and 75th percentiles in parentheses (all such values); [4] *P*-values were obtained using the Kruskal-Wallis test to compare all tertile groups. Differences between groups are denoted by each letter.

Table 3. Daily food group consumption during pregnancy for participants in the WATCH Study with plausible dietary data, by tertile of the protein to non-protein ratio (n = 149) [1,2].

Food group servings [3]	Recommended food group servings	Low P:NP ratio 0.21 (0.19, 0.22) [4] n = 50		Medium P:NP ratio 0.24 (0.23, 0.25) n = 50		High P:NP ratio 0.28 (0.27, 0.30) n = 49		P [5]
		Median	IQR	Median	IQR	Median	IQR	
Breads/cereals (servings/day)	4–6	2.7	2.0–3.2	2.6	2.2–3.4	2.5	1.9–2.9	
Fruit (servings/day)	4	2.6	1.4–3.3	2.7 [a]	2.0–3.5	1.7 [a]	1.0–2.8	<0.01 [a]
Vegetables (servings/day)	5–6	1.8 [a]	1.2–2.5	2.4 [a]	1.8–3.0	2.3	1.9–2.7	<0.01 [a]
Dairy (servings/day)	2	1.8 [a,b]	1.3–2.2	2.0 [a]	1.7–2.6	2.1 [b]	1.7–2.8	<0.01 [a,b]
Meat and alternatives (servings/day)	1.5	1.4 [a]	0.9–1.8	1.6	1.4–2.0	2.0 [a]	1.5–2.5	<0.001 [a]
Extras (servings/day)	0–2.5	4.6 [a]	3.6–5.8	4.3	3.1–5.6	3.6 [a]	2.6–5.5	<0.01 [a]
Sweet (servings/day)		1.5 [a]	1.1–2.1	1.2	0.7–1.8	1.2 [a]	0.6–2.0	<0.01 [a]
Savory (servings/day)		2.6	2.0–3.4	2.6	1.9–3.6	2.1	1.8–2.9	
Alcohol (servings/day)		0.02	0.0–0.05	0.03	0.0–0.11	0.03	0.0–0.18	

P:NP: protein to non-protein; IQR: interquartile range; %E: percentage of total energy; FFQ: food frequency questionnaire; [1] Plausible data is defined as energy intakes ≥4.5 and ≤20.0MJ/d; [2] The proportion of protein (%E) to carbohydrate (%E) and fat (%E), was used to create P:NP tertiles; [3] Serve size (FFQ categories) (a) Breads & Cereals: bread 60 g, cereal 40 g, cooked porridge 230 g, muesli 65 g, cooked rice/pasta/noodles (including lasagna) 180 g, dry biscuits 40 g; (b) Fruit: fruit whole (including canned fruit) 150 g, fruit juice 125 mL; (c) Vegetables: vegetable whole (including potatoes cooked without fat) 75 g; avocado 30, lettuce/endive/salad greens 36 g, tomato sauce/paste 20 g; (d) Dairy: milk 250 mL, cheese 40 g, yogurt 200 g, flavored milk 250 mL; (e) Meat & Alternatives: beef/veal/chicken/lamb/pork 85 g, fish (steamed/grilled/baked/canned) 100 g, ham 100 g, baked beans/tofu/soy beans/soy bean curd/other beans (including chickpeas, lentils, *etc.*) 80 g, nuts 40 g, eggs 100 g; (f) Extras: sweet biscuit 35 g, cakes/sweet pies/tarts/other sweet pastries 40 g, meat pies/pasties/quiche/other savory pies 60 g, pizza 60 g, hamburger 60 g, chocolate 25 g, peanut butter 25 g, potato crisps/corn chips/Twisties® 30 g, jam/marmalade/honey/syrups 45 g, Vegemite®/Marmite®/Promite® 100 g, ice-cream 50 g, bacon 50 g, corned beef/luncheon meats/salami 110 g, sausages/frankfurters 55 g, fried fish 65 g, fat spread 20 g, sugar 40 g, fries 60 g, light beer 600 mL, heavy beer 400 mL, wine (including sparkling wines) 200 mL, spirits/liqueurs 60 mL, fortified wines/port/sherry 60 mL; [4] Median; 25th and 75th percentiles in parentheses (all such values); [5] P-values were obtained using the Kruskal-Wallis test to compare all tertile groups. Differences between groups are denoted by each letter.

The percentage of NRV recommendations for vitamins and minerals that were achieved by pregnant women are summarized in Figures 1 and 2, respectively. Median daily intakes of vitamin A, thiamine, riboflavin, niacin, vitamin C, calcium, phosphorus, sodium and zinc were above 100% of the NRVs in each tertile. Magnesium and potassium intakes only achieved NRV recommendations in the medium P:NP ratio group and the medium and high P:NP ratio groups, respectively. Folate, vitamin E and iron intakes were suboptimal in all tertiles, with less than 60% of recommendations achieved for folate or iron and 75%–95% of NRVs met for vitamin E. Median daily intakes were the highest in the medium P:NP ratio group for all micronutrients, except vitamin C and calcium.

Figure 1. The percentage of Australian Nutrient Reference Value (NRV) recommendations for vitamins that were achieved during pregnancy by women in the WATCH Study who reported plausible dietary data (n = 149) by tertile of the protein to non-protein (P:NP) ratio. Plausible data is defined as energy intakes ≥4.5 and ≤20.0 MJ/day. The proportion of protein (%E) to carbohydrate (%E) and fat (%E) was used to create P:NP tertiles. The P:NP ratio for each tertile: Low P:NP ratio group 0.21 (0.19, 0.22), n = 50; Medium P:NP ratio group 0.24 (0.23, 0.25), n = 50; high P:NP ratio group 0.28 (0.27, 0.30), n = 49. Nutrient Reference Values recommended for pregnancy: Vitamin A = 550 µg, Thiamine = 1.2 mg, Riboflavin = 1.2 mg, Niacin = 14 mg NE, Folate = 520 µg, Vitamin C = 40 mg, Vitamin E = 7 mg [30]. * $P < 0.01$.

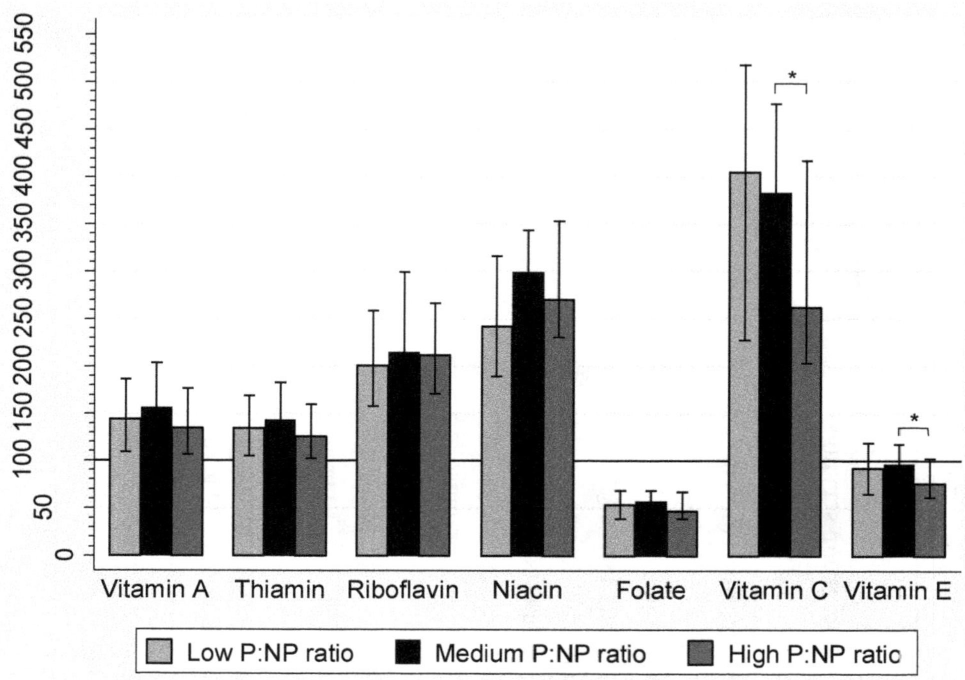

Figure 2. The percentage of Australian Nutrient Reference Value (NRV) recommendations for minerals that were achieved during pregnancy by women in the WATCH Study who reported plausible dietary data (n = 149) by tertile of the protein to non-protein (P:NP) ratio. Plausible data is defined as energy intakes ≥4.5 and ≤20.0 MJ/d. The proportion of protein (%E) to carbohydrate (%E) and fat (%E) was used to create P:NP tertiles. The P:NP ratio for each tertile: Low P:NP ratio group 0.21 (0.19, 0.22), n = 50; Medium P:NP ratio group 0.24 (0.23, 0.25), n = 50; high P:NP ratio group 0.28 (0.27, 0.30), n = 49. Nutrient Reference Values recommended for pregnancy: Calcium = 840 mg, Magnesium = 290 mg, Iron = 22 mg, Phosphorus = 580 mg, Sodium = 920 mg, Potassium = 2800 mg, Zinc = 9 mg [30]. * $P < 0.01$; IQR: interquartile range.

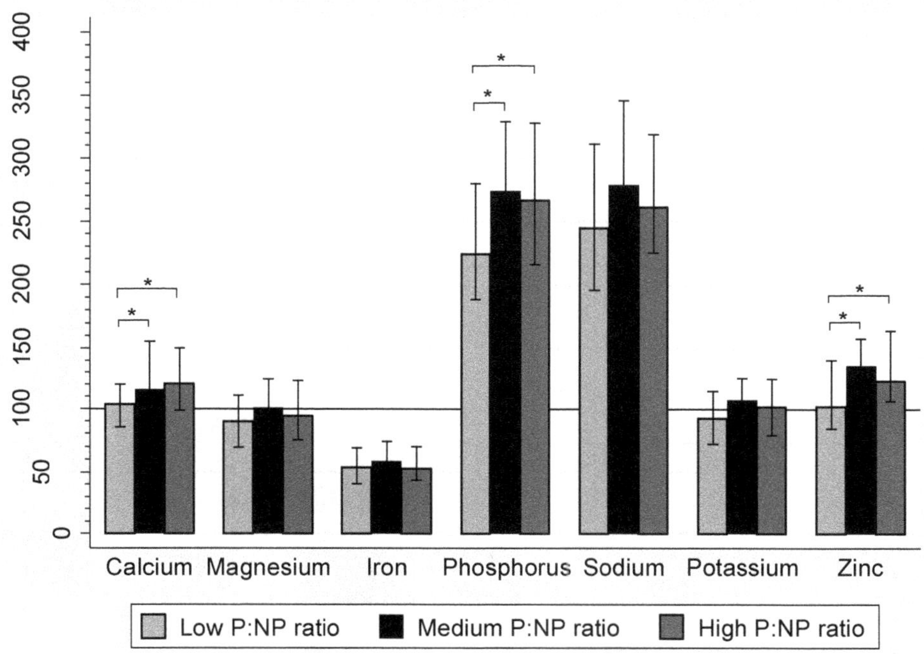

Figure 3 summarizes the percentage of AGHE recommendations achieved by pregnant women according to tertile of the P:NP ratio. None of the women in any tertile achieved the AGHE recommendations for all food groups. The highest adherence rates were for dairy and meat food groups. Pregnant women in the medium and high P:NP ratio groups reported median daily servings of dairy and meat that were above minimum recommendations, while 88.1% and 92.4% of women in low P:NP ratio group met the recommendations, respectively. When food patterns in the low P:NP ratio group were compared to the high P:NP ratio group, adherence rates for dairy (88.1% *vs.* 104.5%; $P = 0.001$) and meat (92.4% *vs.* 132.2%; $P < 0.001$) food groups were lower, and for fruit (64.6% *vs.* 42.1; $P = 0.014$), higher for women in the low P:NP ratio group. Similar adherence rates were found for the bread and cereals food group. Servings of extra foods were compared to the maximum AGHE recommendation of 2.5 servings per day. Despite an inverse association between extra food servings and the P:NP ratio ($P = 0.003$), women in the high P:NP ratio group still reported intakes 37.3% above the maximum recommendation.

Figure 3. The percentage of Australian Guide to Healthy Eating (AGHE) food group recommendations achieved during pregnancy by women in the WATCH Study who reported plausible dietary data, by tertile of the protein to non-protein (P:NP) ratio. Plausible data is defined as energy intakes ≥4.5 and ≤20.0 MJ/day. The proportion of protein (%E) to carbohydrate (%E) and fat (%E) was used to create P:NP tertiles. The P:NP ratio for each tertile: Low P:NP ratio group 0.21 (0.19, 0.22), n = 50; Medium P:NP ratio group 0.24 (0.23, 0.25), n = 50; high P:NP ratio group 0.28 (0.27, 0.30), n = 49. AGHE minimum daily serving recommendations for pregnancy: Bread/Cereals = 4 servings, Fruit = 4 servings, Vegetables = 5 servings, Dairy = 2 servings and Meat = 1.5 servings. The maximum AGHE serving recommendation was used for the Extras food group = 2.5 servings [26]. * $P < 0.01$; ** $P < 0.001$; IQR: interquartile range.

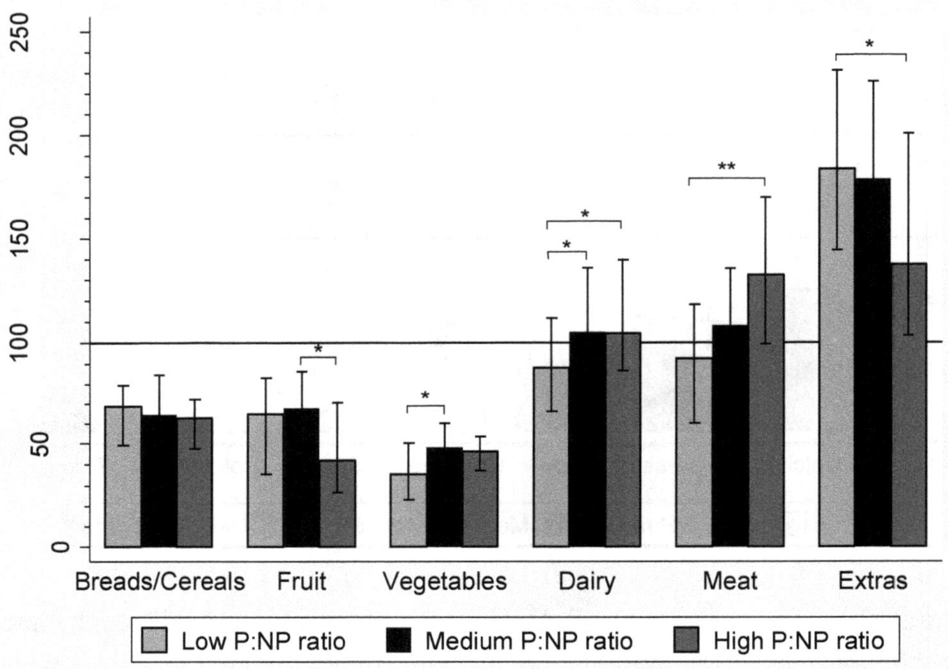

Response surfaces for the effects of maternal macronutrient intake during pregnancy on selected micronutrient intakes (folate, iron, vitamin E, calcium, magnesium and zinc) are presented in Figure 4. Folate and iron intakes were maximized with low protein (<16%E), intermediate fat (30%E) and high carbohydrate (>54%E) intakes. Intakes of all remaining micronutrients (including those not shown) were optimized with a maternal diet of intermediate protein (18%E–20%E), intermediate fat (28%E–30%E) and intermediate carbohydrate (50%E–54%E).

Figure 4. Effects of maternal macronutrient intakes during pregnancy on selected maternal micronutrient intakes. In these plots, known as right-angled mixture triangles [35], fat and protein (% of energy) increase along their respective axes in the normal way, and % carbohydrate decreases with distance from the origin. The negatively sloped dashed lines show the % carbohydrate, as labeled in the first graph. Plotted onto arrays of maternal dietary macronutrient composition points are fitted surfaces for the six response variables (folate, iron, vitamin E, calcium, magnesium and zinc). The isoclines for the micronutrient intakes rise in elevation from dark blue to dark red. Therefore, low micronutrient intakes are represented in the dark blue shading and increase to high micronutrient intakes in the red shading. Micronutrient intakes were generally optimized with a maternal diet of intermediate protein (18%E–20%E), intermediate fat (28%E–30%E) and intermediate carbohydrate (50%E–54%E) in comparison to Nutrient Reference Values (n = 149). Folate and iron intakes were maximized with low protein (<16%E), intermediate fat (30%E) and high carbohydrate (>54%E) intakes. Nutrient Reference Values recommended for pregnancy: Folate = 520 μg, Iron = 22 mg, Vitamin E = 7 mg, Calcium = 840 mg, Magnesium = 290 mg, Zinc = 9 mg [30].

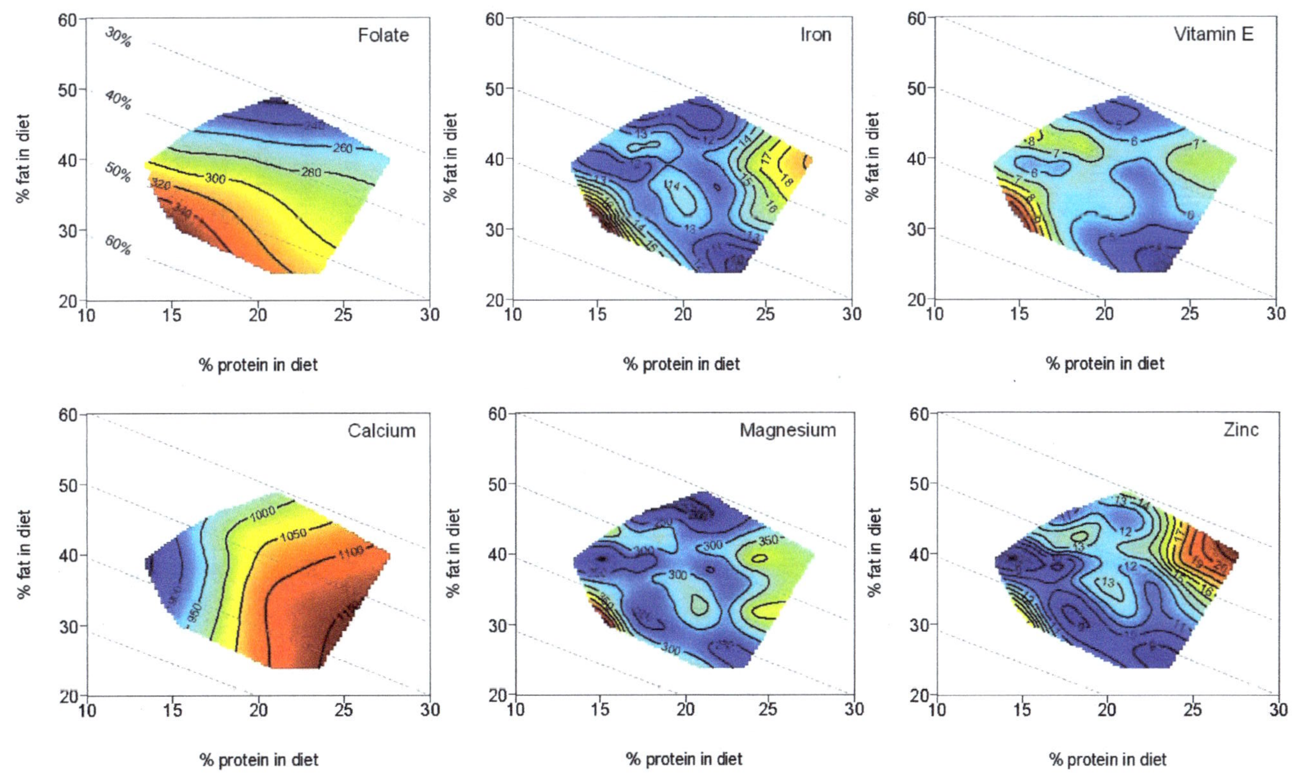

4. Discussion

This study provides the first insight into the eating patterns adopted by pregnant women by tertile of the P:NP ratio and compares patterns to Australian diet and nutrient recommendations. Pregnant women increased their P:NP ratio by an increased protein and reduced carbohydrate intake, as opposed to any changes in total fat intake. The P:NP ratio was positively associated with median daily servings of dairy and meat food groups and inversely associated with the extras food groups. While nutritional adequacy of micronutrient intakes did not significantly improve with increased P:NP tertile, women in the medium P:NP ratio group reported the highest median daily intake for all micronutrients, except vitamin C and calcium.

There was no evidence that a high P:NP ratio improved nutritional adequacy in pregnant women. The dietary patterns reported in this study were similar to those reported by a nationally representative sample of pregnant women in Australia [36]. Previous studies have reported a mismatch between the eating patterns of Australian women during pregnancy and food group recommendations [36], but suggest that an increased fruit and dairy intake may assist women to meet the NRVs for key nutrients important for childbearing (calcium, folate, iron, zinc and fiber) [36]. Results from the present study indicate that women in the medium P:NP ratio group (~18%E–19%E protein) consumed the highest median fruit intake, in conjunction with more vegetables, dairy and a trend towards more meat, compared to women in the low P:NP ratio group (~16%E–17%E protein); whereas women in the high P:NP ratio group (~21%E–22%E protein) consumed less fruit and extras, but more meat compared to those in medium P:NP ratio group. The reduced intake of energy dense, nutrient poor foods in the extras food group by women in the high P:NP ratio group may be beneficial for both maternal [37] and offspring body composition [7]. Plus, reduced intake of these extra foods may reduce offspring risk of obesity through the development of favorable alterations within the central neural network for appetite regulation [38]. However, a reduction of fruit intake without an equivalent increase in vegetable intake may be detrimental for micronutrient intakes, particularly folate. Fruits and vegetables contain many biologically active phytochemicals that have additive and synergistic effects that promote health and prevent chronic disease [39]. These properties are likely to have an important influence during critical windows of fetal development and may consequently affect offspring risk of disease later in life [1]. No significant differences in total fat, saturated fat or sugars were found between women in the medium and high P:NP ratio groups. Therefore, a moderate protein content, such as that adopted by women in medium P:NP ratio group (~18%E–19%E), may allow women to consume the largest variety of nutrients across all food groups. Further research to identify the optimal macronutrient composition during pregnancy and the implications on health in animal models and long-term epidemiological cohorts is required before dietary recommendations can be formulated for pregnant women.

The micronutrients at highest risk of deficiency during pregnancy in developed countries are folate and iron [40]. In this study, folate and iron intakes were well below recommendations in all tertiles of the P:NP ratio, despite higher intakes being visualized with lower protein contents. Results for folate were in agreement with those conducted in women where there was no relationship with diet composition [41]. But interestingly, iron intakes did not improve with increased P:NP ratio and the associated increased meat intake. This is likely to be because the decreased consumption of breads/cereals, fruit and extras servings reported with increased P:NP ratio reduced iron intakes by a similar magnitude. While some cross-sectional studies have reported a positive association between iron status and meat intake [42–44], recent data from a nationally representative sample in the United Kingdom have shown that iron fortified cereals were the largest contributors of iron intake in all age groups [45]. Iron fortified cereals were not specifically quantified by the FFQ used in this study. However, most Australian cereals now contain added iron, and this information was included in the nutrient composition database that was used to provide nutrient intakes in this study. Our results support these findings and indicate that women report inadequate intakes of folate and iron during pregnancy, regardless of whether they consume a protein-rich or carbohydrate-rich diet. While it is possible for pregnant women to achieve nutrient recommendations through food intake alone [36], pregnant women commonly report suboptimal nutrient intakes and may require dietary supplementation. No information was collected on vitamin supplementation in this study, because the purpose was to focus on nutrients supplied from food only. Thus, the nutritional adequacy of contemporary eating patterns across all food groups is as important as macronutrient balance in ensuring micronutrient intakes during pregnancy meet nutrient recommendations.

Our findings contribute to understanding the nutritional impact of maternal protein intake during pregnancy. The mechanisms connecting protein in maternal diet to obesity and metabolic disease in offspring are not fully elucidated, but are believed to involve changes in gene expression through epigenetic alterations, such as DNA methylation [46]. Research in experimental animal models has provided compelling evidence to support a role for glucocorticoids in this process [11,20]. Both maternal protein restriction and protein excess has been linked to increased glucocorticoid sensitivity in offspring, while increased glucocorticoid sensitivity in offspring has been associated with an increased risk of metabolic disease [11,20]. Experimental rodent models have also demonstrated that restriction of maternal micronutrients during pregnancy (multivitamin, multimineral and/or singular nutrients) can lead to an increase in offspring adiposity [20]. The specific phenotypic changes reported by rodent studies include an overall increase in percentage body fat, greater visceral/central fat accumulation, elevated expression of genes related to adiposity and modifications in adipose tissue function and lipid metabolism [20]. Results suggest there may be an optimal proportion of protein in maternal diet to maximize micronutrient adequacy during pregnancy. However, before an optimal macronutrient range can be recommended, research investigating the implications of these contemporary eating patterns on the offspring's expected postpartum developmental environment is required.

Limitations include the use of self-reported FFQ data to measure dietary intake. Dietary data is strengthened by the similarities between the daily mean energy intake reported in our study (8070 kJ/day) and that reported in a representative sample of pregnant women in the Australian Longitudinal Study on Women's Health (7795 kJ/day) in 2003 [47]. Macronutrient distributions were also similar to the Australian data [47]. No information was collected on vitamin supplementation, however, the main purpose was to focus on nutrients supplied from food only. Lastly, the WATCH study contained a higher proportion of women with post-school qualifications, socio-economic advantage and in a married or *de facto* relationship, but had a similar proportion of overweight/obesity and indigenous ethnicity compared to the Australian population. Therefore, care should be taken in extrapolating results at the population level.

5. Conclusions

This study provides evidence that there may be a target maternal macronutrient composition that optimizes micronutrient intakes during pregnancy. Despite eating patterns failing to meet food selection guide recommendations, micronutrient intakes for most nutrients were optimized at intermediate protein (18%E–20%E), intermediate fat (28%E–30%E) and intermediate carbohydrate (50%E–54%E) intakes. Further research is required to understand how contemporary eating behaviors can optimize micronutrient and macronutrient intakes during pregnancy to maximize the health of the mother and developing fetus.

Acknowledgments

The authors would like to thank all WATCH Study participants who have generously volunteered their time and personal information. We thank Patrick McElduff of the University of Newcastle for his advice and guidance with the statistical analyses, and Trish Engel and Therese Finnegan (Midwives) for their involvement in the recruitment process. All authors helped design the study and directed its implementation, including quality assurance and control. MB worked on the statistical analyses and was responsible for the project's implementation, including the preparation of the manuscript. All authors have made a significant contribution to the research and the development of the manuscript.

This work was supported by a PhD scholarship provided by the University of Newcastle and Newcastle Permanent Charitable Foundation, New South Wales, Australia (MB). CEC is supported by a National Health and Medical Research Council Career Development Fellowship Award. DR is part-funded by the National Research Centre for Growth and Development, New Zealand.

References

1. McMillen, I.C.; Robinson, J.S. Developmental origins of the metabolic syndrome: Prediction, plasticity, and programming. *Physiol. Rev.* **2005**, *85*, 571–633.
2. Fall, C.H.D. Evidence for the intra-uterine programming of adiposity in later life. *Ann. Hum. Biol.* **2011**, *38*, 410–428.
3. Rehfeldt, C.; Lang, I.S.; Gors, S.; Hennig, U.; Kalbe, C.; Stabenow, B.; Brussow, K.P.; Pfuhl, R.; Bellmann, O.; Nurnberg, G.; *et al.* Limited and excess dietary protein during gestation affects growth and compositional traits in gilts and impairs offspring fetal growth. *J. Anim. Sci.* **2011**, *89*, 329–341.
4. Zambrano, E.; Bautista, C.J.; Deas, M.; Martinez-Samayoa, P.M.; Gonzalez-Zamorano, M.; Ledesma, H.; Morales, J.; Larrea, F.; Nathanielsz, P.W. A low maternal protein diet during pregnancy and lactation has sex- and window of exposure-specific effects on offspring growth and food intake, glucose metabolism and serum leptin in the rat. *J. Physiol.* **2006**, *571*, 221–230.
5. McCurdy, C.E.; Bishop, J.M.; Williams, S.M.; Grayson, B.E.; Smith, M.S.; Friedman, J.E.; Grove, K.L. Maternal high-fat diet triggers lipotoxicity in the fetal livers of nonhuman primates. *J. Clin. Investig.* **2009**, *119*, 323–335.

6. Bayol, S.A.; Farrington, S.J.; Stickland, N.C. A maternal "junk food" diet in pregnancy and lactation promotes an exacerbated taste for "junk food" and a greater propensity for obesity in rat offspring. *Br. J. Nutr.* **2007**, *98*, 843–851.
7. Blumfield, M.L.; Hure, A.J.; MacDonald-Wicks, L.; Smith, R.; Simpson, S.J.; Giles, W.B.; Raubenheimer, D.; Collins, C.E. Dietary balance during pregnancy is associated with fetal adiposity and fat distribution. *Am. J. Clin. Nutr.* **2012**, *96*, 1032–1041.
8. Sebert, S.; Sharkey, D.; Budge, H.; Symonds, M.E. The early programming of metabolic health: Is epigenetic setting the missing link? *Am. J. Clin. Nutr.* **2012**, *94*, 1953S–1958S.
9. Maurer, A.D.; Reimer, R.A. Maternal consumption of high-prebiotic fibre or -protein diets during pregnancy and lactation differentially influences satiety hormones and expression of genes involved in glucose and lipid metabolism in offspring in rats. *Br. J. Nutr.* **2011**, *105*, 329–338.
10. Buckley, A.J.; Jaquiery, A.L.; Harding, J.E. Nutritional programming of adult disease. *Cell Tissue Res.* **2005**, *322*, 73–79.
11. Almond, K.; Bikker, P.; Lomax, M.; Symonds, M.E.; Mostyn, A. The influence of maternal protein nutrition on offspring development and metabolism: The role of glucocorticoids. *Proc. Nutr. Soc.* **2012**, *71*, 198–203.
12. Simpson, S.J.; Raubenheimer, D. Obesity: The protein leverage hypothesis. *Obes. Rev.* **2005**, *6*, 133–142.
13. Heppolette, C.A.A.; Palmer, D.; Ozanne, S.E. Experimental models of low birth weight—Insight into the developmental programming of metabolic health, aging and immune function. In *Perinatal Programming: The State of the Art*; Plagemann, A., Ed.; Walter de Gruyter: Berlin, Germany, 2012; pp. 11–25.
14. Hales, C.N.; Barker, D.J. Type 2 (non-insulin-dependent) diabetes mellitus: The thrifty phenotype hypothesis. *Diabetologia* **1992**, *35*, 595–601.
15. Petry, C.J.; Dorling, M.W.; Pawlak, D.B.; Ozanne, S.E.; Hales, C.N. Diabetes in old male offspring of rat dams fed a reduced protein diet. *Int. J. Exp. Diabetes Res.* **2001**, *2*, 139–143.
16. Desai, M.; Crowther, N.J.; Ozanne, S.E.; Lucas, A.; Hales, C.N. Adult glucose and lipid metabolism may be programmed during fetal life. *Biochem. Soc. Trans.* **1995**, *23*, 331–335.
17. Barker, D.J. Adult consequences of fetal growth restriction. *Clin. Obstet. Gynecol.* **2006**, *49*, 270–283.
18. Andreasyan, K.; Ponsonby, A.L.; Dwyer, T.; Morley, R.; Riley, M.; Dear, K.; Cochrane, J. Higher maternal dietary protein intake in late pregnancy is associated with a lower infant ponderal index at birth. *Eur. J. Clin. Nutr.* **2007**, *61*, 498–508.
19. Metzler-Zebeli, B.U.; Lang, I.S.; Gors, S.; Brussow, K.P.; Hennig, U.; Nurnberg, G.; Rehfeldt, C.; Otten, W.; Metges, C.C. High-protein-low-carbohydrate diet during pregnancy alters maternal plasma amino acid concentration and placental amino acid extraction but not fetal plasma amino acids in pigs. *Br. J. Nutr.* **2012**, in press.
20. Rao, K.R.; Padmavathi, I.J.; Raghunath, M. Maternal micronutrient restriction programs the body adiposity, adipocyte function and lipid metabolism in offspring: A review. *Rev. Endocr. Metab. Disord.* **2012**, *13*, 103–108.

21. Ramakrishnan, U.; Grant, F.; Goldenberg, T.; Zongrone, A.; Martorell, R. Effect of women's nutrition before and during early pregnancy on maternal and infant outcomes: A systematic review. *Paediatr. Perinat. Epidemiol.* **2012**, *26*, 285–301.
22. Hure, A.J.; Smith, R.; Collins, C.E. A recruiting failure turned success. *BMC Health Serv. Res.* **2008**, *8*, 64.
23. Hure, A.J.; Collins, C.E.; Giles, W.B.; Paul, J.W.; Smith, R. Greater maternal weight gain during pregnancy predicts a large but lean phenotype: A prospective cohort study. *Matern. Child Health J.* **2012**, *16*, 1374–1384.
24. Hure, A.J.; Collins, C.E.; Giles, W.B.; Wright, I.M.R.; Smith, R. Protocol for the women and their children's health (WATCH) study: A cohort of pregnancy and beyond. *J. Epidemiol.* **2012**, *22*, 267–275.
25. Hodge, A.; Patterson, A.J.; Brown, W.J.; Ireland, P.; Giles, G. The Anti Cancer Council of Victoria FFQ: Relative validity of nutrient intakes compared with weighed food records in young to middle-aged women in a study of iron supplementation. *Aust. N. Z. J. Public Health* **2000**, *24*, 576–583.
26. Smith, A.; Kellett, E.; Schmerlaib, Y. *The Australian Guide to Healthy Eating: Background Information for Nutrition Educators*; Commonwealth of Australia: Canberra, Australia, 1998.
27. Food Standards Australia New Zealand. *NUTTAB 2006: Australian Food Composition Tables*; Australian Government Publishing Service: Canberra, Austalia, 2006.
28. Research Institute for Gender and Health. *Women's Health Australia: Databook for Survey 1 of the Australian Longitudinal Study on Women's Health*; University of Newcastle: Newcastle, New South Wales, Australia, 1997.
29. National Health and Medical Research Council. *Dietary Guidelines for Australians*; Australian Government Publishing Service: Canberra, Austalia, 1992.
30. National Health and Medical Research Council. *Nutrient Reference Values for Australia and New Zealand*; Commonwealth of Australia: Canberra, Austalia, 2006.
31. Meltzer, H.M.; Brantsaeter, A.L.; Ydersbond, T.A.; Alexander, J.; Haugen, M. Methodological challenges when monitoring the diet of pregnant women in a large study: Experiences from the norwegian mother and child cohort study (MoBa). *Matern. Child Nutr.* **2008**, *4*, 14–27.
32. Blows, M.W. Measuring nonlinear selection. *Am. Nat.* **2003**, *162*, 815–820.
33. StataCorp. *Stata Statistical Software: Release 11*; StataCorp LP: College Station, Texas, USA, 2009.
34. R Development Core Team. *R: A Language and Environment for Statistical Computing*; R Foundation for Statistical Computing: Vienna, Austria, 2011.
35. Raubenheimer, D. Toward a quantitative nutritional ecology: The right-angled mixture triangle. *Ecol. Monogr.* **2011**, *81*, 407–427.
36. Blumfield, M.L.; Hure, A.J.; MacDonald-Wicks, L.K.; Patterson, A.J.; Smith, R.; Collins, C.E. Disparities exist between national food group recommendations and the dietary intakes of women. *BMC Women's Health* **2011**, *11*, 37.

37. Ostbye, T.; Peterson, B.L.; Krause, K.M.; Swamy, G.K.; Lovelady, C.A. Predictors of postpartum weight change among overweight and obese women: Results from the active mothers postpartum study. *J. Women's Health* **2012**, *21*, 215–222.
38. Ong, Z.Y.; Muhlhausler, B.S. Maternal "junk-food" feeding of rat dams alters food choices and development of the mesolimbic reward pathway in the offspring. *FASEB J.* **2011**, *25*, 2167–2179.
39. Liu, R.H. Potential synergy of phytochemicals in cancer prevention: Mechanism of action. *J. Nutr.* **2004**, *134*, 3479S–3485S.
40. Blumfield, M.L.; Collins, C.; MacDonald-Wicks, L.; Hure, A.J.; Smith, R. A systematic review and meta-analysis of micronutrient intakes during pregnancy in developed countries. *Nutr. Rev.* **2012**, in press.
41. Noakes, M.; Keogh, J.B.; Foster, P.R.; Clifton, P.M. Effect of an energy-restricted, high-protein, low-fat diet relative to a conventional high-carbohydrate, low-fat diet on weight loss, body composition, nutritional status, and markers of cardiovascular health in obese women. *Am. J. Clin. Nutr.* **2005**, *81*, 1298–1306.
42. Galan, P.; Yoon, H.C.; Preziosi, P.; Viteri, F.; Valeix, P.; Fieux, B.; Briancon, S.; Malvy, D.; Roussel, A.M.; Favier, A.; *et al.* Determining factors in the iron status of adult women in the SU.VI.MAX study (SUpplementation en VItamines et Mineraux Antioxydants). *Eur. J. Clin. Nutr.* **1998**, *52*, 383–388.
43. Gibson, S.A. Iron intake and iron status of preschool children: Associations with breakfast cereals, vitamin C and meat. *Public Health Nutr.* **1999**, *2*, 521–528.
44. Heath, A.L.; Skeaff, C.M.; Williams, S.; Gibson, R.S. The role of blood loss and diet in the aetiology of mild iron deficiency in premenopausal adult new zealand women. *Public Health Nutr.* **2001**, *4*, 197–206.
45. Geissler, C.; Singh, M. Iron, meat and health. *Nutrients* **2011**, *3*, 283–316.
46. Altmann, S.; Murani, E.; Schwerin, M.; Metges, C.C.; Wimmers, K.; Ponsuksili, S. Maternal dietary protein restriction and excess affects offspring gene expression and methylation of non-SMC subunits of condensin I in liver and skeletal muscle. *Epigenetics* **2012**, *7*, 239–252.
47. Hure, A.; Young, A.; Smith, R.; Collins, C. Diet and pregnancy status in Australian women. *Public Health Nutr.* **2009**, *12*, 853–861.

3

Altered Fetal Skeletal Muscle Nutrient Metabolism Following an Adverse *In Utero* Environment and the Modulation of Later Life Insulin Sensitivity

Kristyn Dunlop [1], Megan Cedrone [2], James F. Staples [2] and Timothy R.H. Regnault [1,3,4,5,*]

[1] Department of Physiology and Pharmacology, Western University, London, ON N6A-5C1, Canada; E-Mail: kdunlo@uwo.ca

[2] Department of Biology, Western University, London, ON N6A 5B7, Canada; E-Mails: mcedrone@uwo.ca (M.C.); jfstaple@uwo.ca (J.F.S.)

[3] Department of Obstetrics and Gynecology, Western University, London, ON N6H-5W9, Canada

[4] Lawson Health Research Institute, London, ON N6C-2R5, Canada

[5] Children's Health Research Institute, London, ON N6C-2V5, Canada

* Author to whom correspondence should be addressed; E-Mail: tim.regnault@uwo.ca

---

Abstract: The importance of the *in utero* environment as a contributor to later life metabolic disease has been demonstrated in both human and animal studies. In this review, we consider how disruption of normal fetal growth may impact skeletal muscle metabolic development, ultimately leading to insulin resistance and decreased insulin sensitivity, a key precursor to later life metabolic disease. In cases of intrauterine growth restriction (IUGR) associated with hypoxia, where the fetus fails to reach its full growth potential, low birth weight (LBW) is often the outcome, and early in postnatal life, LBW individuals display modifications in the insulin-signaling pathway, a critical precursor to insulin resistance. In this review, we will present literature detailing the classical development of insulin resistance in IUGR, but also discuss how this impaired development, when challenged with a postnatal Western diet, may potentially contribute to the development of later life insulin resistance. Considering the important role of the skeletal muscle in insulin resistance pathogenesis, understanding the *in utero* programmed origins of skeletal muscle deficiencies in insulin sensitivity and how they may interact with an adverse postnatal environment, is an important step in highlighting potential therapeutic options for LBW offspring born of pregnancies characterized by placental insufficiency.

Keywords: IUGR; hypoxia; obese; insulin sensitivity; skeletal muscle; mitochondria; β-oxidation; fats; acylcarnitine; oxygen

1. Introduction

Recent clinical, epidemiological and animal studies have highlighted an association between an altered, adverse *in utero* environment and growth, and the subsequent propensity of these offspring to develop hallmarks of the metabolic syndrome [1–3]. The metabolic syndrome is a cluster of factors indicative of altered metabolism, including hypertension, visceral obesity, glucose intolerance and dyslipidemia, that predispose the patient to the development of comorbidities such as cardiovascular disease, non-alcoholic fatty liver disease and type 2 diabetes [4]. Decreased insulin sensitivity, or insulin resistance, is a critical precursor of the metabolic syndrome, as it is typically evident before other overt symptoms are apparent; and therefore it may represent an early, key step in the pathophysiological progression towards the metabolic syndrome [4].

It has been postulated that the origins of the metabolic syndrome, and insulin resistance specifically, originate during fetal development and early postnatal life [5]. As such, an adverse *in utero* environment has the potential to influence the relative risk of the offspring to the development of aberrant nutrient metabolism in later life, independently of postnatal diet. An adverse *in utero* environment, often characterized by suboptimal nutrient transfer to the fetus, culminates in intrauterine growth restriction (IUGR). IUGR is the endpoint of a continuum of conditions that result in the failure of the fetus to attain its inherent growth potential, which can be diagnosed using ultrasonography during pregnancy [6]. Clinically, IUGR often results in a baby born with a weight or length below the 10th percentile for gestational age [6,7].

The etiology of IUGR is multifactorial, with adverse environmental or genetic and epigenetic factors likely playing a role in the abnormal growth and development of the fetus. One of the most important environmental factors regulating fetal growth, is nutrient delivery to the fetus via placental diffusion and transport [7]. A reduced functional capacity of the placenta, or placental insufficiency, is typically associated with poor placental vascular development, which prevents adequate nutrition and oxygen from reaching the developing fetus, resulting in a hypoxic, nutrient deprived *in utero* environment. Interestingly, it should be noted that, independent of reductions in nutrient supply, hypoxia alone has been shown to have a significant impact on fetal growth, emphasizing hypoxia as a key contributor to impaired fetal growth and potentially IUGR [8].

With exposure to a hypoxic *in utero* environment, the fetus undergoes some key adaptations to ensure survival. A key component of this adaptation in the acute setting has been considered a redistribution of fetal cardiac output towards essential organs such as the brain, heart and adrenal glands, at the expense of other organ systems, including the lungs, kidney, liver and skeletal muscle [9–11]. With prolonged hypoxia, animal and human studies have highlighted a redistribution of blood flow toward the brain, as well as increased blood flow towards adrenal glands [12–15], and it is inferred from this redistribution that the brain continues to receive sufficient perfusion and nutrient supply to maintain relative growth. This brain sparing effect is visible at birth, with the size of the fetal head being larger than that of the abdomen, giving rise to an observable asymmetrical growth restriction. Concurrent with the overall reduction in body weight and brain sparing effect, fetuses exposed to hypoxic *in utero* environments also display a reduced muscle mass compared with normal birth weight offspring [16,17], and are predisposed to altered insulin sensitivity [1,3,5,18]. Furthermore, rodent models of low birth weight have also demonstrated a decrease in skeletal muscle mass [19], similar to the altered muscle to fat ratio observed in older men who were born low birth weight [20]. With this altered development there are metabolic changes to the offspring, resulting in what has been proposed as a "thrifty phenotype" [1,18]. The "thrifty phenotype" encompasses a collection of metabolic adaptations initiated to aid in fetal survival when challenged with nutrient deprivation *in utero* [21]. While the "thrifty phenotype" represents the observable phenotype associated with IUGR, theories of fetal programming postulate that altered oxygen and nutrient transfer during critical windows of development, when the fetus is most sensitive to its environment, are associated with permanent alterations in structure and metabolism, and a fixed functional capacity of vital organs in postnatal life [1]. Since the plasticity of the organs *in utero* is lost in postnatal life, adaptations to these metabolic organs initiated *in utero* may persist into adulthood, increasing the propensity for these offspring to develop metabolic disease with age [1,22].

Markers of altered fetal growth (including low weight at birth and asymmetric growth) are most widely used as indicators of IUGR or a hypoxic *in utero* environment. However, more subtle adaptations at the physiological level may be the drivers underlying the observable later life phenotypes, such as changes in skeletal muscle metabolic function and anabolic capacity, and overall oxygen consumption. Once the organs have fully developed *in utero,* the IUGR fetus faced with a postnatal environment characterized by nutrient excess, a highly prevalent and easily accessible diet in modern society, may develop long-term adverse metabolic consequences [1,5,18]. Unfortunately, the mechanisms underlying these alterations in the metabolic capacity of the IUGR fetus and their propensity towards the development of later life insulin resistance and the metabolic syndrome remain poorly defined.

2. Skeletal Muscle Insulin Signaling and IUGR

Skeletal muscle is the primary location for insulin-stimulated glucose uptake, accounting for up to 70% of whole body glucose disposal [23], and is a key regulator of whole body energy metabolism [24], with other metabolic organs, including liver, adipose tissue and pancreas also involved in the insulin response and pathogenesis of insulin resistance. The primary metabolic objective in the skeletal muscle is production of ATP for contractile purposes; however, skeletal muscle is also responsible for the production and storage of glycogen, an insulin dependent process that provides the cells with glucose for ATP production when circulating levels are low. β-oxidation, a process whereby free fatty acids are broken down to provide muscle with carbon chain substrates, is also important for skeletal muscle ATP production. Since the skeletal muscle is a critical producer of ATP and an important location for glucose and fat metabolism, determining the propensity of skeletal muscle towards developing insulin resistance is a key determinant in the pathophysiological progression towards metabolic syndrome.

Depressed insulin sensitivity, or insulin resistance, is a metabolic state in which peripheral tissues, such as skeletal muscle, are no longer responsive to the anabolic effects of insulin, thereby reducing insulin-stimulated glucose uptake and perpetuating a state of hyperglycemia. Insulin resistance at the level of the skeletal muscle has been associated with a modulation of the serine/threonine phosphorylation status of insulin receptor substrates (IRS) [25–27]. A relative increase in the serine phosphorylation of IRS-1, the predominant isoform in skeletal muscle [28], at Ser^{307} reduces its ability to activate or complex with phosphatidylinositol 3-kinase (PI3-kinase). This activation failure impairs downstream phosphorylation of protein kinase B (Akt) at Ser^{473}, and Akt Substrate of 160 kDa (AS160) at Thr^{642}, ultimately leading to a reduction in glucose uptake into skeletal muscle cells through glucose transporter 4 (GLUT4) transporters [25,27,29].

A hypoxic *in utero* environment, commonly associated with IUGR, is known to negatively influence the fetus during critical periods of development [1,5,18]. Interestingly, IUGR offspring in animal models display improved insulin sensitivity in very early postnatal life, as assessed by intravenous glucose tolerance challenge; however, a shift towards impaired glucose clearance and decreased insulin sensitivity is evident as these offspring age [30–32]. The timing of this shift in insulin sensitivity appears to be sex-specific, with insulin action being impaired earlier in males and later in females [30]. These animal studies highlight that sexually dimorphic effects occur with adverse *in utero* environments, and in the case of insulin resistance, studies suggest males appear to be more susceptible to a programmed later life insulin resistance [30,33].

Interestingly however, this sex-specific programming of insulin resistance may not exist in humans. In a mixed cohort of offspring aged 25 who were growth restricted *in utero*, a significantly lower insulin-stimulated glucose uptake was observed compared to controls, as well as a higher plasma insulin concentration, suggesting the development of insulin resistance. Of note, these observations were in conjunction with a normal glucose tolerance challenge, thus representing an early phase in the pathogenesis to insulin resistance and the metabolic syndrome [34]. However, by age 64, men who were born small exhibited a strong link with impaired glucose tolerance and type 2 diabetes [35], while data concerning women born small is not widely available. Therefore, understanding the early steps in the progression towards insulin resistance in the low birth weight population, and any sex-specific effects, is of critical importance for mitigating the risk of these offspring to the development of later life type 2 diabetes.

Animal models of IUGR, as well as some human studies, have also been used in order to identify the molecular changes occurring at the level of the insulin-signaling cascade that may be underlying the reduced insulin sensitivity in this population [29,36]. In early postnatal life, expression of the insulin receptor is increased in low birth weight sheep, as a compensatory mechanism for the low insulin and glucose levels experienced *in utero* [37]. However, the expression of the insulin receptor is no different to normal birth weight controls in skeletal muscle of older low birth weight rodent offspring, highlighting that the later life alterations in insulin sensitivity are likely due to a defect down-stream of the receptor that affects the ability of GLUT4 to translocate to the membrane and take glucose into the cell [36]. Analysis of key intermediates in the insulin signaling cascade has demonstrated sex-specific alterations that may be responsible for altered GLUT4 expression and reduced glucose uptake that is associated with states of insulin resistance [17,29,36,38].

In rodent models of placental insufficiency, young adolescent male offspring show altered GLUT4 transport in conjunction with an increased phosphorylation of IRS-1 [29], which is known to blunt the physiological response to insulin [27] by reducing the coupling efficiency of the insulin receptor and IRS-1 [39]. IRS-1 is also known to complex with PI3-kinase, and in young male low birth weight offspring, reduced expression of the p85 regulatory subunit and p110β catalytic subunit of

PI3K has also been observed in rodent, as well as larger animal (e.g., sheep) models of placental insufficiency [31,36,37]. Downstream of IRS-1, the total Akt levels were not altered by insulin infusion in growth restricted males [29,36]; however, phosphorylation of this intermediate was increased by insulin, suggesting a compensatory mechanism may be at play to maintain this physiological response to exogenous insulin [29]. Although Akt's involvement in the insulin cascade appears to be unaffected, downstream AS160 shows reduced phosphorylation in response to insulin [29], suggesting a functional impairment that impacts GLUT4 translocation to the plasma membrane [40].

In young adolescent female rodent offspring, the phosphorylation status of Akt is higher in the basal state, and insulin infusion is still able to increase the phosphorylation further. Additionally, there are no changes in the phosphorylation of protein kinase C isoforms and an increased phosphorylation of phosphoinositide-dependent kinase (PDK), all of which point to programming of heightened insulin sensitivity [38]. This heightened sensitivity is in accordance with the early improvement observed in sheep models [30], and may represent a protective response initiated to maintain whole body insulin sensitivity at this early age [38]. However, despite this enhanced sensitivity during the growth phase, with age these offspring exhibited a decrease in insulin sensitivity and progression towards an insulin resistant phenotype [41].

Human data has suggested similar molecular alterations are present in young males born low birth weight, including reduced expression of the p85 and p110β subunits of PI3-kinase and reduced skeletal muscle GLUT4 content [16,36]. These alterations occur in conjunction with a blunted phosphorylation of Akt in response to insulin infusion, but with maintenance of glucose tolerance and whole body insulin sensitivity [16,36]. Taken together, changes in the molecular expression of key insulin signaling intermediates in skeletal muscle of low birth weight offspring may precede development of whole body insulin resistance and glucose intolerance, representing an early defect in metabolism that could be indicative of future metabolic disease [36]. However, the mechanisms by which the *in utero* environment may be modulating these changes in insulin sensitivity remain ill defined.

3. Fiber Type, Oxygen Consumption and IUGR

Skeletal muscle has a high demand for energy in order to perform its contractile function, with most of its energy requirement being met through oxidative phosphorylation (OXPHOS). While OXPHOS produces greater amounts of adenine triphosphate (ATP) than glycolysis, it is an aerobic process requiring oxygen, conducted within the Krebs cycle and electron transport system of the mitochondria. The density of mitochondria is the primary determinant of oxidative capacity, and this is ultimately set by fiber type and fiber distribution within the skeletal muscle bed. There are a number of different skeletal muscle fiber types distinguished primarily by their oxidative capacity. Type Ia (slow oxidative) fibers are the most mitochondria-rich fibers, and type IIb (fast glycolytic) fibers have the least mitochondria and thus the lowest oxidative capacity. Types IIa and IIx (fast oxidative) fibers have an intermediate number of mitochondria and oxidative capacity [42]. Maximal rates of OXPHOS is dictated by mitochondrial number and consequently directly related to fiber type composition [43,44].

OXPHOS is adversely affected in skeletal muscle of growth-restricted animals [19,45,46], in conjunction with decreased mitochondrial number [19]. These factors, combined with a lowered ATP production are associated with the development of insulin resistance [47,48]. The individual OXPHOS complexes, including ATPase activity, have been studied using respirometry, a technique measuring oxygen consumption using a number of substrates that are metabolized by individual complexes within a closed cell chamber. The rate of oxygen consumption is measured in "states", where state 1 represents baseline respiration, state 2 follows the addition of malate and glutamate, malate and pyruvate (metabolized as NADH at complex 1) or rotenone and succinate (rotenone inhibiting complex 1 and succinate metabolized at complex 2). State 3 respiration follows the addition of ADP (measuring ATPase activity) and state 4 follows the addition of oligomycin (inhibiting ATPase activity). The ratio of state 3/state 4 respiration rates, termed the respiratory control ratio (RCR), is commonly used to measure mitochondrial dysfunction. Generally, a low RCR is associated with mitochondrial dysfunction as it measures how tightly respiration and phosphorylation are coupled. In rats, IUGR skeletal muscle state 3 was decreased irrespective of substrate used, compared to controls.

In addition to impaired OXPHOS reported in IUGR rats, reduced fetal glucose oxidation is observed in the heat stress ovine IUGR model [49]. These changes may reflect in the *in utero* determination of skeletal muscle fiber type composition of low birth weight offspring later in life [17,19,50]. In human studies, low birth weight is associated with an increase in type II fibers and no change in type I fibers at 19 years of age [17], and an increased proportion of glycolytic fibers are reported to precede insulin resistance in the *vastus lateralis* of low birth weight males [17]. In rodent studies, IUGR offspring exhibit a lower proportion of type Ia muscle fibers [19] and a shift towards more glycolytic (type IIb) fibers [17], ultimately altering the oxidative capacity and GLUT4 content of the muscle fibers. The results of these adverse *in utero* associated changes however, is not always consistent. For instance, in IUGR piglet studies, the proportion of type I fibers increase in the hind-limb muscles, but the proportion of type IIb were not reported due to methodological difficulties [51,52]. These conflicting conclusions may lie, in part, to species differences, age of fiber collection, but also may be due to the different muscle groups studied.

It is interesting to note that the alterations in skeletal muscle fiber composition and function early in life in low birth weight, IUGR offspring as reported above, appear similar to those observed in later life obese and type 2 diabetic individuals [53,54]. This similarity potentially highlights possible similar mechanisms at play in low birth weight offspring as those at work in patients with a propensity to develop insulin resistance and subsequent type 2 diabetes with age, independent of birth weight and an adverse *in utero* environment. Understanding these similarities will help define the mechanisms underlying altered fiber type distribution and oxygen utilization changes in these various disease states.

4. The Impact of IUGR and Later Life Impaired Skeletal Muscle Fat Metabolism upon the Progression of Insulin Resistance

A key traditional factor identified in the development of insulin resistance has been poor diet. The increasing prevalence of a "Western", or energy-dense, high-fat diet has been implicated as a key-contributing factor in the pathogenesis of insulin resistance, promoting accumulation of fat within the skeletal muscle and impacting mitochondrial function [55–57], leading to a diminished mitochondrial fatty acid oxidation capacity [58]. Consumption of this diet generates a surplus of free fatty acids, ultimately leading to ectopic lipid accumulation in non-adipose tissues such as skeletal muscle [59]. Once in the skeletal muscle, excess fatty acids are activated to form their acyl-CoA derivatives, which can be esterified into diacylglycerol (DAG), metabolized into ceramide, or conjugated to acylcarnitine for entry into the mitochondria to undergo β-oxidation [60]. Excess lipids may also be stored in lipid droplets as triacylglycerols, generating a pool of substrates termed intramyocellular triglycerides (IMTG) [56]. IMTG content is known to increase with percentage body fat, and to be elevated in obese or type 2 diabetic individuals. IMTGs are broken down by lipases to undergo oxidation, however disturbances in the rate of breakdown or oxidation may lead to accumulation of toxic lipid intermediates and subsequent insulin resistance [56,61]. The type of triglyceride (saturated *vs.* unsaturated) that make up the skeletal muscle lipid pool is also important, since unsaturated triglycerides may be destined to accumulate as IMTG, whereas saturated triglycerides may be broken down into DAGs [62]. Additionally, a higher proportion of saturated fatty acids within this lipid pool has recently been associated with insulin resistance [62]. Skeletal muscle relies heavily on fatty acid β-oxidation to generate energy, using this method to provide up to 90% of its total energy demand [58]. Therefore, any alterations in fatty acid oxidation may impair skeletal muscle metabolic capacity. Certainly in rodent IUGR studies, muscle oxidative ability is adversely affected in growth-restricted animals [19,45], and as such could set the stage for impaired mitochondrial function when challenged with a postnatal Western diet.

In rodent lipid infusion studies, insulin resistance develops, and increased concentrations of long-chain acyl CoAs have been associated with insulin resistant skeletal muscle [25]. This increased lipid availability has been associated with reduced levels of skeletal muscle β-oxidation [63,64], leading to accumulation of toxic lipid metabolites including DAG [25] and ceramide [65]. While specific changes in long-chain acyl CoA levels have not been reported in IUGR/low birth weight offspring, reductions in enzymes involved in β-oxidation have [66], suggesting that accumulation of long-chain acyl CoAs secondary to a reduction in oxidative capacity may be involved in the pathogenesis of insulin resistance. Accumulation of these lipid metabolites in the skeletal muscle has been associated with increases in stress-induced kinases, such as protein kinase C (PKC)-θ or ε, isoforms known to act upstream of c-Jun N-terminal kinase (JNK) and IκB (inhibitor of NFκB) kinase (IKKβ). Notably, JNK and IKKβ are two central serine/threonine kinases mediating phosphorylation of IRS-1 at Ser^{307}, a subsequent reduction in Ser^{473} phosphorylation of Akt, and reduced insulin-stimulated glucose uptake [25,60,65,67], similar to the molecular alterations that have been observed in the insulin signaling pathway in skeletal muscle of the low birth weight population [29,36]. PKC-θ activation itself (translocation from the cytosol to the plasma membrane) has also been reported to occur during a state of lipid overload in skeletal muscle, and may represent an alternative pathway mediating alterations in the serine/threonine phosphorylation status of key insulin signaling intermediates [25,61]. Direct evidence that these changes may be happening in low birth weight IUGR offspring as they age is still lacking, but if occurring, presents a potential pathway where *in utero* induced changes in fatty acid oxidation may play a contributing role to later life insulin resistance when challenged with a postnatal high fat diet.

While the concept of reduced fatty acid oxidation has been held as a corner stone of the development of insulin resistance, new studies now suggest excessive, rather than diminished, fatty acid oxidation in skeletal muscle mitochondria may be the root cause. Evidence for this new concept comes from rodent studies, where animals were fed high-fat diets and subsequently display a metabolic phenotype associated with mitochondrial overload, a situation in which an increase in fatty acid uptake and β-oxidation rate is stimulated, but later steps of metabolism, including the tricarboxylic acid (TCA) cycle or the electron transport chain, remain unaltered [26,58]. This mismatch between subsequent steps of oxidation allows accumulation of acylcarnitine intermediates that are indicative of incomplete oxidation or partial fatty acid degradation [26,58]. Incomplete oxidation occurs during mitochondrial overload because the high rates of β-oxidation generates excessive intermediates that overwhelm the TCA cycle, preventing further oxidation and allowing accumulation of acylcarnitines [26,58]. The recent interest in metabolomics has allowed for profiling of these acylcarnitine intermediates, highlighting a method that allows for further investigation of the relationship between incomplete β-oxidation and the pathogenesis of insulin resistance. High-fat feeding in rodents has been shown to induce a lipid profile high in even-chain acylcarnitines. Accumulation of these even-chain acylcarnitine species ranging in length from C6-C22 indicates that a large proportion of the fatty acids entering the mitochondria are only partially degraded for use as metabolic substrates [26,68]. Of interest, recent evidence has suggested that one even-chain acylcarnitine in particular, L-C14 carnitine, which can accumulate with incomplete β-oxidation, has the ability to activate pro-inflammatory pathways, as well as an induction of JNK which may modulate the serine/threonine phosphorylation status of insulin signaling intermediates, perpetuating a state of insulin resistance [67,69]. Mitochondrial overload has also been observed in rodent models of diabetes, including the Zucker Diabetic Fatty rat, further supporting the idea that incomplete fatty acid oxidation and accumulation of acylcarnitine intermediates may be implicated in the pathogenesis of insulin resistance [26,70]. The impact of high fat feeding in low birth weight IUGR offspring upon acylcarnitine production and mitochondrial overload has not been reported. However, short-term high fat feeding trials in human low birth weight offspring show that low birth weight is associated with a reduced degree of plasticity [71], suggesting that changes to β-oxidation and the TCA cycle, in conjunction with postnatal high fat ingestion, may be different in low birth weight offspring and potentially exacerbated.

The regulation of mitochondrial fatty acid oxidation rate is also an important determinant of the propensity for mitochondrial overload to occur when skeletal muscle is faced with excess free fatty acids. Ingestion of a fatty diet appears to alter the activity of an important family of nuclear transcription factors regulating mitochondrial oxidative capacity, known as the peroxisome proliferator-activated receptors (PPARs). The PPARα isoform is mainly expressed in highly oxidative tissues, including skeletal muscle, liver and heart, with activation of this transcription factor promoting an increase in fatty acid uptake and β-oxidation [58,72]. Interestingly, overexpression of PPARα in skeletal muscle of transgenic mice has been associated with increases of lipid-oxidative genes, yet with the development of glucose intolerance [73], lending support to the notion that over-activation of PPARα in skeletal muscle is detrimental to insulin sensitivity [58]. While it appears that increasing fatty acid oxidation in skeletal muscle during periods of high-fat feeding through activation of PPARα should promote fat clearance by increasing fatty acid oxidation, evidence has suggested that only the genes related to fatty acid oxidation and uptake have been increased, with no changes in the downstream steps of oxidation [68,70]. In addition to detrimental changes in PPARα activity, a chronic high fat diet has been associated with a decrease in skeletal muscle levels of peroxisome proliferator-activated receptor-γ co-activator 1α (PGC1α). PGC1α plays an important role in regulating mitochondrial biogenesis and is a critical component of the PPARα-activated transcriptional machinery [68]. Decreases in PGC1α lead to a reduction in the coupling efficiency between β-oxidation and TCA cycle, preventing the mitochondria from completely oxidizing fatty acids in response to high lipid availability [68]. This decrease in PGC1α levels with consumption of a Western diet would contribute to the mismatch of β-oxidation and TCA cycle activity observed in mitochondrial overload. Recent studies have also reported reduced mRNA levels of PGC1α [74,75] and reduced PGC1α protein levels in the soleus [75] and gastrocnemius [76] muscle of young adolescent low birth weight offspring. Additionally, alterations in the methylation status of the PGC1α promoter have been observed in both rodent [76] and human [77] models of IUGR, highlighting a potential epigenetic link with altered fat storage and metabolism in postnatal life. Therefore, reductions in PGC1α due to consumption of a Western diet, combined with a low birth weight situation could promote further incomplete oxidation and the potential for acylcarnitine intermediates to accumulate in the skeletal muscle and potentiate alterations in the phosphorylation status of insulin signaling molecules through the actions of stress-induced kinases. These emerging studies in the low birth weight population highlight a new area of investigation that is working to better characterize the epigenetic modifications to those genes involved in mitochondrial function and β-oxidation, which is a new and expanding field in understanding the development of insulin resistance in offspring of adverse intrauterine pregnancies.

Collectively, new studies suggest there are alterations in the storage and metabolism of fat in the skeletal muscle of low birth weight offspring. However, the nature of the specific alterations, their degree of plasticity, and their underlying contribution to insulin resistance, when challenged with an adverse postnatal diet as these offspring age, remains to be fully elucidated.

5. Conclusions

Infants of an adverse *in utero* environment represent a unique population who appear to be at a greater risk for the development of insulin resistance and subsequent metabolic disease [1,5,18]. Adaptive programmed changes in skeletal muscle metabolic development and function (*i.e.*, changes in insulin signaling, fiber type distribution, oxygen consumption, and oxidative capacity) due to an adverse *in utero* environment, lead to structural and metabolic deficits later in life. Further, and more concerning are recent studies suggesting that these low birth weight offspring are unable lose weight as efficiently as normal birth weight offspring when placed on a calorie restricted diet [19], and that PGC1α deficiencies associated with IUGR appear resistant to exercise intervention [78]. These studies highlight that these unique offspring, while being at a higher risk of developing aspects of metabolic syndrome, may be resistant, or lack plasticity to respond, to current intervention practices. When these infants with programmed alterations in skeletal muscle development are faced with a postnatal environment of nutrient excess, they appear to be at greater risk for aberrant skeletal muscle function. Definitive studies examining the interactive linkages between *in utero* programmed insulin resistance and postnatal environmental challenges, and those investigating the distinct mechanisms underlying the developmental origins of insulin resistance, and a lack of plasticity to later life challenges in low birth weight offspring are needed. With these data, the therapeutic options for this unique population can be better delineated.

Acknowledgments

This work was funded by the Canadian Institutes of Health Research (MOP Grant #209113).

Author Contributions

K.D. and M.C. have contributed to writing and editing the manuscript drafts. J.F.S. and T.R.H.R. have contributed to the editing of the manuscript drafts. All authors have approved the final version of the manuscript.

References

1. Osmond, C.; Barker, D.J. Fetal, infant and childhood growth are predictors of coronary heart disease, diabetes, and hypertension in adult men and women. *Environ. Health Perspect.* **2000**, *108*, 545–553.
2. Kind, K.L.; Clifton, P.M.; Grant, P.A.; Owens, P.C.; Sohlstrom, A.; Roberts, C.T.; Robinson, J.S.; Owens, J.A. Effect of maternal feed restriction during pregnancy on glucose tolerance in the adult guinea pig. *Am. J. Physiol. Regul. Integr. Comp. Physiol.* **2003**, *284*, R140–R152.
3. Leger, J.; Levy-Marchal, C.; Bloch, J.; Pinet, A.; Chevenne, D.; Porquet, D.; Collin, D.; Czernichow, P. Reduced final height and indications for insulin resistance in 20 year olds small for gestational age: Regional cohort study. *BMJ* **1997**, *315*, 341–347.
4. Eckel, R.H.; Grundy, S.M.; Zimmet, P.Z. The metabolic syndrome. *Lancet* **2005**, *365*, 1415–1428.
5. Barker, D.J. The developmental origins of insulin resistance. *Horm. Res.* **2005**, *64* (Suppl. 3), 2–7.
6. Pollack, R.N.; Divon, M.Y. Intrauterine growth retardation: Definition, classification and etiology. *Clin. Obsetrics Gynecol.* **1992**, *35*, 99–107.
7. Bamberg, C.; Kalache, K.D. Prenatal diagnosis of fetal growth restriction. *Semin. Fetal Neonatal Med.* **2004**, *9*, 387–394.
8. Giussani, D.A.; Salinas, C.E.; Villena, M.; Blanco, C.E. The role of oxygen in prenatal growth: Studies in the chick embryo. *J. Physiol.* **2007**, *585*, 911–917.
9. Arbeille, P. Fetal arterial doppler-iugr and hypoxia. *Eur. J. Obstetrics Gynecol. Reprod. Biol.* **1997**, *75*, 51–53.
10. Baschat, A.A. Fetal responses to placental insufficiency: An update. *BJOG Int. J. Obstetrics Gynaecol.* **2004**, *111*, 1031–1041.
11. Rurak, D.W.; Richardson, B.S.; Patrick, J.E.; Carmichael, L.; Homan, J. Blood flow and oxygen delivery to fetal organs and tissues during sustained hypoxemia. *Am. J. Physiol.* **1990**, *258*, 1116–1122.
12. Dubiel, M.; Breborowicz, G.H.; Gudmundsson, S. Evaluation of fetal circulation redistribution in pregnancies with absent or reversed diastolic flow in the umbilical artery. *Early Hum. Dev.* **2003**, *71*, 149–156.
13. Dubiel, M.; Breborowicz, G.H.; Marsal, K.; Gudmundsson, S. Fetal adrenal and middle cerebral artery doppler velocimetry in high-risk pregnancy. *Ultrasound Obstetrics Gynecol.* **2000**, *16*, 414–418.
14. Salihagic-Kadic, A.; Medic, M.; Jugovic, D.; Kos, M.; Latin, V.; Kusan Jukic, M.; Arbeille, P. Fetal cerebrovascular response to chronic hypoxia—Implications for the prevention of brain damage. *J. Mater. Fetal Neonatal Med.* **2006**, *19*, 387–396.

15. Poudel, R.; McMillen, I.C.; Dunn, S.L.; Zhang, S.; Morrison, J.L. Impact of chronic hypoxemia on blood flow to the brain, heart and adrenal gland in the late gestation iugr sheep fetus. *Am. J. Physiol. Regul. Integr. Comp. Physiol.* **2014**, doi:10.1152/ajpregu.00036.2014.
16. Jensen, C.B.; Martin-Gronert, M.S.; Storgaard, H.; Madsbad, S.; Vaag, A.; Ozanne, S.E. Altered pi3-kinase/akt signalling in skeletal muscle of young men with low birth weight. *PLoS One* **2008**, *3*, e3738, doi:10.1371/journal.pone.0003738
17. Jensen, C.B.; Storgaard, H.; Madsbad, S.; Richter, E.A.; Vaag, A.A. Altered skeletal muscle fiber composition and size precede whole-body insulin resistance in young men with low birth weight. *J. Clin. Endocrinol. Metab.* **2007**, *92*, 1530–1534.
18. Barker, D.J.; Hales, C.N.; Fall, C.H.; Osmond, C.; Phipps, K.; Clark, P.M. Type 2 (non-insulin-dependent) diabetes mellitus, hypertension and hyperlipidaemia (syndrome X): Relation to reduced fetal growth. *Diabetologia* **1993**, *36*, 62–67.
19. Beauchamp, B.; Ghosh, S.; Dysart, M.W.; Kanaan, G.N.; Chu, A.; Blais, A.; Rajamanickam, K.; Tsai, E.C.; Patti, M.E.; Harper, M.E. Low birth weight is associated with adiposity, impaired skeletal muscle energetics and weight loss resistance in mice. *Int. J. Obes.* **2014**, doi:10.1038/ijo.2014.120.
20. Kensara, O.A.; Wootton, S.A.; Phillips, D.I.; Patel, M.; Jackson, A.A.; Elia, M.; Hertfordshire Study, G. Fetal programming of body composition: Relation between birth weight and body composition measured with dual-energy X-ray absorptiometry and anthropometric methods in older englishmen. *Am. J. Clin. Nutr.* **2005**, *82*, 980–987.
21. Thorn, S.R.; Rozance, P.J.; Brown, L.D.; Hay, W.W., Jr. The intrauterine growth restriction phenotype: Fetal adaptations and potential implications for later life insulin resistance and diabetes. *Semin. Reprod. Med.* **2011**, *29*, 225–236.
22. Gluckman, P.D.; Hanson, M.A.; Spencer, H.G.; Bateson, P. Environmental influences during development and their later consequences for health and disease: Implications for the interpretation of empirical studies. *Proc. Biol. Sci. R. Soc.* **2005**, *272*, 671–677.
23. DeFronzo, R.A.; Jacot, E.; Jequier, E.; Maeder, E.; Wahren, J.; Felber, J.P. The effect of insulin on the disposal of intravenous glucose: Results from indirect calorimetry and hepatic and femoral venous catheterization. *Diabetes* **1981**, *30*, 1000–1007.
24. Zurlo, F.; Nemeth, P.M.; Choksi, R.M.; Sesodia, S.; Ravussin, E. Whole-body energy metabolism and skeletal muscle biochemical characteristics. *Metab. Clin. Exp.* **1994**, *43*, 481–486.
25. Yu, C.; Chen, Y.; Cline, G.W.; Zhang, D.; Zong, H.; Wang, Y.; Bergeron, R.; Kim, J.K.; Cushman, S.W.; Cooney, G.J.; *et al.* Mechanism by which fatty acids inhibit insulin activation of insulin receptor substrate-1 (IRS-1)-associated phosphatidylinositol 3-kinase activity in muscle. *J. Biol. Chem.* **2002**, *277*, 50230–50236.
26. Koves, T.R.; Ussher, J.R.; Noland, R.C.; Slentz, D.; Mosedale, M.; Ilkayeva, O.; Bain, J.; Stevens, R.; Dyck, J.R.; Newgard, C.B.; *et al.* Mitochondrial overload and incomplete fatty acid oxidation contribute to skeletal muscle insulin resistance. *Cell Metab.* **2008**, *7*, 45–56.
27. Shulman, G.I. Cellular mechanisms of insulin resistance. *J. Clin. Investig.* **2000**, *106*, 171–176.

28. Zierath, J.R.; Krook, A.; Wallberg-Henriksson, H. Insulin action and insulin resistance in human skeletal muscle. *Diabetologia* **2000**, *43*, 821–835.
29. Blesson, C.S.; Sathishkumar, K.; Chinnathambi, V.; Yallampalli, C. Gestational protein restriction impairs insulin regulated glucose transport mechanisms in gastrocnemius muscles of adult male offspring. *Endocrinology* **2014**, doi:10.1210/en.2014-1094.
30. Owens, J.A.; Thavaneswaran, P.; De Blasio, M.J.; McMillen, I.C.; Robinson, J.S.; Gatford, K.L. Sex-specific effects of placental restriction on components of the metabolic syndrome in young adult sheep. *Am. J. Physiol. Endocrinol. Metab.* **2007**, *292*, E1879–E1889.
31. De Blasio, M.J.; Gatford, K.L.; Harland, M.L.; Robinson, J.S.; Owens, J.A. Placental restriction reduces insulin sensitivity and expression of insulin signaling and glucose transporter genes in skeletal muscle, but not liver, in young sheep. *Endocrinology* **2012**, *153*, 2142–2151.
32. De Blasio, M.J.; Gatford, K.L.; McMillen, I.C.; Robinson, J.S.; Owens, J.A. Placental restriction of fetal growth increases insulin action, growth, and adiposity in the young lamb. *Endocrinology* **2007**, *148*, 1350–1358.
33. Sugden, M.C.; Holness, M.J. Gender-specific programming of insulin secretion and action. *J. Endocrinol.* **2002**, *175*, 757–767.
34. Jaquet, D.; Gaboriau, A.; Czernichow, P.; Levy-Marchal, C. Insulin resistance early in adulthood in subjects born with intrauterine growth retardation. *J. Clin. Endocrinol. Metab.* **2000**, *85*, 1401–1406.
35. Hales, C.N.; Barker, D.J.; Clark, P.M.; Cox, L.J.; Fall, C.; Osmond, C.; Winter, P.D. Fetal and infant growth and impaired glucose tolerance at age 64. *BMJ* **1991**, *303*, 1019–1022.
36. Ozanne, S.E.; Jensen, C.B.; Tingey, K.J.; Storgaard, H.; Madsbad, S.; Vaag, A.A. Low birthweight is associated with specific changes in muscle insulin-signalling protein expression. *Diabetologia* **2005**, *48*, 547–552.
37. Thorn, S.R.; Regnault, T.R.; Brown, L.D.; Rozance, P.J.; Keng, J.; Roper, M.; Wilkening, R.B.; Hay, W.W., Jr.; Friedman, J.E. Intrauterine growth restriction increases fetal hepatic gluconeogenic capacity and reduces messenger ribonucleic acid translation initiation and nutrient sensing in fetal liver and skeletal muscle. *Endocrinology* **2009**, *150*, 3021–3030.
38. Oak, S.A.; Tran, C.; Pan, G.; Thamotharan, M.; Devaskar, S.U. Perturbed skeletal muscle insulin signaling in the adult female intrauterine growth-restricted rat. *Am. J. Physiol. Endocrinol. Metab.* **2006**, *290*, E1321–E1330.
39. Copps, K.D.; White, M.F. Regulation of insulin sensitivity by serine/threonine phosphorylation of insulin receptor substrate proteins irs1 and IRS2. *Diabetologia* **2012**, *55*, 2565–2582.
40. Karlsson, H.K.; Zierath, J.R.; Kane, S.; Krook, A.; Lienhard, G.E.; Wallberg-Henriksson, H. Insulin-stimulated phosphorylation of the AKT substrate as160 is impaired in skeletal muscle of type 2 diabetic subjects. *Diabetes* **2005**, *54*, 1692–1697.
41. Holemans, K.; Verhaeghe, J.; Dequeker, J.; van Assche, F.A. Insulin sensitivity in adult female rats subjected to malnutrition during the perinatal period. *J. Soc. Gynecol. Investig.* **1996**, *3*, 71–77.
42. Stein, J.M.; Padykula, H.A. Histochemical classification of individual skeletal muscle fibers of the rat. *Am. J. Anat.* **1962**, *110*, 103–123.

43. Leary, S.C.; Lyons, C.N.; Rosenberger, A.G.; Ballantyne, J.S.; Stillman, J.; Moyes, C.D. Fiber-type differences in muscle mitochondrial profiles. *Am. J. Physiol. Regul. Integr. Comp. Physiol.* **2003**, *285*, R817–R826.
44. Peter, J.B.; Barnard, R.J.; Edgerton, V.R.; Gillespie, C.A.; Stempel, K.E. Metabolic profiles of three fiber types of skeletal muscle in guinea pigs and rabbits. *Biochemistry* **1972**, *11*, 2627–2633.
45. Selak, M.A.; Storey, B.T.; Peterside, I.; Simmons, R.A. Impaired oxidative phosphorylation in skeletal muscle of intrauterine growth-retarded rats. *Ame. J. Physiol. Endocrinol. Metab.* **2003**, *285*, E130–E137.
46. Peterside, I.E.; Selak, M.A.; Simmons, R.A. Impaired oxidative phosphorylation in hepatic mitochondria in growth-retarded rats. *Am. J. Physiol. Endocrinol. Metab.* **2003**, *285*, 1258–1266.
47. Albrecht, E.; Lembcke, C.; Wegner, J.; Maak, S. Prenatal muscle fiber development and bundle structure in beef and dairy cattle. *J. Anim. Sci.* **2013**, *91*, 3666–3673.
48. St-Pierre, J.; Lin, J.; Krauss, S.; Tarr, P.T.; Yang, R.; Newgard, C.B.; Spiegelman, B.M. Bioenergetic analysis of peroxisome proliferator-activated receptor gamma coactivators 1alpha and 1beta (PGC-1alpha and PGC-1beta) in muscle cells. *J. Biol. Chem.* **2003**, *278*, 26597–26603.
49. Limesand, S.W.; Rozance, P.J.; Smith, D.; Hay, W.W., Jr. Increased insulin sensitivity and maintenance of glucose utilization rates in fetal sheep with placental insufficiency and intrauterine growth restriction. *Am. J. Physiol. Endocrinol. Metab.* **2007**, *293*, E1716–E1725.
50. Bauer, R.; Walter, B.; Brust, P.; Füchtner, F.; Zwiener, U. Impact of asymmetric intrauterine growth restriction on organ function in newborn piglets. *Eur. J. Obstetrics Gynecol. Reprod. Biol.* **2003**, *110*, S40–S49.
51. Wank, V.; Bauer, R.; Walter, B.; Kluge, H.; Fischer, M.S.; Blickhan, R.; Zwiener, U. Accelerated contractile function and improved fatigue resistance of calf muscles in newborn piglets with IUGR. *Am. J. Physiol. Regul. Integ. Comp. Physiol.* **2000**, *278*, R304–R310.
52. Bauer, R.; Gedrange, T.; Bauer, K.; Walter, B. Intrauterine growth restriction induces increased capillary density and accelerated type I fiber maturation in newborn pig skeletal muscles. *J. Perinat. Med.* **2006**, *34*, 235–242.
53. He, J.; Watkins, S.; Kelley, D.E. Skeletal muscle lipid content and oxidative enzyme activity in relation to muscle fiber type in type 2 diabetes and obesity. *Diabetes* **2001**, *50*, 817–823.
54. Oberbach, A.; Bossenz, Y.; Lehmann, S.; Niebauer, J.; Adams, V.; Paschke, R.; Schon, M.R.; Bluher, M.; Punkt, K. Altered fiber distribution and fiber-specific glycolytic and oxidative enzyme activity in skeletal muscle of patients with type 2 diabetes. *Diabetes Care* **2006**, *29*, 895–900.
55. Reusch, J.E.; Bridenstine, M.; Regensteiner, J.G. Type 2 diabetes mellitus and exercise impairment. *Rev. Endocr. Metab. Disord.* **2013**, *14*, 77–86.
56. Badin, P.M.; Langin, D.; Moro, C. Dynamics of skeletal muscle lipid pools. *Trends Endocrinol. Metab. TEM* **2013**, *24*, 607–615.
57. Abdul-Ghani, M.A.; DeFronzo, R.A. Pathogenesis of insulin resistance in skeletal muscle. *J. Biomed. Biotechnol.* **2010**, *2010*, 476279, doi:10.1155/2010/476279.

58. Zhang, L.; Keung, W.; Samokhvalov, V.; Wang, W.; Lopaschuk, G.D. Role of fatty acid uptake and fatty acid beta-oxidation in mediating insulin resistance in heart and skeletal muscle. *Biochim. Biophys. Acta* **2010**, *1801*, 1–22.
59. Storlien, L.H.; Jenkins, A.B.; Chisholm, D.J.; Pascoe, W.S.; Khouri, S.; Kraegen, E.W. Influence of dietary fat composition on development of insulin resistance in rats: Relationship to muscle triglyceride and ω-3 fatty acids in muscle phospholipid. *Diabetes* **1991**, *40*, 280–289.
60. Kewalramani, G.; Bilan, P.J.; Klip, A. Muscle insulin resistance: Assault by lipids, cytokines and local macrophages. *Curr. Opin. Clin. Nutr. Metabo. Care* **2010**, *13*, 382–390.
61. Dziewulska, A.; Dobrzyn, P.; Jazurek, M.; Pyrkowska, A.; Ntambi, J.M.; Dobrzyn, A. Monounsaturated fatty acids are required for membrane translocation of protein kinase C-theta induced by lipid overload in skeletal muscle. *Mol. Memb. Biol.* **2012**, *29*, 309–320.
62. Lee, J.S.; Pinnamaneni, S.K.; Eo, S.J.; Cho, I.H.; Pyo, J.H.; Kim, C.K.; Sinclair, A.J.; Febbraio, M.A.; Watt, M.J. Saturated, but not n-6 polyunsaturated, fatty acids induce insulin resistance: Role of intramuscular accumulation of lipid metabolites. *J. Appl. Physiol.* **2006**, *100*, 1467–1474.
63. Kelley, D.E.; Goodpaster, B.; Wing, R.R.; Simoneau, J.-A. Skeletal muscle fatty acid metabolism in association with insulin resistance, obesity and weight loss. *Endocrinol. MeTable* **1999**, *40*, E1130–E1141.
64. Malenfant, P.; Joanisse, D.; Theriault, R.; Goodpaster, B.; Kelley, D.; Simoneau, J.-A. Fat content in individual muscle fibers of lean and obese subjects. *Int. J. Obes.* **2001**, *25*, 1316–1321.
65. Barucci, N.; Bell, K.; Cline, G.W.; Goodyear, L.J.; Griffin, M.E.; Kraegen, E.W.; Lee, D.; Marcucci, M.J.; Shulman, G.I.; White, M.F. Free fatty acid-induced insulin resistance is associated with activation of protein kinase C (theta) and alterations in the insulin signaling cascade. *Diabetes* **1999**, *48*, 1270–1274.
66. Germani, D.; Puglianiello, A.; Cianfarani, S. Uteroplacental insufficiency down regulates insulin receptor and affects expression of key enzymes of long-chain fatty acid (LCFA) metabolism in skeletal muscle at birth. *Cardiovasc. Diabetol.* **2008**, *7*, 14, doi:10.1186/1475-2840-7-14.
67. Henstridge, D.C.; Bruce, C.R.; Pang, C.P.; Lancaster, G.I.; Allen, T.L.; Estevez, E.; Gardner, T.; Weir, J.M.; Meikle, P.J.; Lam, K.S.; *et al.* Skeletal muscle-specific overproduction of constitutively activated c-Jun *N*-terminal kinase (JNK) induces insulin resistance in mice. *Diabetologia* **2012**, *55*, 2769–2778.
68. Koves, T.R.; Li, P.; An, J.; Akimoto, T.; Slentz, D.; Ilkayeva, O.; Dohm, G.L.; Yan, Z.; Newgard, C.B.; Muoio, D.M. Peroxisome proliferator-activated receptor-gamma co-activator 1alpha-mediated metabolic remodeling of skeletal myocytes mimics exercise training and reverses lipid-induced mitochondrial inefficiency. *J. Biol. Chem.* **2005**, *280*, 33588–33598.
69. Rutkowsky, J.M.; Knotts, T.A.; Ono-Moore, K.D.; McCoin, C.S.; Huang, S.; Schneider, D.; Singh, S.; Adams, S.H.; Hwang, D.H. Acylcarnitines activate proinflammatory signaling pathways. *Am. J. Physiol. Endocrinol. Metab.* **2014**, *306*, E1378–E1387.
70. Muoio, D.M.; Koves, T.R. Skeletal muscle adaptation to fatty acid depends on coordinated actions of the ppars and PGC1 alpha: Implications for metabolic disease. *Appl. Physiol. Nutr. Metab.* **2007**, *32*, 874–883.

71. Jacobsen, S.C.; Gillberg, L.; Bork-Jensen, J.; Ribel-Madsen, R.; Lara, E.; Calvanese, V.; Ling, C.; Fernandez, A.F.; Fraga, M.F.; Poulsen, P.; *et al.* Young men with low birthweight exhibit decreased plasticity of genome-wide muscle DNA methylation by high-fat overfeeding. *Diabetologia* **2014**, *57*, 1154–1158.
72. Sugden, M.C.; Caton, P.W.; Holness, M.J. PPAR control: It's sirtainly as easy as PGC. *J. Endocrinol.* **2010**, *204*, 93–104.
73. Finck, B.N.; Bernal-Mizrachi, C.; Han, D.H.; Coleman, T.; Sambandam, N.; LaRiviere, L.L.; Holloszy, J.O.; Semenkovich, C.F.; Kelly, D.P. A potential link between muscle peroxisome proliferator- activated receptor-alpha signaling and obesity-related diabetes. *Cell Metab.* **2005**, *1*, 133–144.
74. Liu, J.; Chen, D.; Yao, Y.; Yu, B.; Mao, X.; He, J.; Huang, Z.; Zheng, P. Intrauterine growth retardation increases the susceptibility of pigs to high-fat diet-induced mitochondrial dysfunction in skeletal muscle. *PLoS One* **2012**, *7*, e34835, doi:10.1371/journal.pone.0034835.
75. Lane, R.H.; Maclennan, N.K.; Daood, M.J.; Hsu, J.L.; Janke, S.M.; Pham, T.D.; Puri, A.R.; Watchko, J.F. Iugr alters postnatal rat skeletal muscle peroxisome proliferator-activated receptor-gamma coactivator-1 gene expression in a fiber specific manner. *Pediatr. Res.* **2003**, *53*, 994–1000.
76. Zeng, Y.; Gu, P.; Liu, K.; Huang, P. Maternal protein restriction in rats leads to reduced PGC-1alpha expression via altered DNA methylation in skeletal muscle. *Mol. Med. Rep.* **2013**, *7*, 306–312.
77. Brons, C.; Jacobsen, S.; Nilsson, E.; Ronn, T.; Jensen, C.B.; Storgaard, H.; Poulsen, P.; Groop, L.; Ling, C.; Astrup, A.; *et al.* Deoxyribonucleic acid methylation and gene expression of PPARGC1A in human muscle is influenced by high-fat overfeeding in a birth-weight-dependent manner. *J. Clin. Endocrinol. Metab.* **2010**, *95*, 3048–3056.
78. Laker, R.C.; Wlodek, M.E.; Wadley, G.D.; Gallo, L.A.; Meikle, P.J.; McConell, G.K. Exercise early in life in rats born small does not normalize reductions in skeletal muscle PGC-1alpha in adulthood. *Am. J. Physiol. Endocrinol. Metab.* **2012**, *302*, E1221–E1230.

4

Impacts of Maternal Nutrition on Vascularity of Nutrient Transferring Tissues during Gestation and Lactation

Kimberly A. Vonnahme [1,*], Caleb O. Lemley [2], Joel S. Caton [1] and Allison M. Meyer [3]

[1] Department of Animal Sciences, North Dakota State University, Fargo, ND 58102, USA; E-Mail: Joel.Caton@ndsu.edu

[2] Department of Animal and Dairy Sciences, Mississippi State University, Mississippi State, MS 39762, USA; E-Mail: CLemley@ads.msstate.edu

[3] Division of Animal Sciences, University of Missouri, Columbus, MO 65210, USA; E-Mail: MeyerAll@missouri.edu

* Author to whom correspondence should be addressed; E-Mail: Kim.Vonnahme@ndsu.edu

Abstract: As the demand for food increases with exponential growth in the world population, it is imperative that we understand how to make livestock production as efficient as possible in the face of decreasing available natural resources. Moreover, it is important that livestock are able to meet their metabolic demands and supply adequate nutrition to developing offspring both during pregnancy and lactation. Specific nutrient supplementation programs that are designed to offset deficiencies, enhance efficiency, and improve nutrient supply during pregnancy can alter tissue vascular responses, fetal growth, and postnatal offspring outcomes. This review outlines how vascularity in nutrient transferring tissues, namely the maternal gastrointestinal tract, the utero-placental tissue, and the mammary gland, respond to differing nutritional planes and other specific nutrient supplementation regimes.

Keywords: mammary gland; placenta; small intestine; uterine blood flow

1. Introduction

The world's population reached 7 billion in 2012, and is projected to be greater than 9 billion by 2050 [1]. Continued economic and population growth in developing countries is expected to increase world-wide demand for meat, milk, and eggs [2]. Increased demand will require rapid development of new technologies to improve food animal production systems in the face of limited land and water, competition with bioenergy, and increasing environmental and animal welfare regulations. With this in mind, it is imperative that we enhance livestock production efficiency by optimizing the function of nutrient transferring tissues, namely the gastrointestinal tract, placenta, and mammary gland. Large animal research ensures food safety and improves the quality and affordability of meat and milk, as well as serve as biomedical models. Understanding nutrient transferring tissue efficiency is critical, not only for the growth and development of the dam, but also for the offspring. Animal models are particularly important to human health in the area of developmental programming. Maternal delivery of nutrients to the fetus can be reduced by decreased placental function, just as poor neonatal nutrient delivery is impaired by poor mammary gland development. Both the placenta and mammary gland are dependent upon the maternal gastrointestinal tract to adequately extract and deliver dietary nutrients. While it is well known that the gastrointestinal tract, placenta, and mammary gland adapt to different nutritional stimuli, how these tissues adapt to different nutritional stressors (*i.e.*, inappropriate nutrient supply, conditional increases in nutrient demand, specific nutrient imbalances, *etc.*) may be keys for enhancement of nutrient transfer efficiency.

The area of developmental programming and the study of nutrient exchange in tissues is of interest to both agriculture and human health. Obviously, research done in agriculturally relevant species such as the cow, sheep, and pig will directly relate to those species. However, these large domesticated animals are also a primary model for human research. The advantages of domesticated animal models are important for moving concepts from the laboratory to human health applications (http://adsbm.msu.edu/) [3]. In particular, sheep have been used as a relevant model for biomedical research for humans because there is a large body of data on reproductive function, including pregnancy, available [4–12]. A variety of animal species, from laboratory rodents to domestic ruminants and non-human primates, have been used to study pregnancy. This review will highlight how nutrient transferring tissues are affected in several domesticated animals, with more data presented from sheep. While no animal model truly recapitulates processes happening in the human, the sheep model has some resemblances with human reproduction which include: 1) a relatively long gestation length (*i.e.*, ~150 days); 2) generally carries singleton or twin fetuses; and 3) the villous tree of the sheep cotyledon is structurally similar to the human placenta. Furthermore, the ewe is a robust model allowing for surgical manipulations for repeated maternal and fetal sampling/data collection to determine how both maternal and fetal tissues respond to physiological stimuli (such as nutritional manipulations). Moreover, there is a wealth of information in the sheep as it has been used extensively over the past 40 years as a model of human pregnancy [9]. Additional appreciable features of the sheep model which are relatively comparable to human fetal development include: neonatal thermoregulation, metabolic regulation, specific organ growth rate, fetal protein turnover, maturity of hypothalamic-pituitary-thyroid-adrenal axis and others, as summarized by Symonds *et al.* [6]. Furthermore, a sheep model allows for performing controlled studies using a greater number of animals, and for obtaining a large amount of tissues from the relevant physiological states.

How Pregnancy Alters Physiology and Metabolism

During pregnancy, maternal physiologic state is associated with significant but reversible modulations to meet metabolic demand as well as alterations to the endocrine and cardiovascular systems. Endocrine secretions from the conceptus allows for communication between the maternal endometrium and fetal membranes of the placenta during mid- to late-gestation, helping to ensure proper nutrient and waste exchange during exponential growth of the fetus. Moreover, it is evident that pregnancy alters vascularity of the small intestine [13] allowing for greater uptake of nutrients. Maternal cardiovascular capacity also changes dramatically during pregnancy, with decreases in systemic arterial blood pressure and vascular resistance and increases in cardiac output, heart rate, heart stroke volume, and blood volume [14]. Mean arterial pressure decreases in early pregnancy and persists throughout gestation in several mammalian species. The decrease in arterial pressure (~5%–10% decrease) is minor compared to the approximate 20%–30% decrease in total peripheral vascular resistance. Maternal cardiac output has been shown to increase as much as 30%–40% in pregnant *vs.* non-pregnant ruminants [14]. Therefore, the increase in cardiac output is associated with a fall in systemic vascular resistance, allowing researchers to characterize pregnancy as a state of systemic vasodilation resulting in profound increases in total systemic flows to all vascular beds. In addition to the changes in the maternal cardiovascular system during pregnancy, it is also noteworthy to point out that the majority of mammals will return to the non-pregnant levels of cardiovascular function 2–5 weeks postpartum indicating that vascularity is important during involution and repair of the uterus.

Two important contributors to the alterations in the cardiovascular system include vascular endothelial growth factor (VEGF) and nitric oxide (NO). Vascular endothelial growth factor and its receptors are distributed widely throughout adult and fetal tissues [15–19]. While many angiogenic factors are associated with fetal development, VEGF is one of the most potent factors associated with fetal and placental vascular growth in many species including sheep [17,18,20–22], cow [23,24], and pig [25,26]. While changes in VEGF in the maternal circulation do not appear to change in cattle or sheep (Table 1), there is an increase in fetal circulation in swine [26]. Moreover, VEGF mRNA increases in the pig placenta, but is not altered in ruminants as gestation advances. In addition to VEGF stimulating angiogenesis, VEGF upregulates nitric oxide (NO) production by endothelial cells [27–30]. While NO metabolites increase as gestation advances in the ewe [22] and cow ([31]; Table 1), similar information has not been reported for pigs. Moreover, while endothelial nitric oxide synthase (eNOS) mRNA expression does not appear to significantly change as gestation advances, it is known that several NO mediated vascular events are occurring in the placenta [32–35] and the mesenteric arteries [36,37].

Table 1. Changes in VEGF protein and placental mRNA as well as nitric oxide metabolite (NOx) and eNOS mRNA from mid- to late-gestation in cattle, sheep, and swine.

	In Circulation	mRNA in Fetal Placenta	mRNA in Maternal Placenta
VEGF			
Cow	Maternal: No change [23]	8% increase [38],*	43% decrease [38],*
Sheep	Maternal: No change [22]	36% increase [21],*	14% decrease [21],*
Pig	Fetal: 83% increase [26]	50% increase [26]	18% increase [26]
Nitric Oxide	NOx	eNOS	eNOS
Cow	210% increase [31]	29% increase [38],*	49% increase [38],*
Sheep	260% increase [22]	37% increase [21],*	42% increase [21],*
Pig	**	**	**

*Not significant at $p \leq 0.05$; ** Unknown.

While there are many reviews that focus on how different maternal nutritional levels impact the growth and development of the offspring, this review will focus on how differing maternal nutritional levels impact nutrient transferring tissues. We hypothesize that in order to develop potential therapeutics that could spare negative influences on the offspring, functions of the small intestine, placenta and/or the mammary gland must become more efficient at nutrient delivery. Core mechanisms that regulate vascularization and blood flow within key nutrient transferring tissues are beginning to be understood, and likely are a major determinant of animal growth and nutrient utilization.

2. Maternal Gastrointestinal Tract during Pregnancy

The maternal gastrointestinal tract is critical for nutrient acquisition but is also a major nutrient sink during pregnancy. In ruminants, the liver and gut consume approximately 40% of maintenance energy demands [39,40]. Within the gastrointestinal tract, which consumes approximately 20% of maintenance energy [41,42], a majority of these nutrient resources are consumed by ion transport, protein turnover, enzyme secretion, and active transport [43,44]. The dam needs to maintain functional capacity of the gastrointestinal tract, even though a decrease in nutrient use by this tissue may be necessary, especially in cases of gestational nutrient restriction. Pregnancy [13,45], stage of gestation [46–48], and nutrient intake (Table 2) affect intestinal tissue mass and growth indices. Alternatively, some studies revealed minimal or no differences in small intestinal mass in response to pregnancy [46], stage of gestation [49], or nutrient intake (Table 3), leading us to hypothesize that changes are influenced by species, age/parity, previous nutritional plane, diet type, and other potential metabolic mechanisms.

Table 2. Histological measurements to assess vascularity of nutrient transferring tissues.

Measure	Calculation	Used to Assess
Capillary Area Density (**CAD**)	total capillary area ÷ tissue area	blood flow
Capillary Surface Density (**CSD**)	total vascular surface ÷ tissue area	nutrient exchange
Capillary Number Density (**CND**)	total number of vessels ÷ tissue area	vascular branching
Area Per Capillary (**APC**)	total capillary area ÷ number of vessels	capillary size
Total Vascularity	CAD × tissue mass	total vascular bed of tissue

The small intestine, which has a high degree of plasticity, is a focus of research during pregnancy because of its role in nutrient acquisition, nutrient utilization, and immunocompetence. Interestingly, the similarities in nutrient-transferring functions associated with the small intestine and the placenta have allowed many research techniques to be adapted and shared across tissues and within studies, including vascular perfusion and histological measures of vascularity (Table 2). In the small intestine, most measures have focused on the proximal jejunum, where both digestion and absorption occur. As with the placenta, these measures of vascularity have been responsive to pregnancy, stage of gestation, and nutritional status during pregnancy. Capillary area density and total vascularity of the jejunum increased in pregnant multiparous ewes, and total vascularity increased from mid- to late gestation [49]. In another study, jejunal capillary surface density and size increased from mid- to late gestation, while capillary number density decreased from early to late gestation in primiparous ewes [47]. Jejunal capillary area density and total vascularity also decreased from early to mid-gestation, then increased from mid- to late-gestation, possibly due to the maternal transition from the anabolic to catabolic state of pregnancy [47]. Additionally, capillary area density of the jejunum also increased from mid- to late-pregnancy in beef cattle [48]. These studies suggest that vascularity of the small intestine may play more of a role as the nutrient demand of fetal growth increases during late gestation. We hypothesize that we are observing increases in vasodilation, which would decrease resistance to blood flow, and allow for increased nutrient acquisition.

Overall, small intestinal size and function, including vascularity, are an active component of maternal physiological adaptations during pregnancy. These adaptations occur in response to increasing metabolic demands of advancing gestation, altered nutritional plane, and inappropriate levels of specific nutrients (Table 2). This should come as no surprise given that the small intestine is responsive to changes in intake and metabolic demand [50].

Vascularization of the Maternal Small Intestine in Response to Different Nutritional Treatments

Effects of nutrient intake in the face of pregnancy demands in ruminants (especially sheep) have been studied extensively by our group, and vascular changes due to nutrient intake, including nutrient restriction, overnutrition, and supranutritional selenium diets, are summarized in Table 2. Jejunal vascularity is not affected by gestational nutrition in beef cows [48], but it has been variable in sheep. Vascularity measures have increased, decreased, or not been affected by nutrient restriction during pregnancy in sheep, even though the mass of the small intestine is generally decreased by nutrient restriction (Table 2). Interestingly, mature ewes undergoing nutrient restriction have increased jejunal capillary area density as the mass of their small intestine decreases, allowing for similar total vascularity of the small intestine in restricted compared with adequately nourished ewes [49]. This phenomenon is not observed in ewe lambs (~8.5 month age at breeding) which demonstrated both decreased capillary area density and small intestinal mass, resulting in a decrease of total vascularity [51]. Because young females are still growing, pregnancy may slow intestinal growth and affect development, resulting in decreased mass and angiogenesis during times of combined physiological and nutritional stress. More studies need to be conducted in order to determine how age, parity, and stage of pregnancy contribute to vascular changes in the small intestine.

Overfeeding ewes during gestation affects vascularity of the small intestine less often than nutrient restriction, despite an increase in mass of the small intestine (Table 2). The increased mass associated with increased feed intake may allow for enough of an increase in overall vascularity [52] that increased vascularity per unit of tissue is not necessary in these instances to meet increased nutrient demand associated with pregnancy.

Factors affecting regulatory mechanisms of vascularity of the small intestine are not well understood. Nutrient intake appears to be a major factor, as growing steers with greater feed intake have increased capillary area, number, and surface densities as well as total vascularity [53]. This suggests that vascularity of the small intestine may follow nutrient intake to allow for greater nutrient absorption, which seems logical. In general, our studies with sheep support this notion, although fetal and placental signals likely complicate this relationship during pregnancy. The VEGF and NO systems play a role in modulating changes in vascularity and they are affected by nutritional plane during gestation (Table 4). In general, expression of VEGF and its receptors within intestinal tissues are altered more than eNOS or soluble guanylate cyclase (GUCY1B3). Additionally, expression of VEGF receptors are down regulated by supranutritional levels of selenium during pregnancy [52,54], whereas even within supranutritional selenium, VEGF is increased with dietary selenium (15 ppm > 3 ppm; 50). *In vitro* systems have demonstrated that VEGF delivery to the small intestine increases vascularity [55]. In our studies, vascularity of the small intestine and expression of genes for angiogenic factors change coordinately [52]. or, at times, in opposite directions [51,52,54]. Additionally, gene expression is not always altered at the same time as a change in vascularity, and *vice versa* (Tables 3 and 4). This could be due to the time of sampling of tissues, or differences in mRNA and protein expression.

The small intestine exhibits a high degree of plasticity and responds to nutrient presence in the lumen, immunomodulatory factors, hormones, growth factors, local cell communication, and microbial and host interactions [56–59]. Thus, changes in the vascularity and size of the small intestine in pregnant animals could be due to increased intake (which is typical when food is consumed ad libitum in most species), increased nutrient demand and resulting hormone and growth factor signals, and signals coming directly from the placenta or fetus. For example, estradiol-17β implants alter jejunal capillary number density and crypt cell proliferation and interact with dietary linseed meal (contains diphenolic compounds with estrogenic-like activity) and results in changes in impact mRNA expression of VEGF receptors and GUCY1B3 in ovariectomized ewes [60]. Additionally, blood flow to the small intestine increases with estradiol-17β infusion [14]. Thus, estradiol during pregnancy may be one of the contributing factors in adaptation of the intestine to pregnancy.

Proper and efficient function of the small intestine is necessary for the dam to acquire and deliver nutrients to the fetus during pregnancy. In all of our sheep studies, nutrient restriction in mid- and late-gestation reduces fetal growth (Table 3). The overall decrease in the nutrient transferring capacity of the small intestine due to changes in mass, vascularity, or other factors likely plays a role in decreased fetal growth. Although the maternal small intestine appears to increase vascularity during nutrient restriction in some studies [49], this has not occurred in all experiments. It is possible that successful maternal adaptation of the gut during nutrient restriction is able to prevent a decrease in nutrient delivery to the fetus in some animals, but more research is necessary. While the maternal gastrointestinal tract has the first opportunity to utilize nutrients after consumption, most data from stable isotope studies indicate [61]. that the gut is a highly competitive tissue, deriving the majority of its amino acids from arterial compared with luminal supplies. Maternal nutrient sourcing (arterial or luminal) has not been well studied during advancing pregnancy. If additional nutrients are used by the small intestine due to poor adaptation to nutrient restriction or pregnancy, decreased nutrients would be available for delivery to the fetus. Additionally, if the gastrointestinal tract is increasing in mass due to overnutrition during gestation (Table 3), this may also divert nutrients from fetal growth.

Table 3. Vascularity and mass of the maternal small intestine in ovine and bovine models for investigating the interrelationships of nutrition and reproduction.

Treatment	Stage	Impact on Vascularity *	Impact on Actual Mass	Impact on Production
Cattle—Gestation				
Control (CON) *vs.* Restricted (RES) Day 30 to 125 gestation [48]	Mid gestation (Day 125)	NS [1]	NS	Fetal weight: NS
Control (CON) *vs.* Restricted (RES) and realimented RES: Day 30 to 125, Realimented: Day 125 to 245 gestation [48]	Late gestation (Day 245)	NS	NS	Fetal weight: NS
Sheep—Gestation				
Control (CON) *vs.* Restricted (RES) Day 50 to 90 gestation [45,49]	Mid gestation (Day 90)	CAD: RES greater than CON	CON > RES	Fetal weight: NS
Control (CON) *vs.* Restricted (RES) Day 50 to 130 gestation [45,49]	Late gestation (Day 130)	CAD: RES greater than CON	CON > RES	Fetal weight: CON greater than RES
Control (CON) *vs.* Restricted (RES) Day 64 to 135 gestation [51]	Late gestation (Day 135)	CAD 17% less, APC 16% less, and total vascularity 35% less in RES *vs.* CON	20% less in RES *vs.* CON	Fetal weight 10% less in RES *vs.* CON
Control (CON) *vs.* RES-CON [2] Day 50 to 132 of gestation [62]	Late gestation (Day 132)	NS	NS	Fetal weight: NS
Control (CON) *vs.* CON-RES [2] Day 50 to 132 of gestation [62]	Late gestation (Day 132)	NS	17% less in CON-RES *vs.* CON	Fetal weight 13% less in CON-RES *vs.* CON
Control (CON) *vs.* RES-RES [2] Day 50 to 132 of gestation [62]	Late gestation (Day 132)	NS	13% less in RES-RES *vs.* CON	Fetal weight 14% less in RES-RES *vs.* CON
Control (CON) *vs.* Restricted (RES) Day 40 gestation to parturition [52,63]	Within 24 h post-partum	CSD 19% less in RES *vs.* CON	NS	Birth weight 9% less in RES *vs.* CON
Control (CON) *vs.* Overnourished (HIGH) Day 0 to 50 gestation [47]	Early gestation (Day 50)	NS	19% greater in HIGH *vs.* CON	Fetal weight: NS
Control (CON) *vs.* Overnourished (HIGH) Day 0 to 90 gestation [47]	Mid gestation (Day 90)	NS	43% greater in HIGH *vs.* CON	Fetal weight: NS
Control (CON) *vs.* Overnourished (HIGH) Day 0 to 130 gcstation [47]	Late gestation (Day 130)	NS	NS	Fetal weight 11% less in HIGH *vs.* CON

Table 3. *Cont.*

Treatment	Stage	Impact on Vascularity *	Impact on Actual Mass	Impact on Production
Sheep—Gestation				
Control (CON) *vs.* Overnourished (HIGH) Day 40 gestation to parturition [52,63]	Within 24 h post-partum	Total vascularity 38% greater in HIGH *vs.* CON	28% greater in HIGH *vs.* CON	Birth weight: NS
Adequate Se (ASe; 0.3 ppm) vs. High Se (HSe; 3 ppm) Day 0 to 135 gestation [51]	Late gestation (Day 135)	NS	10% greater in HSe *vs.* ASe	Fetal weight 10% greater in HSe *vs.* ASe
Adequate Se (ASe; 0.3 ppm) *vs.* High Se (HSe; 3 ppm) Day 0 to 132 gestation [62]	Late gestation (Day 132)	NS	NS	Fetal weight: NS
Adequate Se (ASe; 0.3 ppm) *vs.* High Se (HSe; 3 ppm) Day 0 gestation to parturition [52,63]	Within 24 h post-partum	NS	17% less in ASe *vs.* HSe	Birth weight: NS
Adequate Se (ASe; 0.14 ppm) *vs.* High Se (HSe; 3 or 15 ppm) Day 50 to 134 gestation [64]	Late gestation (Day 134)	APC 33% less in HSe *vs.* ASe	NS	Fetal weight: NS
High-Se wheat *vs.* Sodium selenate (3 ppm) Day 50 to 134 gestation [64]	Late gestation (Day 134)	CND 25% greater and CSD 73% greater in selenate *vs.* wheat	NS	Fetal weight: NS
3 ppm *vs.* 15 ppm of Se (both sodium selenate) Day 50 to 134 gestation [64]	Late gestation (Day 134)	NS	NS	Fetal weight: NS
Sheep—Lactation				
Control (CON) *vs.* Restricted (RES) Day 40 gestation to parturition [3] [52,65]	Early lactation (21 day)	CSD 5% greater in CON *vs.* RES	NS (both increased post-partum)	Milk production 22% less in RES *vs.* CON
Control (CON) *vs.* Overnourished (HIGH) Day 40 gestation to parturition [3] [52,65]	Early lactation (21 day)	Total vascularity 13% greater in HIGH *vs.* CON	NS (both increased post-partum)	Milk production: NS
Adequate Se (ASe; 0.3 ppm) *vs.* High Se (HSe; 3 ppm) Day 0 gestation to parturition [3] [52,65]	Early lactation (21 day)	APC 23% greater in HSe *vs.* ASe	NS (both increased post-partum)	Milk production 10% greater for HSe *vs.* ASe

* Vascularity measurements are included in Table 3. CAD = capillary area density; CSD = capillary surface density; CND = capillary number density; APC = area per capillary; [1] NS = not significant; [2] RES-CON = RES from Day 50 to 90 of gestation, CON from Day 90 to 132 of gestation; CON-RES = CON from Day 50 to 90 of gestation, RES from Day 90 to 132 of gestation; RES-RES = RES from Day 50 to 132 of gestation; [3] Fed to meet NRC requirements for lactation with adequate Se post-partum.

Table 4. Expression of VEGF and NO system mRNAs in the small intestine of ewes.

Treatment	Stage	Gene Expression [2]
Sheep—Gestation		
Control (CON) *vs.* Restricted (RES) Day 64 to 135 gestation [51,54]	Late gestation (Day 135)	VEGF, FLT1, KDR: RES > CON
Control (CON) *vs.* Restricted (RES) Day 40 gestation to parturition [52,63]	Within 24 h post-partum	FLT1: RES > CON
Control (CON) *vs.* Overnourished (HIGH) Day 40 gestation to parturition [52,63]	Within 24 h post-partum	VEGF, FLT1, and NOS3: HIGH > CON
Adequate Se (ASe; 0.3 ppm) *vs.* High Se (HSe; 3 ppm) Day 0 to 135 gestation [51,54]	Late gestation (Day 135)	NS [3]
Adequate Se (ASe; 0.3 ppm) *vs.* High Se (HSe; 3 ppm) Day 0 gestation to parturition [52,63]	Within 24 h post-partum	FLT1: ASe > HSe
Adequate Se (ASe; 0.14 ppm) *vs.* High Se (HSe; 3 or 15 ppm) Day 50 to 134 gestation [54,64]	Late gestation (Day 134)	[4] KDR: ASe > HSe
High-Se wheat *vs.* Sodium selenate (3 ppm) Day 50 to 134 gestation [54,64]	Late gestation (Day 134)	[4] NS
3 ppm *vs.* 15 ppm of Se (both sodium selenate) Day 50 to 134 gestation [54,64]	Late gestation (Day 134)	[4] VEGF: 15 ppm > 3 ppm
Sheep—Lactation		
Control (CON) *vs.* Restricted (RES) Day 40 gestation to parturition [52,64,65]	Early lactation (21 day)	NS
Control (CON) *vs.* Overnourished (HIGH) Day 40 gestation to parturition [52,64,65]	Early lactation (21 day)	NS
Adequate Se (ASe; 0.3 ppm) *vs.* High Se (HSe; 3 ppm) Day 0 gestation to parturition [1]	Early lactation (21 day)	NS

[1] Fed to meet NRC requirements for lactation with adequate Se post-partum; [2] FLT1 = fms-related tyrosine kinase 1 (VEGF receptor 1), KDR = kinase insert domain receptor (VEGF receptor 2), GUCY1B3 = soluble guanylate cyclase (NO receptor); [3] NS = not significant; [4] NOS3 and GUCY1B3 were not measured.

3. Placenta

Unlike most eutherians, livestock have non-invasive placentas. Gross morphology of the ruminant placenta is termed cotyledonary, and pigs and horses have a diffuse type of placentation. Microscopically, livestock species have epitheliochorial placentation, with six cellular layers separating maternal and fetal blood. Some argue that ruminant placentas are better classified as syndesmochorial due to their formation of giant trophoblast cells by chorionic and uterine epithelia [66–68]. In swine, the diffuse placenta has chorionic villi attachment distributed over the entire surface of the chorion. The presence of primary and secondary rugae increases the relative surface area of attachment between the endometrium and the fetal membranes [69]. Within the large white breeds of domestic pigs, placental area of attachment continues to increase as gestation advances [70,71] and vascular development of the placenta, as measured by the density of larger blood vessels (*i.e.*, arterioles), increases ~200% in the fetal portion of the placenta [71] with maternal vascular density remaining similar [26,71] from mid- to late-gestation. In ruminants, the fetal placenta attaches to discrete sites on the uterine wall called caruncles, which are aglandular sites appearing as knobs along the uterine luminal surface of non-pregnant animals [72]. The placental membranes attach at these sites via chorionic villi in areas termed cotyledons. The caruncular-cotyledonary unit is called a placentome and is the primary functional area of physiological exchanges between mother and fetus. In the ewe, the growth of the cotyledonary mass is exponential during the first 70–80 days of pregnancy, thereafter slowing markedly until term [73]. In contrast, the placental growth in the cow progressively increases throughout gestation [24,74]. Perhaps, these alterations in growth patterns in the sheep and cow placenta help explain the change of capillary area density (*i.e.*, a blood flow related measure; [21]) that exist from mid- to late-gestation [75]. While sheep placentas remain relatively similar in weight from mid- to late-gestation, there caruncular and cotyledonary capillary area density increase ~200 and 400%, respectively [21,75]. Bovine placentas exhibit relatively modest changes in capillary area density (compared to sheep) from mid- to late-gestation with capillary area density in caruncular tissue decreasing ~30% and cotyledonary tissue increasing ~190%, with caruncular and cotyledonary tissue weights increasing ~530% and ~650%, respectively [24].

3.1. Vascularity of the Placenta and Utero-Placental Blood Flow in Response to Different Nutritional Treatments

Several authors have established that many of the models of placental insufficiency are, in part, due to reduced placental vascularity and uterine or umbilical blood flows (reviewed in [76–78]). When placental growth is restricted in ewes, umbilical and uterine blood flows are reduced, limiting fetal growth [79]. Recently, in our laboratories, we have investigated if placental vascularity and uterine/umbilical blood flows are impacted by different maternal dietary treatments. In sheep, while we have observed reductions in umbilical blood flow [80] and increases in arterial indices of resistance [81], we have not observed alterations in placental capillary densities [82,83]. After 30 days whereby a 40% reduction in intake was applied (*i.e.*, on Day 50), umbilical blood flow of singleton fetuses was reduced compared to adequately fed control ewes [80]. This reduction remains through late gestation (Day 130). In beef cattle, we initially hypothesized that, similar to sheep, reductions in intake would lead to reductions in uterine blood flow. In contrast, we observed that during a 110 day nutrient restriction (*i.e.*, 40% of the control diet), uterine blood flows were similar [84]. Interestingly, upon realimentation, blood flow to the ipsilateral horn increases [84]. While our work has been done with global nutrient restriction and realimentation, Perry *et al.* [85] reported that protein restriction during the first trimester of pregnancy followed by increased protein concentration during the second trimester enhances placental development and fetal growth. Increased dry matter intake has been linked to enhanced maternal insulin-like growth factor-1 during late pregnancy [86]. If exogenous insulin-like growth factor-1 is administered to the dam, there is increased glucose and amino acid uptake by both fetal and maternal tissues [87]. Uteroplacental blood flow is undoubtedly associated with fetal growth and development; however, specific nutrient transport across the feto-placental unit rely not only on adequate blood flow but also on adequate nutrient transporter densities.

For our beef cattle studies, color Doppler ultrasonography was utilized. Prior to our studies, others have used this non-invasive technique which has been used to measure uterine blood flow and arterial indices of resistance in cattle [88–90]. Foundational uterine blood flow work in beef cattle has been conducted utilizing more invasive techniques such as electromagnetic blood flow transducers [91] or infusion of deuterium water [92]. By using color Doppler ultrasonography to assess uterine blood flow and vascular resistance throughout gestation in pregnant beef cows, we were able to examine the same animal continuously throughout gestation with no surgical preparation and with minimal interference to dam. Similarly, Bollwein *et al.* [88] measured uterine blood flow in cows during the estrous cycle. They suggested that Doppler ultrasonography was a reliable method to determine uterine blood flow and did not require use of blood flow probes and/or chronically catheterized animals. Moreover, findings from this study and others suggest that the use of Doppler ultrasonography as the technique to investigate uterine blood flow during pregnancy may also constitute a reliable method. In several breeds of cattle, when Doppler ultrasonography assessed uterine hemodynamics throughout gestation (*i.e.*, Day 30–270) resistance index decreased and uterine blood flow increased exponentially with increased blood flow in ipsilateral *vs.* contralateral horns [89,93]. Moreover, resistance index was negatively correlated to uterine blood flow [93].

The hypothesis that during nutrient restriction total uterine blood flow would be reduced was rejected. Moreover, while total uterine blood flow was similar after realimentation, ipsilateral uterine blood flow was enhanced in cows that were previously restricted. In many sheep models investigated to date [76,80], nutrient restriction results in reduced uterine and/or umbilical blood flow. This could be innate species differences, or also due to parity or age of the dam. Regardless, until more beef cattle work is performed to confirm our results, caution should be used when comparing data acquired in sheep as it may not be directly applicable to beef cattle. Inanition in swine during mid-pregnancy (Day 50–90; gestation length = 114 days) resulted in no change to uterine blood flow, similar to our findings in the beef cow, and resulted in no change in weight of the total uterine mass [94]. Despite this lack of change in uterine blood flow, Hard and Anderson [94] further demonstrated that blood volume was reduced during inanition, but increased by 24% within 20 days of realimentation. Unfortunately, how realimentation influenced uterine blood flow was not measured in the Hard and Anderson study. In women experiencing hyperemesis gravidarum, uterine blood flow per 100 g of fetus is increased compared to control women [95], but the authors were unable to locate information on how normal intakes may have impacted uterine blood flow in those pregnancies. While there is a paucity of information on how restriction and/or realimentation impacts uterine blood flow, it appears most pregnant females alter their body reserves to allow continuation of adequate blood flow for the developing conceptus. However, to our knowledge, uterine blood flow in models of nutrient restriction has not been measured upon realimentation in any species.

3.2. Utero-Placental Amino Acids

Uteroplacental and fetal uptake of amino acids can be primarily divided into two areas of interest focusing on either metabolic pathways or transport systems [77,96,97]. From a metabolic standpoint, research has shown consistent uterine and fetal uptakes of essential amino acids [98]. However, there is evidence that amino acid derivatives, such as creatine, which is actively transported across the placenta, may provide beneficial impacts to the fetus [99]. Focusing on essential amino acids, previous research has shown net uteroplacental consumption of isoleucine, leucine, and valine, while methionine was the only essential Amino Acid (AA) showing a net uteroplacental release [98]. The uteroplacental consumption of branched-chain amino acids to their respective keto acids contributes extensively to placental glutamate production via α-ketoglutarate. This relationship allows for the establishment of a feto-placental glutamate–glutamine shuttle, whereby the fetus is dependent on this exogenous supply of glutamine from the placenta [100–102], which could be altered by placental insufficiency [103,104]). The ovine placenta expresses glutamine synthetase, which catalyzes the condensation of glutamate and ammonia into glutamine [98].

Branched-chain amino acids regulate mammalian target of rapamycin (mTOR), which has been implicated as a nutritional sensor, that regulates cell growth and protein synthesis via increased rates of mRNA translation through the phosphorylation of eukaryotic initiation factor 4E-binding protein 1 (4E-BP1) and the ribosomal protein S6 kinase 1 [105–107]. Moreover, supplementation of branched-chain amino acids to dams on a protein deficient diet can restore fetal growth and minimize the decreases in fetal organ mass and carcass fat, which is associated with increased mTOR signaling in the fetus [108]. Recent evidence in human placental cell cultures as well as choriocarcinoma cell lines indicate that amino acid transporter expression and/or activity may be regulated by mTOR signaling pathways [109]. Specifically, treatment of the BJAB cell line with rapamycin (an inhibitor of mTOR complex 1) decreases mRNA expression of multiple amino acid transporters [110]. In human primary trophoblast cell cultures, inhibition of mTOR by rapamycin reduces the activity of system A, system L, and taurine amino acid transporters; however, mTOR inhibition does not change amino acid protein expression. Therefore, amino acid transporter activation is independent of increased protein synthesis.

Multiple animal models of intrauterine growth restriction have been used to examine amino acid concentrations and flux across the uteroplacenta. Table 5 summarizes maternal and offspring measurements of branched-chain amino acids following nutrient or protein restriction in various animal models. Using a mid- to late-gestation ovine model of intrauterine growth restriction, we examined branched-chain amino acid exchange via the uteroplacenta [111]. For this experiment, singleton pregnant ewes were provided 100% (control) or 60% (restricted) of nutrient recommendations from Day 50–130 of gestation. On Day 130 of gestation, ewes were anesthetized and concurrent blood samples were collected from a catheterized maternal saphenous artery and the gravid uterine vein. Immediately following this collection, the gravid uterine horn was dissected and concurrent blood samples were collected from the umbilical vein and umbilical artery. This concurrent blood sampling procedure was used to calculate gravid uterine flux of nutrients, which is equal to uterine blood flow multiplied by the maternal arterial-venous concentration difference (maternal saphenous artery–gravid uterine vein) of any given substance. Fetal flux of nutrients was calculated by taking umbilical blood flow multiplied by the fetal venous-arterial concentration difference (umbilical vein-umbilical artery) of any given substance [111]. In this experimental model, we observed a decrease in both umbilical artery and uterine artery blood flow (Table 5). Uterine and fetal uptakes of isoleucine were decreased by nutrient restriction. Interestingly, similar uterine uptakes of leucine and valine were observed between dietary treatments; however, fetal uptake of both leucine and valine were decreased in nutrient restricted *vs.* control fed ewes.

Table 5. Maternal and offspring measurements of branched-chain amino acid (BCAA).

Dietary Treatment	Dependent Variable	Response
Ovine model of nutrient restriction from Day 50 to 130 [80,111]	Fetal weight (Day 130)	Decreased 15% to 20%
	Placental weight (Day 130)	Similar
	Umbilical blood flow (Day 50–110)	Decreased 20%
	Uterine blood flow (Day 130)	Decreased 20%
	Uteroplacental nutrient flux (Day 130)	
	Uterine uptake of isoleucine	Decreased 42%
	Fetal uptake of isoleucine	Decreased 37%
	Uterine uptake of leucine	Similar
	Fetal uptake of leucine	Decreased 60%
	Uterine uptake of valine	Similar
	Fetal uptake of valine	Decreased 69%
Ovine model of nutrient restriction from Day 28 to 135 [112]	Fetal weight (Day 135)	Decreased 15%
	Maternal and fetal plasma BCAA	
	Maternal concentration of isoleucine	Decreased 19%
	Fetal concentration of isoleucine	Decreased 28%
	Maternal concentration of leucine	Decreased 41%
	Fetal concentration of leucine	Decreased 38%
	Maternal concentration of valine	Decreased 43%
	Fetal concentration of valine	Decreased 35%
Ovine model of metabolizable protein restriction from Day 100 to 130 [113]	Fetal weight (Day 130)	Decreased 20% to 45%
	Placental weight (Day 130)	Similar
	Umbilical blood flow (Day 50–110)	Similar
	Uterine blood flow (Day 130)	Increased 50% to 80% ***NS**
	Maternal and Fetal BCAA (Day 130)	
	Maternal concentration of leucine	Similar
	Fetal concentration of leucine	Decreased 40% to 50%
	Maternal concentration of valine	Similar
	Fetal concentration of valine	Decreased 30% to 50%
Porcine model of protein restriction from mating to Day 60 [114]	**Maternal artery and umbilical vein BCAA**	
	Maternal artery concentration of isoleucine	Similar
	Umbilical concentration of isoleucine	Decreased 19%
	Maternal artery concentration of leucine	Similar
	Umbilical concentration of leucine	Decreased 29%
	Maternal artery concentration of valine	Similar
	Umbilical concentration of valine	Decreased 20%
Porcine model of isocaloric diets with high or low protein compared to standard diet [115]	Litter weights; litter sizes	Similar
	Maternal and umbilical/fetal BCAA	
	Maternal venous concentration of isoleucine	Decreased 32%
	Umbilical/fetal concentrations of isoleucine	Similar
	Maternal venous concentration of valine	Decreased 73%
	Umbilical/fetal concentrations of valine	Similar
	Maternal venous concentration of leucine	Decreased 21%
	Umbilical/fetal concentrations of leucine	Similar

Table 5. *Cont.*

	Newborn pup weights	Decreased 9% to 18%
	Maternal and newborn BCAA	
	Maternal concentration of isoleucine	Decreased 36%
[6] **Rodent model of protein restriction from Day 1 to term** [108]	Newborn concentration of isoleucine	Decreased 59%
	Maternal concentration of leucine	Decreased 43%
	Newborn concentration of leucine	Decreased 60%
	Maternal concentration of valine	Decreased 52%
	Newborn concentration of valine	Decreased 68%

* NS = not statistically different at $p < 0.05$.

Other ovine models of nutrient or protein restriction have shown comparable decreases in fetal weight and branched-chain amino acid profiles (Table 5). For example, Kwon *et al.* [112] observed similar decreases in maternal and fetal concentrations of isoleucine, leucine, and valine following maternal nutrient restriction from Day 28–135 of pregnancy. Using an ovine metabolizable protein restriction model where samples were simultaneously collected, Lekatz and Vonnahme [113] showed a decrease in fetal concentrations of leucine and valine; however, maternal concentrations of leucine and valine were not different between dietary treatments. Similar to the ovine metabolizable protein restriction model, Wu *et al.* [114] observed decreased fetal concentrations of branched-chain amino acids with no difference in maternal concentrations of branched-chain amino acids following protein restriction from early to mid-pregnancy in pigs. Metzler-Zebeli *et al.* [115] observed maternal venous changes, but no differences in umbilical or fetal blood of branch-chained amino acids (Table 5). Pregnant rats which were protein restricted from Day 1 to term had a decrease (36%–68%) in both maternal and newborn concentrations of branched-chain amino acids [108]. In addition to these observations, this study also identified a critical role for branched-chain amino acid supplementation in partially rescuing fetal growth restriction induced by maternal dietary protein restriction.

In conclusion, we have made interesting observations of branched chain amino acids in several sheep models of nutrient intake; however, more research is needed to determine how the placenta adapts to other maternal stressors that impact nutrient delivery, including amino acids, fatty acids, and sugars.

4. How Pregnancy Prepares the Dam for Lactation

The growth and development of the mammary gland from fetal life through involution in livestock has been reviewed recently and sets the stage for the discussion below [116]. As mentioned above, dramatic changes occur within the maternal cardiovascular system during pregnancy [14] and maternal energy consumption and metabolism also are altered [117] to nourish the growing conceptus and to prepare the mammary gland for lactation. Although, lactating high producing non-pregnant dairy cattle will show a substantial increase in cardiac output compared to their non-pregnant non-lactating counterparts [118,119], this redistribution of blood flow during the transition period from the uteroplacental vasculature towards the mammary gland is still a phenomenal physiological feat to allow for peak lactation shortly after parturition.

Mammary gland growth, milk yield, and mammary tissue DNA content was influenced by energy and protein intake in sows during lactation [120]. Moreover, increased dietary lipids in peripubertal ewe lambs results in increased mammogenesis [121]. While we have observed no effects of nutrition on mammary gland growth in our beef cow models [122], we do observe differences in ewes. Development of the mammary gland is unique to ewes and unlike other livestock, sheep do not exhibit post-parturient growth of the mammary gland [123]. Our laboratory has recently reported that maternal selenium supplementation as well as differing levels of maternal nutrition during mid- to late-gestation alters colostrum yield and mammary gland microanatomy [65,124–126]. Mammary gland alveolar epithelium has an increased proliferation index in overnourished ewes compared with restricted and adequately fed ewes indicating that the increased level of nutrients stimulated alveolar growth [124]. This increase in alveolar proliferation may be indicative of an earlier differentiation of the gland, due to overnourished ewes exhibiting decreased estradiol-17β and progesterone concentrations in circulation compared to restricted and adequately fed ewes [86,127]. Decreases in estradiol-17β reduce glucocorticoid-binding protein, allowing free cortisol to further complete cellular differentiation in preparation for lactogenesis [128]. Overnourished ewes have elevated levels of cortisol [86,127], potentially allowing for this increase in mammary gland differentiation. Progesterone is also needed for lobular alveolar growth in the mammary gland [128]. While colostrum yield is reduced in both restricted and overnourished ewes [65,124], when ewes are fed similarly throughout lactation, overfed ewes, but not restricted ewes, rebound in their milking ability to yield similar milk weights as CON ewes [65].

Not only does maternal diet impact the milking ability of the ewe, but the milking ability of her offspring and reproductive capacity of her grand-offspring [129]. This postnatal response may be linked to the anatomical differences observed in mammary gland development during fetal life. Fetuses from maintenance fed ewes had larger mammary gland weights at 100 days of fetal life compared to *ad libitum* fed ewes, without impacting mammary duct area or number or fetal weights [130]. Perhaps, this enhanced milk production is due to decreased fat pad hyperplasia and increased abundance of Mitogen-activated protein kinases (MAPK) and mTOR pathway signaling proteins within the fat pad [131].

4.1. Vascularity of the Mammary Gland

The mammary gland is a very dynamic organ that is influenced by gestational nutrition as evidenced by the alveolar proliferation and other cellular activity that may occur. However, it does not appear that maternal nutritional plane during gestation impacts the capillary vascularity of the mammary gland in sheep (Table 6) or beef cattle [122]. Interestingly, our laboratory has demonstrated that supranutritional levels of selenium fed during pregnancy increases mammary gland vascularity at birth, as well as by the end of a 20 day lactation (Table 6). Moreover, enhanced milk yields from ewes supplemented with supranutritional levels of selenium compared to adequately levels of selenium in the diet of ewes have been reported [65]. Investigations are on-going to determine what role enhanced vascularity may be contributing to increased milk yield. While selenium has been reported as an effective breast cancer reducing supplement [132], we hypothesize that the enhanced vascularity of ewe mammary glands resulting from supranutritional selenium supplementation may be advantageous from a milk production and offspring standpoint. While most breast cancers are associated with higher estrogen levels in women [133], we have not observed that supranutritional selenium supplementation alters estradiol-17β concentrations in circulation [86,127]. It is unknown, however, what concentrations of estradiol-17β are within the mammary gland itself.

Table 6. Impacts of maternal diet during pregnancy on vascularity and production of the mammary gland in ewes.

Treatment	Stage	Impact on Vascularity Compared to Control	Colostrum/Milk Production Compared to Control
Nutritional plane	**At birth**		
Control *vs.* nutrient restricted		NS *, [125,126]	Decreased 53%–70% [65,124].
Control *vs.* overnourished		NS *, [125,126]	Decreased 37%–58% [65,124].
	Lactation Day 20		
Control *vs.* nutrient restricted		NS *, [126]	Decreased 28% [65]
Control *vs.* overnourished		NS *, [126]	NS [65]
Level of Selenium (Se) Supplementation			
Control (0.3ppm) *vs.* Supra (3.0 ppm) Se	birth	Increased 20%–25% [125]	NS *, [124]
Control (0.3ppm) *vs.* Supra (3.0 ppm) Se	birth	NS *, [126]	Increased 37% [65]
Control (0.3ppm) *vs.* Supra (3.0 ppm) Se	Lactation Day 20	Increased 22% [126]	Increased 10% [65]

* NS = not significant at $p > 0.05$.

4.2. Maternal Small Intestine during Lactation

The shift from pregnancy to lactation typically includes an increase in voluntary feed intake in addition to the other metabolic and hormonal changes; therefore, the small intestine generally increases in mass during early lactation [52,134–136]. Increased intestinal mass during lactation could result from both increasing metabolic demand and intake. Research with murine models demonstrate the influence of metabolic demand of lactation on the small intestine. In lactating mice that had undergone intestinal resection, small intestinal mass increases 200%–300% to enhance nutrient acquisition, compared with a 60% increase in mass of controls [137]. Little is known about changes in vascularity of the small intestine during early lactation. In ewes, capillary area density decreased by 10% from Day 0–20 post-partum [52]. Because mass of the small intestine also increased by 40% during the first 20 day of lactation, this allowed for similar total vascularity between the two time periods. The decrease in capillary area density may result from a dilution of vascular area caused by the rapid increase in the mass of the small intestine. Furthermore, it appears that the metabolic pressure of lactation may rely less on the vascularity of the small intestine per unit area, and more on the increase in size of the small intestine to increase nutrient absorption capacity.

Few data demonstrate the influence of pre-partum nutrition on small intestinal measures during lactation. It is unknown if any of the changes that gestational nutrition causes on the maternal small intestine program its function long-term. Due to the plastic nature of the tissue, it appears that the small intestine changes rapidly during early lactation, especially in the face of adequate nutrition post-partum. In first parity ewes, we demonstrated that even when vascularity of the small intestine was affected by nutritional plane or supranutritional levels of selenium at parturition, the same measures were similar after being on common diets for 20 day of lactation [52]. In fact, when ewes were fed to meet their nutrient requirements for early lactation post-partum (*i.e.*, all treatments experienced an increase in nutrient intake), mass of the small intestine was similar for all ewes at Day 20 of lactation. Mass of the small intestine rebounds faster than ewe body weight, resulting in ewes that had previously been on a lower plane of nutrition having greater proportional small intestinal mass (g kg^{-1} body weight) than control ewes. This results from a greater increase in crypt cell proliferation in ewes that had been nutrient restricted compared with those that had been adequately fed during gestation [52].

To our knowledge, vascularity of the small intestine during lactation in response to previous plane of nutrition during gestation has only been reported in one study ([52]; Table 3). In this study, ewes that had been nutrient restricted during gestation have increased capillary surface density of the jejunum compared with control ewes at 20 days of lactation. Additionally, ewes previously overnourished during gestation had greater total vascularity compared with control ewes at 20 days of lactation. In both cases, these changes due to nutrition during pregnancy were consistent with those observed at parturition, suggesting that vascularity of the small intestine does not change as quickly as proliferation and mass. Despite this, previous intake of supranutritional selenium during gestation resulted in ewes having greater capillary size in the jejunum at 20 days of lactation when compared with control, even though these treatments had similar capillary size immediately post-partum. This supports the hypothesis that selenium suppresses vascular beds, as capillary size increased after return to an adequate selenium diet, although ewes had not likely yet returned to the selenium status of control. The role of VEGF and NO systems in altering vascular changes of the small intestine during early lactation is not clear. In this study, any differences of divergent treatments from control immediately post-partum subsided by Day 20 of lactation, including gene expression of angiogenic factors ([52]; Table 4).

Nutrient release by the portal-drained viscera (including small intestine) increases with milk production in ewes, suggesting that nutrient absorption by the small intestine increases with milk yield [138,139]. In our previous study, milk production for the first 20 days of lactation did move in a similar direction as vascularity of the small intestine for ewes that were nutrient restricted or fed supranutritional selenium during gestation [52,65]. (Table 3). We hypothesized that the small intestine impacts milk yield differences (decreased milk yield in ewes from lower planes of nutrition during gestation) by altering nutrient acquisition or by diverting nutrients from milk production to the rebuilding of body tissues including the gastrointestinal tract. Perhaps, during these times of high physiological demands, the intestine modulates its ability to secure more nutrients from luminal compared with arterial supplies. Data addressing this question are not available in the literature but would increase our understanding and potentially provide better positioning for management during physiological stress. Additionally, it is not known if small intestinal adaptation pre-partum is partially in preparation for lactation. Because the gastrointestinal tract responds rapidly to changes in nutrient intake, inappropriate nutrient intake pre-partum can alter the magnitude of its adaptation to lactation. Moreover, periparturient changes in the small intestine are necessary for adequate nutrient digestion and absorption to provide for milk yield, so this likely impacts lactation and nutrient availability for offspring during postnatal life.

5. Conclusions

The vascularity of the gastrointestinal tract, placenta, and mammary gland may be able to adapt to different nutritional stimuli, and in some cases, we know that nutrient exchange can be altered. It is imperative that we continue to investigate how the pregnant animal can not only survive under stressful nutritional paradigms (*i.e.*, inappropriate nutrient supply, conditional increased nutrient demand, specific nutrient imbalances, *etc.*), but also how those adaptations may be impacting her ability to deliver nutrients to the developing offspring. Continued effects to understand how vascularity and other factors associated with nutrient extraction may be key for enhancement of nutrient transfer efficiency.

Acknowledgments

The authors wish to thank the following individuals for the contribution to results presented in this review: A. Grazul-Bilska, G. Lardy, S. O'Rourke, D. Redmer, L. Reynolds, C. Schauer, P. Shukla, and K. Swanson; graduate students: L. Camacho, L. Lekatz, and A. Reyaz; staff in the NDSU Animal Nutrition and Physiology Center and Beef Cattle Research Complex as well as technicians in the Physiology, Nutrition, and Pharmacology groups are also recognized. Studies were funded in part by: Agriculture and Food Research Initiative competitive grants 2009-65203-0581 and 2009-35206-05276 and Research Initiative competitive grant 2005-35206-15281 and Postdoctoral Fellowship grant 2011-67012-30683 from the USDA National Institute of Food and Agriculture, National Sciences Foundation grant HRD-0811239, Lalor Foundation, Inc., American Heart Association, and the ND State Board of Agricultural Research and Education.

Author Contributions

All authors were involved in review preparation with K.A.V. and C.O.L. focusing on uteroplacental and mammary gland information and J.S.C. and A.M.M. focusing on the gastrointestinal tract information. All authors read and approved the final version of the manuscript.

References

1. U.N. Department of Economic and Social Affairs, Population Division. World Population Prospects: The 2012 Revision. Available online: http://esa.un.org/unpd/wpp/Excel-Data/population.htm (accessed on 13 December 2013).
2. Food and Agriculture Organization of the U.N. World Livestock 2011: Livestock in Food Security. Available online: http://www.fao.org/docrep/014/i2373e/i2373e.pdf (accessed on 13 December 2013).
3. The Advantages of Domestic Species as Dual Purpose Models. Available online: http://adsbm.msu.edu/ (accessed on 26 December 2014).
4. Roberts, R.M. The place of farm animal species in the new genomics world of reproductive biology. *Biol. Reprod.* **2001**, *64*, 409–417.
5. Symonds, M.E.; Budge, H.; Stephenson, T.; McMillen, I.C. Fetal endocrinology and development—Manipulation and adaptation to long-term nutritional and environmental challenges. *Reproduction* **2001**, *121*, 853–862.
6. Symonds, M.E.; Stephenson, T.; Gardner, D.S.; Budge, H. Long-term effects of nutritional programming of the embryo and fetus: Mechanisms and critical windows. *Reprod. Fert. Develop.* **2007**, *19*, 53–63.
7. Campbell, B.K.; Souza, C.; Gong, J.; Webb, R.; Kendall, N.; Marsters, P.; Robinson, G.; Mitchell, A.; Telfer, E.E.; Baird, D.T. Domestic ruminants as models for the elucidation of the mechanisms controlling ovarian follicle development in humans. *Reproduction* **2003** *61*, 429–443.

8. Wallace, J.M.; Regnault, T.R.H.; Limesand, S.W.; Hay, Jr., W.W.; Anthony. R.V. Investigating the causes of low birth weight in contrasting ovine paradigms. *J. Physiol.* **2005,** *565*, 19–26.
9. Barry, J.S.; Anthony, R.V. The pregnant sheep as a model for human pregnancy. *Theriogenology* **2008**, *69*, 55–67.
10. Ireland, J.J.; Roberts, R.M.; Palmer, G.H.; Bauman, D.E.; Bazer, F.W. A commentary on domestic animals as dual-purpose models that benefit agricultural and biomediçal research. *J. Anim. Sci.* **2008**, *86*, 2797–2805
11. Reynolds, L.P.; Caton, J.S.; Redmer, D.A.; Grazul-Bilska, A.T.; Vonnahme, K.A.; Borowicz, P.P.; Luther, J.S.; Wallace, J.M.; Wu, G.; Spencer, T.E. Evidence for altered placental blood flow and vascularity in compromised pregnancies. *J. Physiol.* **2006**, *572*, 51–58.
12. Reynolds, L.P.; Ireland, J.J.; Seidel, J.; G.E. Editorial: "Brain drain" and loss of resources jeopardize the continued use of domestic animals for agricultural and biomedical research. *J. Anim. Sci.* **2008**, *86*, 1–2.
13. Scheaffer, A.N.; Caton, J.S.; Bauer, M.L.; Redmer, D.A.; Reynolds, L.P. The effect of pregnancy on visceral growth and energy use in beef heifers. *J. Anim. Sci.* **2003**, *81*, 1853–1861.
14. Magness, R.R. *Maternal Cardiovascular and Other Physiologic Responses to the Endocrinology of Pregnancy*; Bazer, F., Ed.; Humana Press: Totowa, NJ, USA, 1998.
15. Shifren, J.L.; Doldi, N.; Ferrara, N.; Mesiano, S.; Jaffe, R.B. In the human fetus, vascular endothelial growth factor is expressed in epithelial cells and myocytes, but not vascular endothelium: Implications for mode of action. *J. Clin. Endocrinol. Metable* **1994**, *79*, 316–322.
16. Ahmed, A.; Li, X.F.; Dunk, C.; Whittle, M.J.; Rushton, D.I.; Rollason, T. Colocalisation of vascular endothelial growth factor and its Flt-1 receptor in human placenta. *Growth Factors* **1995**, *12*, 235–243.
17. Cheung, C.Y. Vascular endothelial growth factor: Possible role in fetal development and placental function. *J. Soc. Gynecol. Investig.* **1997**, *4*, 169–171.
18. Tsoi, S.C.; Wen, Y.; Chung, J.Y.; Chen, D.; Magness, R.R.; Zheng, J. Co-expression of vascular endothelial growth factor and neuropilin-1 in ovine feto-placental artery endothelial cells. *Mol. Cell Endocrinol.* **2002**, *196*, 95–106.
19. Chung, J.Y.; Song, Y.; Wang, Y.; Magness, R.R.; Zheng, J. Differential expression of vascular endothelial growth factor (VEGF), endocrine derived-VEGF and VEGF receptors in human placentas from normal and preeclampsic pregnancies. *J. Clin. Endocrinol. MeTable* **2004**, *89*, 2484–2490.
20. Cheng, C.Y.; Brace, R.A. Developmental expression of vascular endothelial growth factor and its receptors in ovine placenta and fetal membranes. *J. Soc. Gynecol. Investig.* **1999**, *6*, 179–185.
21. Borowicz, P.P.; Arnold, D.R.; Johnson, M.L.; Grazul-Bilska, A.T.; Redmer, D.A.; Reynolds, L.P. Placental growth throughout the last two-thirds of pregnancy in sheep: Vascular development and angiogenic factor expression. *Biol. Reprod.* **2007**, *76*, 259–267.
22. Vonnahme, K.A.; Wilson, M.E.; Li, Y.; Rupnow, H.L.; Phernetton, T.M.; Ford, S.P.; Magness, R.R. Circulating levels of nitric oxide and vascular endothelial growth factor throughout ovine pregnancy. *J. Physiol.* **2005**, *565*, 101–109.
23. Eckternkamp, S.E.; Vonnahme, K.A.; Green, J.A.; Ford, S.P. Increased vascular endothelial growth factor and pregnancy-associated glycoproteins, but not insulin-like growth factor-1, in maternal blood of cows gestating twin fetuses. *J. Anim. Sci.* **2006**, *84*, 2057–2064.

24. Vonnahme, K.A.; Zhu, M.J.; Borowicz, P.P.; Geary, T.W.; Hess, B.W.; Reynolds, L.P.; Caton, J.S.; Means, W.J.; Ford, S.P. Effect of Early Gestational Undernutrition on Angiogenic Factor Expression and Vascularity in the Bovine Placentome. *J. Anim. Sci.* **2007**, *85*, 2464–2472.
25. Vonnahme, K.A.; Ford, S.P. Placental vascular endothelial growth factor receptor system mRNA expression in pigs selected for placental efficiency. *J. Physiol.* **2004**, *554*, 194–201.
26. Vonnahme, K.A.; Ford, S.P. Differential expression of the vascular endothelial growth factor-receptor system in the gravid uterus of Yorkshire and Meishan pigs. *Biol. Reprod.* **2004**, *71*, 163–169.
27. Ahmed, A.; Dunk, C.; Kniss, D.; Wilkes, M. Role of VEGF receptor-1 (Flt-1) in mediating calcium-dependent nitric oxide release and limiting DNA synthesis in human trophoblast cells. *Lab Investig.* **1997**, *76*, 779–791.
28. Asahara, T.; Murohara, T.; Sullivan, A.; Silver, M.; van der Zee, R.; Li, T.; Witzenbichler, B.; Schatteman, G.; Isner, J.M. Isolation of putative progenitor endothelial cells for angiogenesis. *Science* **1997**, *275*, 964–967.
29. Van der Zee, R.; Murohara, T.; Luo, Z.; Zollmann, F.; Passeri, J.; Lekutat, C.; Isner, J.M. Vascular endothelial growth factor/vascular permeability factor augments nitric oxide release from quiescent rabbit and human vascular enotheluim. *Circulation* **1997**, *95*, 1030–1037.
30. Parenti, A.; Morbidelli, L.; Cui, X.L.; Douglas, J.G.; Hood, J.D.; Granger, H.J.; Ledda, F.; Ziche, M. Nitric oxide is an upstream signal of vascular endothelial growth factor-induced extracellular signal-regulated kinase ½ activation in postcapillary endothelium. *J. Biol. Chem.* **1998**, *272*, 4220–4226.
31. Fleming, B.O.; Brockus, K.E.; Hart, C.G.; Lemley, C.O. Effects of dietary melatonin supplementation on total serum nitrites and antioxidant capacity of late gestating Holstein heifers. *J. Anim. Sci.* **2014**, 92, 244.
32. Vonnahme, K.A.; Lemley, C.O.; Skukla, P.; O'Rourke, S.T. 2011 and 2012 Early Career Achievement Awards: Placental programming: How the maternal environment can impact placental function. *J. Anim. Sci.* **2013**, *91*, 2467–2480.
33. Williams, D.J.; Vallance, P.J.; Neild, G.H.; Spencer, J.A.; Imms, F.J. Nitric-oxide mediated vasodilation in human pregnancy. *Am. J. Physiol. Heart Circ. Physiol.* **1997**, *272*, H748–H752.
34. Sladek, S.M.; Magness, R.R.; Conrad, K.P. Nitric oxide and pregnancy. *Am. J. Physiol. Regul. Integr. Comp. Physiol.* **1997**, *272*, R441–R463.
35. Shukla, P.; Lemley, C.O.; Dubey, N.; Meyer, A.M.; O'Rourke, S.T.; Vonnahme, K.A. Effect of maternal nutrient restriction and melatonin supplementation from mid to late gestation on vascular reactivity of maternal and fetal placental arteries. *Placenta* **2014**, *35*, 461–466.
36. Itoh, S.; Brawley, L.; Wheeler, T.; Anthony, F.W.; Poston, L.; Hanson, M.A. Vasodilation to vascular endothelial growth factor in the uterine artery of the pregnant rat is blunted by low dietary protein intake. *Pediatr. Res.* **2002**, *51*, 485–491.
37. Yamamoto, T.; Kajikuri, J.; Watanabe, Y.; Suzuki, Y.; Suzumori, K.; Itoh, T. Chronic nitroglycerine administration reduces endothelial nitric oxide production in rabbit mesenteric resistance artery. *Br. J. Pharmacol.* **2005**, *146*, 534–542.
38. Mordhorst, B.R. Influence of maternal nutrient intake on placental vascular function in pregnant beef cows. Master's Thesis, North Dakota State University, Fargo, ND, USA, April 2014.

39. Huntington, G.B. Energy metabolism in the digestive tract and liver of cattle: Influence of physiological state and nutrition. *Reprod. Fertil. Dev.* **1990**, *30*, 35–47.
40. Ferrell, C.L. Contribution of visceral organs to animal energy expenditures. *J. Anim. Sci.* **1988**, *66*, 23–34.
41. Webster, A.J.F. Bioenergetics, bioengineering and growth. *Livest. Prod.* **1989**, *48*, 249–269.
42. Eisemann, J.H.; Nienaber, J.A. Tissue and whole-body oxygen uptake in fed and fasted steers. *Br. J. Nutr.* **1990**, *64*, 399–411.
43. Gregg, V.A.; Milligan, L.P. In vitro energy costs of Na^+, K^+ ATPase activity and protein synthesis in muscle from calves differing in age and breed. *Br. J. Nutr.* **1982**, *48*, 65–71.
44. Caton, J.S.; Bauer, M.L.; Hidari, H. Metabolic components of energy expenditure in growing beef cattle. *Asian-Aus. J. Anim. Sci.* **2000**, *13*, 702–710.
45. Scheaffer, A.N.; Caton, J.S.; Redmer, D.A.; Reynolds, L.P. The effect of dietary restriction, pregnancy, and fetal type in different ewe types on fetal weight, maternal body weight, and visceral organ mass in ewes. *J. Anim. Sci.* **2004**, *82*, 1826–1838.
46. Scheaffer, A.N.; Caton, J.S.; Bauer, M.L.; Reynolds, L.P. Influence of pregnancy on body weight, ruminal characteristics, and visceral organ mass in beef heifers. *J. Anim. Sci.* **2001**, *79*, 2481–2490.
47. Caton, J.S.; Reed, J.J.; Aitken, R.; Milne, J.S.; Borowicz, P.P.; Reynolds, L.P.; Redmer, D.A.; Wallace, J.M. Effects of maternal nutrition and stage of gestation on body weight, visceral organ mass, and indices of jejunal cellularity, proliferation, and vascularity in pregnant ewe lambs. *J. Anim. Sci.* **2009**, *87*, 222–235.
48. Meyer, A.M.; Reed, J.J.; Vonnahme, K.A.; Soto-Navarro, S.A.; Reynolds, L.P.; Ford, S.P.; Hess, B.W.; Caton, J.S. Effects of stage of gestation and nutrient restriction during early to mid-gestation on maternal and fetal visceral organ mass and indices of jejunal growth and vascularity in beef cows. *J. Anim. Sci.* **2010**, *88*, 2410–2424.
49. Scheaffer, A.N.; Caton, J.S.; Redmer, D.A.; Arnold, D.R.; Reynolds, L.P. Effect of dietary restriction, pregnancy, and fetal type on intestinal cellularity and vascularity in Columbia and Romanov ewes. *J. Anim. Sci.* **2004**, *82*, 3024–3033.
50. Johnson, D.E.; Johnson, K.A.; Baldwin, R.L. Changes in liver and gastrointestinal tract energy demands in response to physiological workload in ruminants. *J. Nutr.* **1990**, *120*, 649–655.
51. Reed, J.J.; Ward, M.A.; Vonnahme, K.A.; Neville, T.L.; Julius, S.L.; Borowicz, P.P.; Taylor, J.B.; Redmer, D.A.; Grazul-Bilska, A.T.; Reynolds, L.P.; *et al.* Effects of selenium supply and dietary restriction on maternal and fetal body weight, visceral organ mass and cellularity estimates, and jejunal vascularity in pregnant ewe lambs. *J. Anim. Sci.* **2007**, *85*, 2721–2733.
52. Meyer, A.M.; Reed, J.J.; Neville, T.L.; Taylor, J.B.; Reynolds, L.P.; Redmer, D.A.; Vonnahme, K.A.; Caton, J.S. Effects of nutritional plane and selenium supply during gestation on visceral organ mass and indices of intestinal growth and vascularity in primiparous ewes at parturition and during early lactation. *J. Anim. Sci.* **2012**, *90*, 2733–2749.
53. Cunningham, H.C. Relationship of feed efficiency and small intestinal biology in beef cattle. Master's Thesis, University of Wyoming, Laramie, WY, USA, August 2014.

54. Neville, T.L.; Redmer, D.A.; Borowicz, P.P.; Reed, J.J.; Ward, M.A.; Johnson, M.L.; Taylor, J.B.; Soto-Navarro, S.A.; Vonnahme, K.A.; Reynolds, L.P.; *et al.* Maternal dietary restriction and selenium supply alters mRNA expression of angiogenic factors in maternal intestine, mammary gland, and fetal jejunal tissues during late gestation in pregnant ewe lambs. *J. Anim. Sci.* **2010**, *88*, 2692–2702.
55. Rocha, F.G.; Sundback, C.A.; Krebs, N.J.; Leach, J.K.; Mooney, D.J.; Ashley, S.W.; Vacanti, J.P.; Whang, E.E. The effect of sustained delivery of vascular endothelial growth factor on angiogenesis in tissue-engineered intestine. *Biomaterials* **2008**, *29*, 2884–2890.
56. Levine, G.M. Regulation of intestinal mucosal growth. In *Growth of the Gastrointestinal Tract: Gastrointestinal Hormones and Growth Factors*; Morisset, J., Solomon, T.E., Eds.; CRC Press: Boca Raton, FL, USA, 1991; pp. 175–189.
57. Ferraris, R.P. Regulation of intestinal nutrient transport. In *Physiology of the Gastrointestinal Tract*; Johnson, L.R., Ed.; Raven Press: New York, NY, USA, 1994; pp. 1821–1844.
58. Trahair, J.F.; Sangild, P.T. Studying the development of the small intestine: Philosophical and anatomical perspectives. In *Biology of the Intestine in Growing Animals*; Zabielski, R., Gregory, P.C., Westrom, B., Eds.; Elsevier Science: Amsterdam, The Netherlands, 2002; pp. 1–54.
59. Burrin, D.G. Trophic factors and regulation of gastrointestinal tract and liver development. In *Fetal and Neonatal Physiology*; Polin, R.A., Fox, W.W., Abman, S.H., Eds.; Saunders: Philadelphia, PA, 2004; pp. 1095–1100.
60. O'Neil, M.R.; Lardy, G.P.; Reynolds, L.P.; Caton, J.S.; Vonnahme, K.A. Impacts of linseed meal and estradiol-17B on mass, cellularity, angiogenic factors, and vascularity of the jejunum. *J. Anim. Sci.* **2008**, *86*, 3014–3022.
61. MacRae, J.C.; Bruce, L.A.; Brown, D.S.; Farningham, D.A.H.; Franklin, M. Absorption of amino acids from the intestine and their net flux across the mesenteric-and portal drained viscera of lambs. *J. Anim. Sci.* **1997**, *75*, 3307–3314.
62. Carlson, D.B.; Reed, J.J.; Borowicz, P.P.; Taylor, J.B.; Reynolds, L.P.; Neville, T.L.; Redmer, D.A.; Vonnahme, K.A.; Caton, J.S. Effects of dietary selenium supply and timing of nutrient restriction during gestation on maternal growth and body composition of pregnant adolescent ewes. *J. Anim. Sci.* **2009**, *87*, 669–680
63. Meyer, A.M.; Reed, J.J.; Neville, T.L.; Taylor, J.B.; Hammer, C.J.; Reynolds, L.P.; Vonnahme, K.A.; Caton, J.S. Effects of plane of nutrition and selenium supply during gestation on ewe and neonatal offspring performance, body composition, and serum selenium. *J. Anim. Sci.* **2010**, *88*, 1786–1800.
64. Neville, T.L.; Ward, M.A.; Reed, J.J.; Soto-Navarro, S.A.; Julius, S.L.; Borowicz, P.P.; Taylor, J.B.; Redmer, D.A.; Reynolds, L.P.; Caton, J.S. Effects of level and source of dietary selenium on maternal and fetal body weight, visceral organ mass, cellularity estimates, and jejunal vascularity in pregnant ewe lambs. *J. Anim. Sci.* **2008**, *86*, 890–901.
65. Meyer, A.M.; Reed, J.J.; Neville, T.L.; Thorson, J.F.; Maddock-Carlin, K.R.; Taylor, J.B.; Reynolds, L.P.; Redmer, D.A.; Luther, J.S.; Hammer, C.J.; *et al.* Nutritional plane and selenium

supply during gestation impact yield and nutrient composition of colostrum and milk in primiparous ewes. *J. Anim. Sci.* **2011**, *89*, 1627–1639.

66. Björkman, N. Fine structure of the ovine placentome. *J. Anat.* **1965**, *99*, 283–297.
67. Hoffman, L.H.; Wooding, F.B.; Owens, J.A.; Falconer, J.; Robinson, J.S. Giant and binucleate trophoblast cells of mammals. *Am. J. Physiol.* **1986**, *250*, R427–R434.
68. Wooding, F.B.P.; Wathes, D.C. Binucleate cell migration in the bovine placentome. *J. Reprod. Fert.* **1980**, *59*, 425–430.
69. Dantzer, V. Scanning electron microscopy of exposed surfaces of the porcine placenta. *Acta. Anat.* **1984**, *118*, 96–106.
70. Knight, J.W.; Bazer, F.W.; Thatcher, W.W.; Franke, D.E.; Wallace, H.D. Conceptus development in intact and unilaterally hysterectomized-ovariectomized gilts: Interrelations among hormonal status, placental development, fetal fluids and fetal growth. *J. Anim. Sci.* **1977**, *44*, 620–637.
71. Vonnahme, K.A.; Wilson, M.E.; Ford, S.P. Relationship between placental vascular endothelial growth factor expression and placental/endometrial vascularity in the pig. *Biol. Reprod.* **2001**, *64*, 1821–1825.
72. Ford, S.P. Cotyledonary placenta. *Encycl. Reprod.* **1999**, *1*, 730–738.
73. Stegeman, J.H.J. Placental development in the sheep and its relation to fetal development. *Bijdr. Tot De Dierkund.* **1974**, *44*, 3–72.
74. Reynolds, L.P.; Ferrell, C.L.; Robertson, D.A.; Klindt, J. Growth hormone, insulin and glucose concentrations in bovine fetal and maternal plasmas at several stages of gestation. *J. Anim. Sci.* **1990**, *68*, 725–733.
75. Funston, R.N.; Larson, D.L.; Vonnahme, K.A. Impacts of maternal nutrition on conceptus growth and offspring performance: Implications for beef cattle production. *J. Anim. Sci.* **2010**, *88*, E205–E215.
76. Reynolds, L.P.; Borowicz, P.P.; Vonnahme, K.A.; Johnson, M.L.; Grazul-Bilska, A.T.; Redmer, D.A.; Caton, J.S. Placental angiogenesis in sheep models of compromised pregnancy. *J. Physiol.* **2005**, *565*, 43–58.
77. Fowden, A.L.; Ward, J.W.; Wooding, F.P.B.; Forhead, A.J.; Constancia, M. Programming placental nutrient transport capacity. *J. Physiol.* **2006**, *572*, 5–15.
78. Burton, G.J.; Fowden, A.L. Review: The placenta and developmental programming: Balancing fetal nutrient demands with maternal resource allocation. *Placenta* **2012**, *33*, S23–S27.
79. Owens, J.A.; Falconer, J.; Robinson, J.S. Effect of restriction on placental growth on umbilical and uterine blood flows. *Am. J. Physiol.* **1986**, *250*, R427–R434.
80. Lemley, C.O.; Meyer, A.M.; Camacho, L.E.; Neville, T.L.; Newman, D.J.; Caton, J.S.; Vonnahme, K.A. Melatonin supplementation alters uteroplacental hemodynamics and fetal development in an ovine model of intrauterine growth restriction (IUGR). *Am. J. Physiol.* **2012**, *302*, R454–R467.
81. Lekatz, L.A.; Luther, J.S.; Caton, J.S.; Vonnahme, K.A. Impacts of maternal nutritional plane on umbilical artery hemodynamics, fetal and placentome growth in sheep. *Anim. Reprod.* **2013**, *10*, 99–105.
82. Lekatz, L.A.; Ward, M.A.; Borowicz, P.P.; Taylor, J.B.; Redmer, D.A.; Grazul-Bilska, A.T.; Reynolds, L.P.; Caton, J.S.; Vonnahme, K.A. Cotyledonary responses to maternal selenium and

dietary restriction may influence alterations in fetal weight and fetal liver glycogen in sheep. *Anim. Reprod. Sci.* **2010**, *117*, 216–225.

83. Eifert, A.W.; Wilson, M.E.; Vonnahme, K.A.; Camacho, L.E.; Borowicz, P.P.; Redmer, D.A.; Romero, S.; Dorsam, S.; Haring, J.; Lemley, C.O. Effect of melatonin or maternal nutrient restriction on vascularity and cell proliferation in the ovine placenta. *Anim. Reprod. Sci.* **2015**, *153*, 13–21.
84. Camacho, L.E.; Lemley, C.O.; Prezotto, L.D.; Bauer, M.L.; Freetly, H.C.; Swanson, K.C.; Vonnahme, K.A. Effects of maternal nutrient restriction followed by re-alimentation during mid-gestation on uterine blood flow in beef cows. *Theriogenology* **2014**, *81*, 1248–1256.
85. Perry, V.E.A.; Norman, S.T; Owens, J.A.; Daniel, R.C.W.; Phillips, N. Low dietary protein during early pregnancy alters bovine placental development. *Anim. Reprod. Sci.* **1999**, *55*, 13–21.
86. Lemley, C.O.; Meyer, A.M.; Neville, T.L.; Hallford, D.M.; Camacho, L.E.; Maddock-Carlin, K.R.; Wilmoth, T.A.; Wilson, M.E.; Perry, G.A.; Redmer, D.A.; *et al*. Dietary selenium and nutritional plane alters maternal endocrine profiles during pregnancy and lactation. *Dom. Anim. Endocrinol.* **2014**, *46*, 1–11.
87. Sferruzzi-Perri, A.N.; Owens, J.A.; Standen, P.; Taylor, R.L.; Keinemann, G.K.; Robinson, J.S.; Roberts, C.T. Early treatment of the pregnant guinea pig with IGFs promotes placental transport and nutrient partitioning near term. *Am. J. Physiol.* **2007**, *292*, E668–E676.
88. Bollwein, H.; Meyer, H.H.; Maierl, J.; Weber, F.; Baumgartner, U.; Stolla, R. Transrectal Doppler sonography of uterine blood flow. *Theriogenology* **2000**, *53*, 1541–1552.
89. Panarace, M.; Garnil, C.; Marfil, M.; Jauregui, G.; Lagioia, J.; Luther, E.; Medina, M. Transrectal Doppler sonography for evaluation of uterine blood flow throughout pregnancy in 13 cows. *Theriogenology* **2006**, *66*, 2113–2119.
90. Herzog, K.; Bollwein, H. Application of Doppler ultrasonography in cattle reproduction. *Reprod. Dom. Anim.* **2007**, *42*, 51–58.
91. Ford, S.P.; Christensen, R.K. Blood flow to uteri of sow during the estrous cycle and early pregnancy: Local effect of the conceptus on the uterine blood supply. *Biol. Reprod.* **1979**, *21*, 617–624.
92. Reynolds, L.P.; Ferrell, C.L. Transplacental clearance and blood flows of bovine gravid uterus at several stages of gestation. *Am. J. Physiol.* **1987**, *253*, 735–739.
93. Bollwein, H.; Baumgartner, U.; Stolla, R. Transrectal Doppler sonography of uterine blood flow in cows during pregnancy. *Theriogenology* **2002**, *57*, 2053–2061.
94. Hard, D.L.; Anderson, L.L. Interaction of maternal blood volume and uterine blood flow with porcine fetal development. *Biol. Reprod.* **1982**, *27*, 79–90.
95. Zubek, L.; Monos, E.; Csepli, J. Significance of blood flow measurement in the cervix uteri on the 1st trimester of pregnancy. *Zentralbl. Gynakol.* **1986**, *108*, 900–905.
96. Battaglia, F.C.; Regnault, T.R.H. Placental transport and metabolism of amino acids. *Placenta* **2001**, *22*, 145–161.
97. Jansson, T. Amino acid transporters in the human placenta. *Pediatr. Res.* **2001**, *49*, 141–147.
98. Chung, M.; Teng, C.; Timmerman, M.; Meschia, G.; Battaglia, F.C. Production and utilization of amino acids by ovine placenta *in vivo*. *Am. J. Physiol. Endocrinol. MeTable* **1998**, *274*, E13–E22.

99. Dickinson, H.; Ellery, S.; Ireland, Z.; LaRosa, D.; Snow, R.; Walker, D.W. Creatine supplementation during pregnancy: Summary of experimental studies suggesting a treatment to improve fetal and neonatal morbidity and reduce mortality in high-risk human pregnancy. *BMC Pregnancy Childbirth.* **2014**, *14*, 150.
100. Neu, J. Glutamine in the fetus and critically ill low birth weight neonate: Metabolism and mechanism of action. *J. Nutr.* **2001**, *131*, 25855–25895.
101. Wu, X.; Xie, C.; Zhang, Y.; Fan, Z.; Yin, Y.; Blachier, F. Glutamate-glutamine cycle and exchange in the placenta-fetus unit during late pregnancy. *Amino Acids* **2015**, *47*, 45–53.
102. Day, P.E.; Cleal, J.K.; Lofthouse, E.M.; Goss, V.; Koster, G.; Postle, A.; Jackson, J.M.; Hanson, M.A.; Jackson, A.A.; Lewis, R.M. Partitioning of glutamine synthesized by the isolated perfused human placenta between the maternal and fetal circulations. *Placenta* **2013**, *34*, 1223–1231.
103. Van der Linden, D.S.; Sciascia, Q.; Sales, F.; McCoard. S.A. Placental nutrient transport is affected by pregnancy rank in sheep. *J. Anim. Sci.* **2013**, *91*, 644–653.
104. Ashworth, C.J.; Dwyer, C.M.; McIlvaney, K.; Werkman, M.; Rooke, J.A. Breed differences in fetal and placental development and feto-maternal amino acid status following nutrient restriction during early and mid pregnancy in Scottish Blackface and Suffolk sheep. *Reprod. Fertil. Dev.* **2011**, *23*, 1024–1033.
105. Lynch, C.J.; Halle, B.; Fujii, H.; Vary, T.C.; Wallin, R.; Damuni, Z.; Hutson, S.M. Potential role of leucine metabolism in the leucine-signaling pathway involving mTOR. *Am. J. Physiol. Endocrinol. MeTable* **2003**, *285*, E854–E863.
106. Wullschleger, S.; Loewith, R.; Hall, M.N. TOR signaling in growth and metabolism. *Cell* **2006**, *124*, 471–484.
107. Rosario, F.J.; Kanai, Y.; Powell, T.L.; Jansson, T. Mammalian target of rapamycin signaling modulates amino acid uptake by regulating transporter cell surface abundance in primary human trophoblast cells. *J. Physiol.* **2013**, *591*, 609–625.
108. Teodoro, G.F.R.; Vianna, D.; Torres-Leal, F.L.; Pantaleao, L.C.; Matos-Neto, E.M.; Donato, J.; Tirapegui, J. Leucine is essential for attenuating fetal growth restriction caused by a protein-restricted diet in rats. *J. Nutr.* **2012**, *142*, 924–930.
109. Edinger, A.L.; Thompson, C.B. Akt maintains cell size and survival by increasing mTOR-dependent nutrient uptake. *Mol. Biol. Cell* **2002**, *13*, 2276–2288.
110. Peng, T.; Golub, T.R.; Sabatini, D.M. The immunosuppressant rapamycin mimics a starvation-like signal distinct from amino acid and glucose deprivation. *Mol. Cell. Biol.* **2002**, *22*, 5575–5584.
111. Lemley, C.O.; Camacho, L.E.; Meyer, A.M.; Kapphahn, M.; Caton, J.S.; Vonnahme, K.A. Dietary melatonin supplementation alters uteroplacental amino acid flux during intrauterine growth restriction in ewes. *Animal* **2013**, *7*, 1500–1507.
112. Kwon, H.; Ford, S.P.; Bazer, F.W.; Spencer, T.E.; Nathanielsz, P.W.; Nijland, M.J.; Hess, B.W.; Wu, G. Maternal nutrient restriction reduces concentrations of amino acids and polyamines in ovine maternal and fetal plasma and fetal fluids. *Biol. Reprod.* **2004**, *71*, 901–908.
113. Lekatz, L.A. The role of maternal protein intake during late gestation on placental vascular function. Ph.D. Thesis, North Dakota State University, Fargo, ND, USA, April 2013.
114. Wu, G.; Pong, W.G.; Ott, T.; Bazer, F.W. Matenral dietary protein deficiency decreases amino acid concentrations in fetal plasma and allantoic fluid of pigs. *J. Nutr.* **1998**, *128*, 894–902.

115. Metzler-Zebeli, B.U.; Lang, I.S.; Gors, S.; Brussow, K.P.; Hennig, U.; Nurnberg, G.; Rehfeldt, C.; Otten, W.; Metges, C.C. High-protein–low-carbohydrate diet during pregnancy alters maternal plasma amino acid concentration and placental amino acid extraction but not fetal plasma amino acids in pigs. *Br. J. Nutr.* **2012**, *108*, 2176–2189.
116. Rowson, A.R.; Daniels, K.M.; Ellis, S.E.; Hovey, R.C. Growth and development of mammary glands of livestock: A veritable barnyard of opportunities. *Semin. Cell Dev. Biol.* **2012**, *23*, 557–566.
117. Freetly, H.C.; Ferrell, C.L. Net flux of nonesterified fatty acids, cholesterol, triacylglycerol, and glycerol across the portal-drained viscera and liver of pregnant ewes. *J. Anim. Sci.* **2000**, *78*, 1380–1388.
118. Collier, R.J. Nutritional, metabolic, and environmental aspects of lactation. In *Lactation*; Larson, B.L., Ed.; The Iowa State University Press: Ames, IA, USA, 1985; pp. 103–110.
119. Davis, S.R.; Collier, R.J.; McNamara, J.P.; Head, H.H.; Sussman, W. Effects of thyroxine and growth hormone treatment of dairy cows on milk yield, cardiac output and mammary blood flow. *J. Anim. Sci.* **1988**, *66*, 70–79.
120. Kim, S.W.; Hurley, W.L.; Han, I.K.; Stein, H.H.; Easter, R.A. Effect of nutrient intake on mammary gland growth in lactating sows. *J. Anim. Sci.* **1999**, *77*, 3304–3315.
121. McFadden, T.B.; Daniel, T.E.; Akers, R.M. Effects of nutrition, growth hormone and unsaturated fat on mammary growth in prepubertal lambs. *J. Anim. Sci.* **1990**, *68*, 3171–3179.
122. Camacho, L.E.; Lemley, C.O.; Haring, J.S.; Borowicz, P.P.; Hallford, D.M.; Swanson, K.C.; Vonnahme, K.A. Maternal nutrient restriction followed by realimentation during early to mid-gestation on mammary gland development in beef cows. *Proc. West. Sec. ASAS* **2013**, *64*, 76–79.
123. Anderson, R.R. Mammary gland growth in sheep. *J. Anim. Sci.* **1975**, *41*, 118–123.
124. Swanson, T.J.; Hammer, C.J.; Luther, J.S.; Carlson, D.B.; Taylor, J.B.; Redmer, D.A.; Neville, T.L.; Reed, J.J.; Reynolds, L.P.; Caton, J.S.; *et al.* Effects of plane of nutrition and selenium supplementation on colostrum quality and mammary development in pregnant ewe lambs. *J. Anim. Sci.* **2008**, *86*, 2415–2423.
125. Vonnahme, K.A.; Wienhold, C.M.; Borowicz, P.P.; Neville, T.L.; Redmer, D.A.; Reynolds, L.P.; Caton, J.S. Selenium Supplementation Increases Mammary Gland Vascularity in Postpartum Ewe Lambs. *J. Dairy Sci.* **2011**, *94*, 2850–2858.
126. Neville, T.L.; Meyer, A.M.; Reyaz, A.; Redmer, D.A.; Borowicz, P.P.; Reynolds, L.P.; Caton, J.S.; Vonnahme, K.A. Effects of dietary selenium and nutritional plane during gestation on mammary gland growth, cellular proliferation, and vascularity in ewe lambs. *J. Anim. Sci. Biotech.* **2013**, *4*, 6.
127. Vonnahme, K.A.; Neville, T.L.; Perry, G.A.; Reynolds, L.P.; Redmer, D.A.; Caton J.S. Maternal diet alters organ mass, and endocrine and metabolic profiles in pregnant ewe lambs. *Anim. Reprod. Sci.* **2013**, *141*, 131–141.
128. Tucker, H.A. Endocrine and neural control of the mammary gland. In *Lactation*; Larson, B.L., Ed.; Iowa State University Press: Ames, IA, USA, 1985; pp. 39–79.
129. Blair, H.T.; Jenkinson, C.M.C.; Peterson, S.W.; Kenyon, P.R.; van der Linden, D.S.; Davenport, L.C.; Mackenzie, D.D.S.; Morris, S.T.; Firth, E.C. Dam and granddam feeding during pregnancy in sheep affects milk supply in offspring and reproductive performance in grand-offspring. *J. Anim. Sci.* **2010**, *88*, E40–E50.

130. Van der Linden, D.S.; Kenyon, P.R.; Blair, H.T.; Lopez-Villalobos, N.; Jenkinson, C.M.C.; Peterson, S.W.; Mackenzie, D.D.S. Effects of ewe size and nutrition on fetal mammary gland development and lactational performance of offspring at their first lactation. *J. Anim. Sci.* **2009**, *87*, 3944–3954.
131. Sciascia, Q.; Sales, F.; van der Linden, D.; Wards, N.; Oliver, M.; Blair, H.; McCoard, S. Nutritional plane of twin-bearing ewes alters fetal mammary gland biochemical composition and mTOR/MAPK pathway signaling. *J. Anim. Sci.* **2015**, *93*, 699–708.
132. Zhang, S.; Li, F.; Younes, M.; Liu, H.; Chen, C.; Yao, Q. Reduced selenium-binding protein 1 in breast cancer correlates with poor survival and resistance to the anti-proliferative effects of selenium. *PLoS ONE* **2013**, *8*, e63702.
133. Yager, J.D.; Davidson, N.E. Estrogen carcinogenesis in breast cancer. *N. Engl. J. Med.* **2006**, *354*, 270–282.
134. Gibb, M.J.; Ivings, W.E.; Dhanoa, M.S.; Sutton, J.D. Changes in body components of autumn-calving Holstein-Friesian cows over the first 29 weeks of lactation. *Anim. Prod.* **1992**, *55*, 339–360.
135. Hammond, K.A. Adaptation of the maternal intestine during lactation. *J. Mammary Gland Biol. Neoplasia.* **1997**, *2*, 243–252.
136. Reynolds, C.K.; Durst, B.; Lupoli, B.; Humphries, D.J.; Beever, D.E. Visceral tissue mass and rumen volume in dairy cows during the transition from late gestation to early lactation. *J. Dairy Sci.* **2004**, *87*, 961–971.
137. Hammond, K.A.; Lam, M.; Kent Lloyd, K.C.; Diamond, J. Simultaneous manipulation of intestinal capacities and nutrient loads in mice. *Am. J. Physiol.* **1996**, *271*, G969–G979.
138. Freetly, H.C.; Ferrell, C.L. Relationship between the consumption of oxygen by portal-drained viscera and liver and milk production in the ewe. *J. Dairy Sci.* **1997**, *80*, 3256–3262.
139. Freetly, H.C.; Ferrell, C.L. Relationship of portal-drained viscera and liver net flux of glucose, lactate, volatile fatty acids, and nitrogen metabolites to milk production in the ewe. *J. Dairy Sci.* **1999**, *82*, 597–604.

5

Dietary Patterns and Maternal Anthropometry in HIV-Infected, Pregnant Malawian Women

Roshan T. Ramlal [1,*], Martin Tembo [2], Caroline C. King [3], Sascha Ellington [3], Alice Soko [2], Maggie Chigwenembe [2], Charles Chasela [2,4], Denise J. Jamieson [3], Charles van der Horst [1], Margaret Bentley [1], Linda Adair [1] and the BAN Study Team

1 University of North Carolina, Chapel Hill, NC 27599, USA;
E-Mails: charles_vanderhorst@med.unc.edu (C.H.); pbentley@unc.edu (M.B.); linda_adair@unc.edu (L.A.)

2 UNC Project Malawi, Tidziwe Center, Mzimba Road, Lilongwe, Malawi;
E-Mails: martintembo@gmail.com (M.T.); asoko@unclilongwe.org (A.S.); mchigwenembe@unclilongwe.org (M.C.); Charles.Chasela@wits.ac.za (C.C.)

3 U.S. Centers for Disease Control and Prevention, 4770 Buford Highway, Atlanta, GA 30341, USA;
E-Mails: ccking@cdc.gov (C.C.K.); sellington@cdc.gov (S.E.); djamieson@cdc.gov (D.J.J.)

4 Division of Epidemiology and Biostatistics, Faculty of Health Sciences, University of Witwatersrand, Johannesburg, 2193, South Africa

* Author to whom correspondence should be addressed; E-Mail: roshan.m.thomas@gmail.com

---

Abstract: Diet is a modifiable factor that can contribute to the health of pregnant women. In a sample of 577 HIV-positive pregnant women who completed baseline interviews for the Breastfeeding, Antiretrovirals, and Nutrition Study in Lilongwe, Malawi, cluster analysis was used to derive dietary patterns. Multiple regression analysis was used to identify associations between the dietary patterns and mid-upper arm circumference (MUAC), arm muscle area (AMA), arm fat area (AFA), and hemoglobin at baseline. Three key dietary patterns were identified: animal-based, plant-based, and grain-based. Women with relatively greater wealth were more likely to consume the animal-based diet, which had the highest intake of energy, protein, and fat and was associated with higher hemoglobin levels compared to the other diets. Women with the lowest wealth were more likely to consume the grain-based diet with the lowest intake of energy, protein, fat, and iron and were more likely to have lower AFA than women on the animal-based and plant-based diets, but higher AMA compared to women on the animal-based diet. Pregnant, HIV-infected women in Malawi could benefit from nutritional support to ensure greater nutrient diversity during pregnancy, when women face increased nutrient demands to support fetal growth and development.

Keywords: maternal diet; nutrition; pregnancy; HIV; anthropometry; Malawi; cluster analysis

---

1. Introduction

Infection with human immunodeficiency virus (HIV) increases resting energy expenditure and may limit dietary intake and reduce nutrient absorption [1]. In addition, nutritional status can influence the progression of HIV disease. Women are disproportionately affected by HIV compared to men. Across all age groups there is a higher rate of HIV prevalence among women than among men. Approximately 60% of adults living with HIV in Malawi are female [2]. HIV-infected pregnant women are particularly at risk since they have additional nutrient demands to support fetal growth and development [3]. Diet during pregnancy is a potentially modifiable factor that can contribute to the health of pregnant women and improve birth outcomes [4].

Women account for an estimated 60% of HIV infections in sub-Saharan Africa, where food availability, malnutrition, and infectious disease morbidity can vary substantially by season due to cycles of rainfall and agricultural production [5,6]. In Malawi, the annual famine season extends from August to March. The typical Malawian diet includes a staple food, such as *Nsima*, a thick maize porridge molded into patties, served with beans, vegetables, or relish for flavor. Most animal-source foods, rich in protein and micronutrients, are expensive and scarce. The current study used cluster analysis to identify three dietary patterns among 577 HIV-positive pregnant women in Lilongwe, Malawi, and compare sociodemographic and anthropometric characteristics of the women across diet patterns.

2. Experimental Section

Dietary recalls were collected from women who enrolled in the Breastfeeding, Antiretrovirals, and Nutrition (BAN) Study from April 2004 to March 2006. The BAN Study recruited women from four antenatal clinics with outreach to all pregnant women in Lilongwe [7]. At the first antenatal visit, consenting women were screened for pre-delivery study inclusion criteria: (1) ≤30 weeks gestation based on last menstrual period or fundal height; (2) ≥14 years of age; (3) confirmed HIV infection; (4) hemoglobin ≥ 7 g/dL; (5) CD4 count ≥ 200 cells/μL; (6) no prior antiretroviral medication use; (7) normal liver function tests (<2.5 times the upper limit of normal); (8) no serious complications of pregnancy; and (9) not previously enrolled in the BAN Study. At the second antenatal visit (referred to as the baseline visit), women completed a standardized interview, physical exam, and specimen collection. All women received prenatal iron folate tablets (200 mg ferrous sulfate and 0.25 mg folic acid) per Malawi standard of care and all women diagnosed with malaria were treated. The BAN Study included up to 5 antenatal visits, a labor and delivery visit, and 14 postpartum visits, with randomization occurring within 1 week of delivery to a 2-arm nutritional intervention to prevent maternal depletion and a 3-arm antiretroviral intervention to prevent HIV transmission during breastfeeding [8,9]. The BAN Study protocol was approved by the Malawi National Health Sciences Research Committee and the institutional review boards at the University of North Carolina at Chapel Hill and the U.S. Centers for Disease Control and Prevention (ClinicalTrials.gov identifier NCT00164762).

From April 2004 to March 2006, 738 women completed baseline interviews and delivered live singletons. Trained BAN Study staff collected 24-h dietary recalls at the baseline visit. Recipes and ingredients of mixed dishes were recorded. Women were asked if the diet recall indicated "typical intake" and were prompted for an explanation if it did not. Food models and utensils were used to help respondents recall portion sizes and proportion of mixed dishes consumed. A Malawi nutrient food composition table (FCT) [10] was used to estimate nutrient intakes. Supplemental nutrient information was obtained from Malawi's Ministry of Health's FCT, a Tanzanian FCT [11], and the USDA nutrient database [12]. The resulting database had nutrient content of individual food items as well as mixed dishes based on standard recipes. Dietary recalls were reviewed for plausible portion sizes and nutrient intakes; 577 recalls were deemed reliable for this analysis. Independent sample t-tests were used to evaluate potential selection bias.

Weight, height, mid-upper arm circumference (MUAC), and triceps skinfold thickness were measured by trained BAN Study staff. Weight was measured to the nearest 100 g at each visit with an electronic scale checked regularly with a standard 5 Kg weight. Height was measured with a wall-mounted stadiometer. At each visit, MUAC was measured at the midpoint between the olecranon and acromion process, to the nearest 0.1 cm using an insertion tape, while the arm hung freely at the side. Triceps skinfold thickness was measured in triplicate at each visit using Lange Calipers. The mean of the three measurements was used with MUAC to derive arm muscle area ($AMA = [MUAC - (\text{triceps skinfold} \times \pi)]^2/4\pi$) and arm fat area ($AFA = MUAC^2/4\pi - AMA$) [29]. Only the initial baseline measure, which was typically in the second trimester, was used in this analysis. Infant weights were measured at delivery or at the first visit post-delivery for home deliveries.

Anemia was defined as mild (<12 g/dL) or moderate (<10 g/dL) in accordance with the 2004 Malawi Demographic Health Survey (MDHS) definitions [13].

Statistical Analysis

To identify dietary patterns, we categorized food items into 12 groups: (1) grains; (2) legumes, groundnuts, seeds and soy; (3) tubers; (4) fruit; (5) leafy green vegetables; (6) fish; (7) meat poultry, and eggs; (8) dairy; (9) fats and oils; (10) sugars, candy, soft drinks; (11) hot beverages; and (12) miscellaneous. Nutrient densities (grams/total calories) of each food group were calculated and daily intake was used in the cluster analysis. Standardization by energy contribution helps to remove dietary variations due to differences in age, body size, and physical activity and to retain the proportional differences in food intake patterns [14,15]. Prior to cluster analysis, values were transformed into sample-specific Z-scores so that food intake differences between clusters could be illustrated and compared. Dietary patterns were generated by K-means cluster analysis [16] based on nutrient densities of each food group. We examined solutions with 2 to 5 clusters to evaluate which set of clusters was more meaningful to define dietary patterns.

The STATA [16] kmeans cluster method was used to group women according to nutrient densities of intake derived from each of the 12 food groups. The three-cluster solution was determined most appropriate based on power requirements and sufficient representation of typical dietary patterns of

Malawian women with nutritionally meaningful variation between clusters. Sociodemographic characteristics, anthropometrics, and macro-nutrient intakes were compared across the three clusters using chi-square tests for categorical variables and a one-factor analysis of variance (ANOVA) for continuous variables. If the global p-value was significant (<0.05), pairwise comparisons were made using a Bonferroni correction for multiple comparisons (p-value considered significant if <0.017). Multivariable linear regression was used to examine associations between dietary patterns and maternal nutritional indicators: MUAC, AMA, AFA, and hemoglobin. The multivariable models included a variable indicating whether or not the 24-h dietary recall reflected the participant's typical diet. Exposure to the famine season, defined by the number of days during the previous month that were spent in the famine season (August-May), was also included as a covariate. A wealth index of five quintiles was derived using principal component analysis of household characteristics: house construction (type of walls, floors, and roof), number of rooms and residents, electricity, refrigeration, sanitation, water source and cooking fuel source [17]. Other covariates included in the regression models were total energy intake, age, parity, education, maternal employment status, height and CD4 count. Multivariable models were assessed for statistically significant interactions ($p < 0.20$) between the dietary patterns and exposure to the famine season and between dietary patterns and wealth status [18].

3. Results

There were no significant differences ($p < 0.05$) in anthropometric, clinical, or seasonal indicators between the 577 women included (Table 1) and those excluded from this study, suggesting no selection bias. The mean daily energy intake was low (1378 kcal, interquartile range: 778, 1813), and over half of the women had mild (32.1%) or moderate (23.7%) anemia. No significant interactions were detected between dietary patterns and exposure to famine season and between dietary patterns and wealth status.

The three diet pattern clusters were labeled: 1) animal-based; 2) grain-based; and 3) plant-based. By definition, Cluster 1 had the highest intake of fish, meat, poultry, fat/oil, eggs and dairy, providing diets rich in energy and micronutrients (Figure 1). A typical meal in this cluster was a meat stew or soup with added oil or dried fish. Cluster 2 represents a grain-based diet of maize, rice, and millet, providing low levels of energy and micronutrients. A typical meal in this cluster was a plate of nsima only. Cluster 3 represents a mostly plant-based diet of leafy vegetables, beans, legumes, tubers, nuts, and fruits providing high levels of protein-rich or micronutrient-rich carbohydrates. A typical meal in this cluster was nsima with mustard greens and groundnut flour.

Table 1. Baseline demographics, nutritional status, caloric intake, and clinical characteristics among 577 pregnant women participating in the BAN Study.

Characteristic	$N = 577$
Age (year) [mean ± SD] [1]	25.9 ± 4.9
Education	
No school (%)	11.3
Primary (%)	52.8
Secondary or higher (%)	35.9

Table 1. *Cont.*

Characteristic	$N = 577$
Occupation Status	
Unemployed (%)	81.3
Employed (%)	18.7
Experienced famine season	
None (%)	39.7
Some (%)	14.6
All (%)	45.7
Parity (live births) [mean ± SD]	1.7 ± 1.3
Gestational age (weeks) [mean ± SD]	25.2 ± 5.4
CD4 count (cells/uL) [range (IQR) [2]]	442 (325–601)
Hemoglobin (g/dL) [mean ± SD]	10.8 ± 1.2
Daily energy total intake (kcal) [mean ± SD]	1378 ± 821
Mid-upper arm circumference (cm) [mean ± SD]	26.4 ± 2.6
Arm muscle area (cm^2) [mean ± SD]	36.6 ± 6.4
Arm fat area (cm^2) [mean ± SD]	19.5 ± 7.8

[1] SD: standard deviation; [2] IQR: interquartile range.

Comparisons across the three clusters indicated that employment status and median CD4 count did not differ significantly but mean age ($p = 0.02$) and education ($p = 0.05$) did. However, in pairwise comparisons with Bonferroni correction, age and education were not significant. The clusters differed by wealth and exposure to the famine season. Significantly more women in the grain-based cluster were in the lowest wealth index quintile compared to women in the animal-based cluster, and more were exposed to the famine season compared to either the animal-based or plant-based clusters (Table 2). Women in the grain-based cluster compared to the animal-based cluster also had a history of more live births. Women in the grain-based diet cluster consumed significantly fewer calories, protein, fat, and iron than women in the animal-based or plant-based diets (Table 2). They also had significantly lower carbohydrate intake than women in the plant-based cluster. In univariate analysis, women in the grain-based cluster had significantly lower AFA compared to women in the plant-based cluster (Table 2). However, in multivariable analysis, the predicted mean difference in AFA was significant comparing the grain-based cluster to both the plant-based (−2.47 cm^2 lower) and animal-based (−2.09 cm^2 lower) clusters (Table 3). Compared to women in the animal-based cluster, women in the grain-based cluster had significantly higher AMA and lower hemoglobin level in both univariate and multivariable analysis. The predicted mean increase in AMA was 1.86 cm^2 and the predicted decrease in hemoglobin level was −0.27 g/dL. The animal-based diet cluster had the highest intake of energy, protein, and fat at levels significantly above those of the plant-based cluster. In contrast, the plant-based diet had the highest intake of carbohydrates at a level significantly above that of the animal-based diet. While there were no differences between in maternal anthropometrics of women in the animal-based and plant-based diet clusters in univariate analysis, in multivariable analysis, the plant-based cluster had a significantly lower predicted mean difference in hemoglobin level (0.32 g/dL) than the animal-based cluster (Table 3). These measures did not have any clinical significance; however, it describes the association between prenatal body composition and dietary profiles. There were no differences in mean MUAC between the clusters in unadjusted (Table 2) or adjusted analysis. Furthermore, there were no differences between the diet clusters in infant weight at delivery.

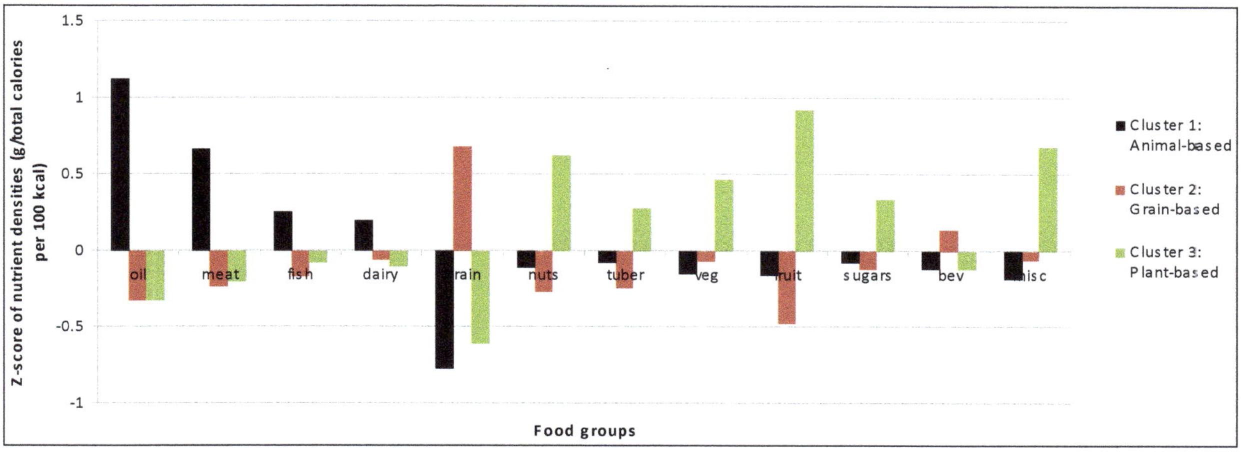

Figure 1. Cluster analysis of dietary patterns among HIV-infected Malawian pregnant women.

Table 2. Demographic, nutrient, and clinical indicators by the 3 diet clusters among 577 pregnant women participating in the BAN Study.

Indicators	Animal-Based [1] (n = 160)	Grain-based [2,3] (n = 254)	Plant-based [4] (n = 163)	*P* value for Pairwise Cluster Comparisons [5] Animal *vs.* Grain	Animal *vs.* Plant	Grain *vs.* Plant
Characteristics [6]						
Age (year) (mean ± SD)	25.0 ± 4.4	26.2 ± 5.1	26.2 ± 4.9	-	-	-
No school (n = 65) [n(%)]	11 (6.9)	37 (14.5)	17 (10.4)	-	-	-
Lowest wealth index (n = 108) [n(%)]	17 (15.7)	63 (58.3)	28 (25.9)	0.001	-	-
Parity > 2 (n = 133) [n(%)]	23(14.3)	67 (26.4)	43 (26.3)	0.014	-	-
Any famine season exposure (n = 348) [n(%)]	83 (51.9)	180 (70.9)	85 (51.2)	<0.001	-	<0.001
Nutrition status						
Daily energy total intake (kcal)	1776.8 ± 859.5	1083.5 ± 672.2	1445.4 ± 818.5	<0.001	<0.001	<0.001
Carbohydrates (g/day)	195.8 ± 116.3	201.1 ± 128.9	237.4 ± 135.3	-	0.010	0.014
Protein (g/day)	69.3 ± 57.1	32.6 ± 28.3	47.1 ± 35 9	<0.001	<0.001	0.001
Total fat (g/day)	82.9 ± 51.2	19.9 ± 18.5	41.2 ± 43 8	<0.001	<0.001	<0.001
Iron (g/day)	10.1 ± 9.9	6.9 ± 5.9	11.3 ± 8.4	<0.001	-	<0.001
Hemoglobin (g/dL)	11.0 ± 1.1	10.7 ± 1.2	10.7 ± 1.1	0.017	-	-
MUAC (cm)	26.3 ± 2.7	26.3 ± 2.6	26.8 ± 2.6	-	-	-
AMA (cm^2)	35.3 ± 6.2	37.3 ± 6.5	37.0 ± 6.3	0.007	-	-
AFA (cm^2)	20.2 ± 8.0	18.7 ± 7.0	20.7 ± 8.5	-	-	0.003
Infant weight at delivery (g)	3058.6 ± 431.4	2976.9 ± 434.4	3053.9 ± 395.2	-	-	-

[1] Food pattern of high fish, meat and oil; [2] Food pattern of high grain and grain-derived foods; [3] Food or food group contributed the relatively lowest mean intake across the 3 clusters; [4] Food pattern of high leafy vegetables, nuts, tubers, fruits; [5] Determined by t tests or chi-square tests (values $p < 0.017$, Bonferroni adjustment for multiple comparisons); [6] CD4 and maternal work status are not included in the table because no significant differences were found when comparing across three clusters (*i.e.*, global p-value > 0.05).

Table 3. Predicted mean difference in arm muscle area (AMA), arm fat area (AFA), and hemoglobin level (Hb) of women in the three clusters of dietary patterns.

Outcome	Mean Difference	95% CI		*p* value
	AMA [1] *(cm^2)*			
Grain (compared to animal)	1.86	0.53	3.19	0.01
Plant (compared to animal)	1.23	−0.14	2.60	0.08
Plant (compared to grain)	−0.63	−1.89	0.63	0.33
	AFA [1] *(cm^2)*			
Grain (compared to animal)	−2.09	−3.75	−0.44	0.01
Plant (compared to animal)	0.38	−1.33	2.08	0.67
Plant (compared to grain)	2.47	0.90	4.03	<0.01
	Hb [1] *(g/dL)*			
Grain (compared to animal)	−0.27	−0.52	−0.01	0.04
Plant (compared to animal)	−0.32	−0.59	−0.07	0.01
Plant (compared to grain)	−0.06	−0.30	0.18	0.62

[1] Adjusted for total energy intake, season, age, parity, education, wealth index, maternal employment status, height and CD4 count.

4. Discussion

To our knowledge, this is the first study to use cluster analysis to examine dietary patterns among pregnant, HIV-infected women in sub-Saharan Africa. This sample represents a young group of HIV-positive Malawian women with low levels of education, high unemployment, low parity and relatively high CD4 counts, indicative of good immune status. The women in our study had relatively healthy values of MUAC, AMA, and AFA that are representative of Malawian women [19–21]. Despite the provision of prenatal iron tablets, women in the study were mildly anemic. However, anemia is common among HIV-infected women in resource-limited areas where nutritional deficiencies are compounded by parasitic infections, compromised immunity, and the hematological consequences of chronic and systemic inflammation [22,23].

Three key dietary patterns were identified and were associated with differences in nutrient quality, sociodemographic characteristics, and nutritional outcomes for the women. Women in the lowest wealth index were more likely to consume grain-based diets with the lowest intake of energy, protein, fat, and iron. A higher proportion of women on grain-based diets were exposed to the famine season, which would be expected to negatively impact nutritional outcomes, and had lower AFA compared to women on the plant-based and animal-based diets [24]. However, women on grain-based diet had a higher AMA compared to women on animal-based diets. The higher lean muscle mass among women consuming grain-based diets may reflect increased manual labor, such as farming. Women on animal-based diets had the highest intake of energy, protein, and fat and had significantly higher mean difference in hemoglobin level compared to women on the plant-based and grain-based diets. In addition, high intake of phytate and low intake of heme-iron results in lower bioavailability of iron, which would further compound low iron intake.

While multiple 24-h recalls would be ideal for analyzing associations between diet and maternal body composition [25], only one 24-h recall was collected in the BAN Study. Although one study suggested that Malawian diets among low-income women have little daily variation [10], another recent study among pregnant, rural Malawian women found high within and between individual variance in energy intakes [19]. As such, our use of only one dietary recall per participant may result in some diet misclassification. Further misclassification may arise due to the use of nutrient content based on the raw ingredients of each dish although several dishes were consumed cooked.

With more than 500 dietary recalls from HIV-infected, pregnant Malawian women, we derived dietary patterns typical of Malawians using cluster analysis and showed that the patterns differed markedly in diet quality. The use of dietary patterns rather than individual nutrients in assessing diet and health relationships has emerged as a method of capturing the total diet [26–29]. This type of evaluation allows for the examination of associations of multiple dietary components with the outcome of interest [15]. Analyzing foods instead of nutrients makes it easier to translate results into intervention messages. Furthermore, seasonal and cultural factors influence diet patterns, which in turn affect nutrient intakes.

Some limitations of the cluster analysis method include inherent subjectivity, which occurs throughout the pattern analysis because investigators must decide how to collapse the data into food groups and how to quantify the contribution of each food group to the total diet [26,30,31]. Additionally, the label attributed to a given diet pattern is a crude and sometimes subjective description, based either on a quantitative measure of the predominant food group consumed or a qualitative measure of health of the diet. To the best of our ability, we objectively used food composition databases and substantial knowledge of Malawian diets to select food groups and clusters most representative of diet patterns of Malawian women.

Although WHO and Malawi guidelines for ART initiation has changed and many of the subjects in this study would be eligible for ART, pregnant, HIV-infected women in Malawi could still benefit from nutritional counseling and food supplementation to ensure greater nutrient diversity during the gestational period, when they face additional nutrient demands to support fetal growth and development.

5. Conclusions

In summary, we identified three patterns of diet among pregnant HIV-infected women in Malawi, and these patterns were related to socioeconomic status as well as nutritional outcomes. A primarily grain-based diet had the least nutrient quality, and women consuming this diet appeared to be the most vulnerable to adverse nutritional outcomes. This study describe typical diets of HIV-infected, pregnant women and highlights poor quality of maternal diets that need to enhanced to meet demands of this particular group of pregnant women, vulnerable to both HIV and malnutrition. Therefore, nutrition interventions and food aid programs tailored to the needs of HIV-infected pregnant women are of great importance, particularly those with low socioeconomic status and those with limited food intake during rainy seasons when food insecurity is at its peak. This analysis also presents a novel way to assess and analyze dietary intake patterns among pregnant women in sub-Saharan Africa.

Acknowledgments

We are grateful to the BAN Study Team at University of North Carolina Chapel Hill, Centers for Disease Control and Prevention, Atlanta, and UNC Project team in Lilongwe. Finally, and most especially, all the women and infants that have agreed to participate in the study.

Author Contributions

R.T. Ramlal, M. Tembo, C. Chasela, D.J. Jamieson, C. van der Horst, M. Bentley and L. Adair designed the study. R.T. Ramlal, M. Tembo, A. Soko, M. Chigwenembe, and C. Chasela collected the data. R.T. Ramlal analyzed the data. R.T. Ramlal, C.C. King, S. Ellington, D.J. Jamieson, C. van der Horst, M. Bentley, and L. Adair interpreted the data. R.T. Ramlal wrote the report and had primary responsibility for the final content. All authors critically reviewed versions of the report and contributed to the intellectual content of the manuscript.

References

1. Scrimshaw, N.; SanGiovanni, J. Synergism of nutrition, infection and immunity: An overview. *Am. J. Clin. Nutr.* **1997**, *66*, 464S–477S.
2. HIV/AIDS JUNPo. *Global report: UNAIDS report on the global AIDS epidemic: 2012*; UNAIDS: Geneva, Switzerland, 2012.
3. Villamor, E.; Msamanga, G.; Spiegelman, D.; Coley, J.; Hunter, D.J.; Peterson, K.E.; Fawzi, W.W. HIV status and sociodemographic correlates of maternal body size and wasting during pregnancy. *Eur. J. Clin. Nutr.* **2002**, *56*, 415–424.
4. Fawzi, W.W.; Hunter, D.J. Vitamins in HIV disease progression and vertical transmission. *Epidemiology* **1998**, *9*, 457–466.
5. Hartikainen, H.M.K.; Kulmala, T.; Ashorn, P. Seasonality of gestational weight gain and fetal growth in rural Malawi. *East Afr. Med. J.* **2005**, *82*, 294–299.
6. Larmarange, J. [HIV prevalence in sub-Saharan Africa: background of an estimation]. *Med. Sci. (Paris)* **2009**, *25*, 87–92.
7. Moses, A.; Zimba, C.; Kamanga, E.; Nkhoma, J.; Maida, A.; Martinson, F.; Mofolo, I.; Joaki, G.; Muita, J.; Spensley, A.; *et al.* Prevention of mother-to-child transmission: Program changes and the effect on uptake of the HIVNET 012 regimen in Malawi. *Aids* **2008**, *22*, 83–87.
8. Van der Horst, C.; Chasela, C.; Ahmed, Y.; Hoffman, I.; Hosseinipour, M.; Knight, R.; Fiscus, S.; Hudgens, M.; Kazembe, P.; Bentley, M.; *et al.* Modifications of a large HIV prevention clinical trial to fit changing realities: A case study of the Breastfeeding, Antiretroviral, and Nutrition (BAN) protocol in Lilongwe, Malawi. *Contemp. Clin. Trials* **2009**, *30*, 24–33.
9. Chasela, C.S.; Hudgens, M.G.; Jamieson, D.J.; Kayira, D.; Hosseinipour, M.C.; Kourtis, A.P.; Martinson, F.; Tegha, G.; Knight, R.J.; Ahmed, Y.I.; *et al.* Maternal or infant antiretroviral drugs to reduce HIV-1 transmission. *N. Engl. J. Med.* **2010**, *362*, 2271–2281.
10. Ferguson, E.L.; Gadowsky, S.L.; Huddle, J.M.; Cullinan, T.R.; Lehrfeld, J.; Gibson, R.S. An interactive 24-h recall technique for assessing the adequacy of trace mineral intakes of rural Malawian women; its advantages and limitations. *Eur. J Clin Nutr* **1995** *49*, 565–578.

11. Lukmanji, Z.H.E.; Mlingi, N.; Assey, V.; Ndossi, G.; Fawzi, W. *Tanzania Food Composition Tables*; MUHAS-TFNC, HSPH: Dar es Salaam, Tanzania, 2008.
12. *USDA National Nutrient Database for Standard Reference, Release 22*. United States Department of Agriculture, Agricultural Research Service: Washington, DC, USA, 2010.
13. National Statistical Office (NSO) [Malawi] aOM: *Malawi Demographic and Health Survey 2004;* NSO: Lilongwe, Malawi, 2005.
14. Chen, H.; Ward, M.H.; Graubard, B.I.; Heineman, E.F.; Markin, R.M.; Potischman, N.A.; Russell, R.M.; Weisenburger, D.D.; Tucker, K.L. Dietary patterns and adenocarcinoma of the esophagus and distal stomach. *Am. J. Clin. Nutr.* **2002**, *75*, 137–144.
15. Newby, P.K.; Tucker, K.L. Empirically derived eating patterns using factor or cluster analysis: A review. *Nutr. Rev.* **2004**, *62*, 177–203.
16. StataCorp. *Stata Statistical Software: Release 9*. StataCorp LP: College Station, TX, USA, 2005.
17. Kolenikov, S.A.G. *The Use of Discrete Data in PCA: Theory, Simulations, and Applications to Socioeconomic Indices*; University of North Carolina at Chapel Hill and Carolina Population Center: Chapel Hill, NC, USA, 2004.
18. Harrell, F.E. *Regression Modeling Strategies: With Application to Linear Models, Logistic Regression and Survival Analysis*; Springer Science+Business Media, Inc: New York, NY, USA, 2001.
19. Huddle, J.M.; Gibson, R.S.; Cullinan, T.R. Is zinc a limiting nutrient in the diets of rural pregnant Malawian women? *Br. J. Nutr.* **1998**, *79*, 257–265.
20. Friis, H.; Gomo, E.; Nyazema, N.; Ndhlovu, P.; Kaestel, P.; Krarup, H.; Michaelsen, K.F. HIV-1 viral load and elevated serum alpha(1)-antichymotrypsin are independent predictors of body composition in pregnant Zimbabwean women. *J. Nutr.* **2002**, *132*, 3747–3753.
21. Friis, H.; Gomo, E.; Nyazema, N.; Ndhlovu, P.; Krarup, H.; Kaestel, P.; Michaelsen, K.F. Maternal body composition, HIV infection and other predictors of gestation length and birth size in Zimbabwe. *Br. J. Nutr.* **2004**, *92*, 833–840.
22. Antelman, G.; Msamanga, G.I.; Spiegelman, D.; Urassa, E.J.; Narh, R.; Hunter, D.J.; Fawzi, W.W. Nutritional factors and infectious disease contribute to anemia among pregnant women with human immunodeficiency virus in Tanzania. *J. Nutr.* **2000**, *130*, 1950–1957.
23. Brocklehurst, P.; French, R. The association between maternal HIV infection and perinatal outcome: A systematic review of the literature and meta-analysis. *Br. J. Obstet. Gynaecol.* **1998**, *105*, 836–848.
24. Ramlal, R.T.; Tembo, M.; Soko, A.; Chigwenembe, M.; Tohill, B.C.; Kayira, D.; King, C.C.; Chasela, C.; Jamieson, D.; van der Horst, C. Patterns of Body Composition Among HIV-Infected, Pregnant Malawians and the Effects of Famine Season. *Matern. Child Health J.* 2013, 17, 265–273.
25. Nyambose, J.; Koski, K.G.; Tucker, K.L. High intra/interindividual variance ratios for energy and nutrient intakes of pregnant women in rural Malawi show that many days are required to estimate usual intake. *J. Nutr.* **2002**, *132*, 1313–1318.
26. Newby, P.K.; Muller, D.; Tucker, K.L. Associations of empirically derived eating patterns with plasma lipid biomarkers: A comparison of factor and cluster analysis methods. *Am. J. Clin. Nutr.* **2004**, *80*, 759–767.

27. Hu, F.B. Dietary pattern analysis: A new direction in nutritional epidemiology. *Curr. Opin. Lipidol.* **2002**, *13*, 3–9.
28. Kant, A.K. Dietary patterns and health outcomes. *J. Am. Diet. Assoc.* **2004**, *104*, 615–635.
29. Panagiotakos, D.B.; Pitsavos, C.; Skoumas, Y.; Stefanadis, C. The association between food patterns and the metabolic syndrome using principal components analysis: The ATTICA Study. *J. Am. Diet. Assoc.* **2007**, *107*, 979–987.
30. Newby, P.K.; Muller, D.; Hallfrisch, J.; Andres, R.; Tucker, K.L. Food patterns measured by factor analysis and anthropometric changes in adults. *Am. J. Clin. Nutr.* **2004**, *80*, 504–513.
31. Newby, P.K.; Muller, D.; Hallfrisch, J.; Qiao, N.; Andres, R.; Tucker, K.L. Dietary patterns and changes in body mass index and waist circumference in adults. *Am. J. Clin. Nutr.* **2003**, *77*, 1417–1425.

6

Lower Protein-to-Carbohydrate Ratio in Maternal Diet is Associated with Higher Childhood Systolic Blood Pressure up to Age Four Years

Michelle L. Blumfield [1,2], Caryl Nowson [3], Alexis J. Hure [4], Roger Smith [5], Stephen J. Simpson [6], David Raubenheimer [6], Lesley MacDonald-Wicks [1,2] and Clare E. Collins [1,2,*]

[1] School of Health Sciences, Faculty of Health and Medicine, University of Newcastle, Callaghan, New South Wales 2308, Australia; E-Mails: Michelle.Blumfield@newcastle.edu.au (M.B.); Lesley.Wicks@newcastle.edu.au (L.M.-W.)

[2] Priority Research Centre in Physical Activity and Nutrition, Faculty of Health and Medicine, University of Newcastle, Callaghan, New South Wales 2308, Australia

[3] School of Exercise and Nutrition Science, Deakin University, Geelong, Victoria 3216, Australia; E-Mail: Caryl.Nowson@deakin.edu.au

[4] School of Medicine and Public Health, Faculty of Health and Medicine, University of Newcastle, Callaghan, New South Wales 2308, Australia; E-Mail: Alexis.Hure@newcastle.edu.au

[5] Mothers and Babies Research Centre, Hunter Medical Research Institute, John Hunter Hospital, Level 3, Endocrinology, Locked Bag 1, Hunter Region Mail Centre, New South Wales 2310, Australia; E-Mail: Roger.Smith@newcastle.edu.au

[6] Charles Perkins Centre, School of Biological Sciences, University of Sydney, Sydney, New South Wales 2006, Australia; E-Mails: Stephen.Simpson@sydney.edu.au (S.J.S.); David.Raubenheimer@sydney.edu.au (D.R.)

* Author to whom correspondence should be addressed; E-Mail: Clare.Collins@newcastle.edu.au

---

Abstract: The prenatal environment can influence development of offspring blood pressure (BP), which tracks into adulthood. This prospective longitudinal study investigated whether maternal pregnancy dietary intake is associated with the development of child BP up to age four years. Data are from 129 mother-child dyads enrolled in the Women and Their Children's Health study. Maternal diet was assessed using a validated 74-item food frequency questionnaire at 18 to 24 weeks and 36 to 40 weeks, with a reference period of the previous three months. Child systolic and diastolic BP were measured at 3, 6, 9, 12, 24, 36 and 48 months, using an automated BP monitor. Using mixed-model regression analyses adjusted for childhood growth indices, pregnancy intakes of percentage of energy (E%) polyunsaturated fat (β coefficient 0.73; 95% CI 0.003, 1.45; $p = 0.045$), E% omega-6 fatty acids (β coefficient 0.89; 95% CI 0.09, 1.69; $p = 0.03$) and protein-to-carbohydrate (P:C) ratio (β coefficient −14.14; 95% CI −27.68, −0.60; $p = 0.04$) were associated with child systolic BP trajectory up to 4 years. Child systolic BP was greatest at low proportions of dietary protein (<16% of energy) and high carbohydrate (>40% of energy) intakes. There may be an ideal maternal macronutrient ratio associated with optimal infant BP. Maternal diet, which is potentially modifiable, may play an important role in influencing offspring risk of future hypertension.

Keywords: maternal; pregnancy; dietary intake; macronutrient; blood pressure; systolic; child; protein; diet; nutrition

---

1. Introduction

The worldwide burden of cardiovascular disease (CVD) has substantially increased, to cause an estimated 17.3 million deaths in 2008 [1]. It is forecast that by 2030, more than 23 million people will die annually from CVDs [2]. Elevated blood pressure (BP) and childhood adiposity are independent predictors of adult hypertension and CVD [3]. Both obesity and hypertension are increasingly prevalent in the pediatric population, with 42 million children under five estimated to be overweight in 2013 and 2% to 5% of children considered hypertensive globally [2]. There is strong evidence across diverse populations for tracking of BP from childhood into adulthood [4]. Even short periods of hypertension in childhood increases the adult risk of hypertension [1]. Thus early prevention of elevated BP is an important global public health goal.

Variations in maternal diet during pregnancy may lead to elevated offspring risk in adulthood for hypertension and obesity. Both human and animal studies provide compelling evidence suggesting a link between maternal nutritional status and offspring cardiovascular function [5]. Animal studies provide indisputable evidence that maternal protein restriction or a global reduction in dietary intake during pregnancy can influence offspring cardiovascular function [5–8]. Studies have mainly focused on interventions in pregnant rodents, although several dietary intervention studies in pregnant sheep suggest commonality among species [5]. Raised blood pressure has frequently been reported in offspring of nutritionally deprived animals and those fed a low protein-to-carbohydrate (P:C) ratio diet during pregnancy [5,9]. Prenatal exposure to protein restriction or dietary global restriction in animal models has produced offspring with abnormalities in vascular function in isolated resistance arteries [5]. However in recent cross-sectional studies of children born in developed countries, associations between changes in diet during pregnancy with childhood BP have been small, or negligible [10]. A recent Finnish study found systolic BP in four year old children was positively associated with maternal pregnancy carbohydrate and fat intakes [11]. The same group also reported a U-shaped relationship between both maternal carbohydrate and monounsaturated fat intakes and infant BP at six months [12].

The escalation in prevalence of maternal and child obesity increases the public health significance of determining the extent to which maternal diet can predict offspring BP [10]. In healthy weight pregnant women exposed to a variety of dietary and/or supplement regimes there was minimal impact on offspring BP, compared to women who experienced lifestyle and nutritional limitations similar to conditions in World War II [12,13]. However, much stronger associations have been reported on later BP when birthweight and/or accelerated postnatal growth were considered, or adjustment for current body weight [13]. This highlights the inter-relationships between childhood growth, current body weight and cardiovascular control.

Our previous work identified that across a wide range of species optimal ratios of macronutrients exist and that protein intake is a critical determinant of total energy intake [14,15]. Animal models confirm that the ratio of dietary P:C impacts on aging and disease, with indirect evidence from human models suggesting the P:C ratio is a primary determinant of health [16]. We have demonstrated a link between maternal dietary ratio of protein to non-protein energy to variations in offspring body composition [15]. In human pregnancy, maternal macronutrient profile was associated with fetal adiposity and fat distribution [14]. Here we have examined the link between maternal macronutrient ratios and childhood blood pressure trajectory. We hypothesized that after adjustment for potential confounders and growth indices, child systolic BP up to age four years would be associated with maternal pregnancy macronutrient intake and protein-to-carbohydrate (P:C) ratio.

2. Experimental Section

2.1. Sample

The sample is from the Women and Their Children's Health (WATCH) study (n = 179). WATCH is a prospective, longitudinal cohort investigating whether maternal nutrition is an important predictor of offspring outcomes including growth, body composition and childhood cognition [17]. The WATCH study was initiated in July 2006 in Newcastle, Australia. Pregnant participants were recruited from the antenatal clinic at the John Hunter Hospital from July 2006 to June 2008. A consent rate of 61% was achieved for pregnant women who were approached [18]. No exclusion criteria were used during recruitment. Women attended study visits during pregnancy at 19, 24, 30, and 36 weeks of gestation. Postnatal follow-up of women and their children occurred at 3-month intervals during the first year after birth and annually thereafter, until age 4 years.

The characteristics of the WATCH cohort have been reported previously [19,20]. The WATCH study contained a higher proportion of women with post-school qualifications and socioeconomic advantage, but a similar proportion of overweight/obese and of indigenous ethnicity as the Australian population [14,20]. Significant differences were also previously found between women with available dietary data (n = 156) and women without dietary data (n = 23). Women without dietary data were less likely to be married or in a de facto relationship (p = 0.03) and more likely to be of socio-economic disadvantage (p = 0.04) and to have had a preterm delivery (p = 0.001) [14].

Dietary and BP data from 129 mother-child dyads were available for the current analysis. All participants gave written informed consent and ethical approval for the study was obtained from the Hunter New England Human Research Ethics Committee (06/05/24/5.06). Recruitment, withdrawals and participant attendance during pregnancy has previously been described [20].

2.2. Data Collection

Details of the data collection have been described elsewhere [20]. Demographic and social data were collected during the first study visit using questions modeled on those in the Women's Health Australia, Australian Longitudinal Study on Women's Health survey. Pre-pregnancy weight was self-reported at either the first antenatal clinic visit at 14 weeks gestation or at the first study visit. Dietary data during pregnancy were collected between 18 to 24 weeks and again at 36 to 40 weeks gestation using a validated 74-item food frequency questionnaire (FFQ), the Dietary Questionnaire for Epidemiological Studies. This tool was previously validated against weighed-food records in young women [21]. The FFQ includes food and beverage data but does not ask about vitamin or mineral supplement use. The dietary intake reference period was the previous three months. Therefore, dietary data collected between 18 to 24 weeks and 36 to 40 weeks gestation referred to a reference period of 6 to 24 weeks gestation (early pregnancy) and 24 to 40 weeks gestation (late pregnancy), respectively. Positive moderate to strong pairwise correlations have been previously reported between all dietary variables in early and late pregnancy ($0.46 < r < 0.78$; $p < 0.001$) [14]. Therefore, maternal dietary intakes during pregnancy were expressed as the mean of intakes during early and late pregnancy.

Child systolic and diastolic BP were measured at each postnatal study visit using an automated DINAMAP PRO 300V2 BP monitor (GE Healthcare, Helsinki, Finland) under standardised conditions. Maternal and child anthropometric measurements were taken at every study visit by a team of Accredited Practising Dietitians, each with Level One Anthropometry certification from the International Society for the Advancement of Kinanthropometry (ISAK). Weight and height were measured in accordance with the ISAK protocol.

2.3. Statistical Analysis

The main outcome measures were child systolic and diastolic BP (mm/Hg). Dietary predictors included maternal intake of energy yielding nutrients (energy, protein, total fat, saturated fatty acids (SFA), monounsaturated fatty acids, polyunsaturated fatty acids (PUFA), omega-3 (*n*-3) fatty acids, omega-6 (*n*-6) fatty acids, total carbohydrate, sugars, starch and fibre) expressed as total intakes (grams), percentage of total energy intake, and the ratio of P:C intake and *n*-6:*n*-3 intake. Nutrient intakes were adjusted for energy using the residual method [22]. Childhood growth indices included birthweight and BMI *z*-score. BMI was converted to *z*-scores using the WHO Child Growth Standards reference data [23].

Normally distributed data were reported as mean ± SD and non-parametric data as median, 25th and 75th percentiles. Comparisons were performed using two-sample *t*-tests, the Kruskal-Wallis test or the chi-squared statistic. Linear mixed-models used longitudinal data to determine whether maternal macronutrient intakes during pregnancy were associated with the development of childhood BP up to 4 years. Independent predictor variables were assessed for colinearity.

In preliminary univariate analyses, maternal age, pre-pregnancy weight, education, parity, smoking status, weight gained during pregnancy, preterm delivery, marital status, ethnicity and child gender were not significant predictors for childhood systolic or diastolic BP ($p < 0.2$) and did not remain in multivariate models (data not shown). Analyses were conducted using: (i) unadjusted data; (ii) data adjusted for maternal energy intake and child birthweight; and (iii) data adjusted for maternal energy intake, birthweight and child BMI *z*-score. All analyses were repeated with and without women who reported diabetes or hypertension during pregnancy. The main findings did not change with the exclusion of women who reported diabetes (n = 8) or hypertension (n = 10) during pregnancy, thus analyses were not adjusted for these conditions. To address potential dietary misreporting, the pregnancy energy cut-off values recommended by Meltzer *et al.* (2008) [24] were applied, by excluding those who reported daily energy intakes <4.5 or >20.0 MJ/day [24].

Parametric response surfaces for mean systolic BP were fitted over macronutrient intake arrays and then visualized by using nonparametric thin-plate splines. This approach allowed the complex relationship between infant systolic BP up to four years and the two major axes of percentage protein and percentage carbohydrate in the maternal diet to be visualized.

All data manipulation and statistical analyses were performed using Intercooled Stata 11.2 (Stata, College Station, Texas, USA). Graphics were performed using *R* software. *p*-Values < 0.05 were considered statistically significant.

3. Results

The final sample included 129 mother and child dyads. Maternal characteristics are presented in Table 1. There were no significant differences between individuals in this sub-study (n = 129) and the total sample of women and children in the WATCH cohort (n = 179).

Table 1. Maternal characteristics of the participants in the Women and Their Children's Health Study.

Characteristic	Women (n = 129)
Age (year)	29.1 ± 5.4 [1]
Height (cm)	165.1 ± 6.5
Born in Australia [n (%)] [2]	120 (93.0)
Aboriginal, not Torres Strait Islander [n (%)]	4 (3.1)
Married or in de facto relationship [n (%)]	114 (88.4)
Education [n (%)] [3]	96 (74.4)
Socioeconomic status, IRSAD [4] decile <= 5 [n (%)] [5]	37 (28.7)
Smoked during pregnancy [n (%)]	15 (11.6)
Prepregnancy weight (kg)	65.0 (58.0, 79.0) [6]
Weight gain during pregnancy (kg)	12.0 (8.9, 17.0)
Nulliparous [n (%)]	59 (45.7)
Preterm delivery before 37 weeks of gestation [n (%)]	9 (7.0)

[1] Mean ± SD (all such values); [2] Other countries include England (n = 3), Belgium (n = 1), Canada (n = 1), Malaysia (n = 1), New Zealand (n = 1), Papua New Guinea (n = 1) and the United States (n = 1); [3] Maternal education level ≥Australian year 12 high school certificate; [4] IRSAD, index of relative socioeconomic advantage and disadvantage; [5] Relative disadvantage and lack of advantage based on postcode (IRSAD decile ≤ 5), ([25]); [6] Median; 25th and 75th percentiles in parentheses (all such values).

The BP and growth characteristics of children are summarized in Table 2. Compared with female children, male children became significantly heavier ($p < 0.01$) and longer ($p < 0.05$) between birth and 24 months, and had a larger BMI between 3 and 12 months ($p < 0.01$). No significant differences were found between child gender and BP measurements.

Table 2. Characteristics of children in the Women and Their Children's Health Study.

Child Characteristics	Males	Females	*P* [1]
Birth			
Gender [*n* (%)]	67 (51.9)	62 (48.1)	0.66
Gestational age (week)	39.5 ± 1.3 [2]	39.3 ± 2.1	0.45
Birthweight (g)	3618.7 ± 552.7	3318.2 ± 591.2	0.003
Length (cm)	51.9 ± 2.8	50.3 ± 4.0	0.01
3 months			
n	64	60	
Weight (kg)	6.5 ± 0.8	5.7 ± 0.7	<0.001
Length (cm)	63.0 ± 2.5	60.6 ± 2.8	<0.001
BMI	16.1 ± 1.5	15.2 ± 1.5	<0.001
BMI *z*-score	−0.5 (−1.2, 0.2)	−0.7 (−1.7, −0.1)	0.26
n	20	21	
Systolic blood pressure (mmHg)	96.0 (82.5, 104.5) [3]	96.0 (86.0, 103.0)	0.77
Diastolic blood pressure (mmHg)	60.0 (34.0, 66.5)	55.0 (47.0, 59.0)	0.68
6 months			
n	61	53	
Weight	8.2 ± 1.1	7.3 ± 1.0	<0.001
Length	69.3 ± 2.9	66.4 ± 3.0	<0.001
BMI	17.0 ± 1.4	16.5 ± 1.5	0.03
BMI *z*-score	−0.2 (−0.9, 0.4)	−0.3 (−0.9, 0.3)	0.72
n	36	36	
Systolic blood pressure (mmHg)	101.0 (96.0, 108.0)	103.0 (95.5, 109.0)	0.78
Diastolic blood pressure (mmHg)	57.0 (51.0, 65.5)	52.5 (45.5, 62.0)	0.30
9 months			
n	54	56	
Weight	9.5 ± 1.4	8.5 ± 1.0	<0.001
Length	73.9 ± 2.9	71.3 ± 2.9	<0.001
BMI	17.1 ± 1.7	16.6 ± 1.2	0.03
BMI *z*-score	−0.1 (−0.9, 0.8)	−0.04 (−0.7, 0.5)	0.76
n	40	48	
Systolic blood pressure (mmHg)	103.0 (98.0, 109.0)	101.5 (93.5, 110.0)	0.78
Diastolic blood pressure (mmHg)	55.5 (49.5, 62.0)	56.5 (46.0, 61.5)	0.54

Table 2. *Cont.*

Child Characteristics	Males	Females	*P* [1]
12 months			
n	57	55	
Weight	10.5 ± 1.3	9.3 ± 1.0	<0.001
Length	78.0 ± 3.3	75.1 ± 2.9	<0.001
BMI	17.1 ± 1.4	16.4 ± 0.9	0.001
BMI *z*-score	0.1 (−0.5, 0.8)	0.1 (−0.5, 0.5)	0.24
n	37	38	
Systolic blood pressure (mmHg)	98.0 (94.0, 106.0)	98.5 (94.0, 108.0)	0.81
Diastolic blood pressure (mmHg)	58.0 (50.0, 66.0)	56.0 (46.0, 62.0)	0.59
24 months			
n	47	44	
Weight	13.5 ± 1.6	12.6 ± 1.8	0.009
Length	89.1 ± 4.9	86.7 ± 4.2	0.02
BMI	17.0 ± 1.3	16.7 ± 1.3	0.37
BMI *z*-score	1.0 (−0.1, 1.4)	0.7 (0.06, 1.2)	0.97
n	35	32	
Systolic blood pressure (mmHg)	100.0 (96.0, 105.5)	98.0 (92.0, 104.0)	0.13
Diastolic blood pressure (mmHg)	61.0 (56.0, 65.0)	61.0 (58.0, 64.5)	0.63
36 months			
n	42	38	
Weight	15.4 ± 1.8	14.4 ± 2.8	0.06
Length	97.4 ± 5.7	95.0 ± 7.3	0.11
BMI	16.1 ± 1.4	15.8 ± 1.5	0.34
BMI *z*-score	0.4 (−0.5, 1.3)	0.2 (−0.3, 0.7)	0.60
n	36	33	
Systolic blood pressure (mmHg)	103.0 (98.5, 111.0)	104.0 (97.0, 113.0)	0.87
Diastolic blood pressure (mmHg)	63.0 (59.5, 66.0)	62.0 (58.0, 67.0)	0.90
48 months			
n	40	45	
Weight	17.7 ± 2.1	17.4 ± 3.0	0.61
Length	105.3 ± 7.4	103.6 ± 5.8	0.24
BMI	15.1 ± 1.3	16.1 ± 2.5	0.61
BMI *z*-score	0.4 (−0.2, 1.3)	0.3 (−1.2, 0.8)	0.69
n	26	28	
Systolic blood pressure (mmHg)	101.0 (95.0, 114.0)	106.0 (94.0, 115.0)	0.72
Diastolic blood pressure (mmHg)	65.0 (59.0, 66.0)	65.0 (58.5, 67.5)	0.89
Systolic blood pressure up to 4 years (mmHg)	101.5 (97.0, 106.3)	101.6 (94.7, 106.3)	0.78
Diastolic blood pressure up to 4 years (mmHg)	60.3 (55.3, 63.5)	57.0 (50.3, 61.0)	0.01

[1] *p* Values were derived by 2-sample *t* tests or the Kruskal-Wallis test; [2] Mean ± SD (all such values); [3] Median; 25th and 75th percentiles in parentheses (all such values).

Maternal dietary composition during pregnancy is summarized in Table 3. Results of the mixed-model regression analyses examining relationships between pregnancy diet and child systolic BP up to age 4 years are summarized in Table 4. The components of maternal diet associated with child systolic

BP included: PUFA (% of energy), specifically n-6 fatty acids (% of energy), and the P:C ratio (Table 4). Median (25p, 75p) P:C ratio was 0.43 (0.38, 0.48). Therefore, for each 0.1 unit decrease in the P:C ratio during pregnancy, child systolic BP increased by 1.41 mmHg (Table 4). Similar findings were observed in the comparison of energy-adjusted values (Table 4). In subgroup analyses, maternal smoking status did not have a significant effect on childhood systolic BP (data not shown). There were no relationships between maternal pregnancy diet and child diastolic BP up to 4 years.

Table 3. Maternal dietary composition during pregnancy (n = 129) [1].

Absolute Values	Grams	% of Energy
Protein	81.4 (64.8, 105.6)	19.1 (17.4, 20.9)
Total fat	73.0 (57.7, 95.8)	37.6 (34.7, 40.0)
SFA	31.1 (23.2, 41.7)	15.9 (13.6, 18.4)
PUFA	11.2 (7.8, 13.7)	5.0 (4.0, 6.2)
n-3 Fatty acids	1.4 (1.0, 1.7)	0.7 (0.6, 0.8)
n-6 Fatty acids	9.2 (6.2, 11.9)	4.2 (3.3, 5.3)
MUFA	25.4 (19.5, 33.2)	13.0 (11.8, 13.9)
Total carbohydrate	185.3 (153.7, 244.0)	41.5 (39.3, 44.4)
Sugars	92.1 (72.2, 115.1)	19.5 (17.0, 22.1)
Starch	99.2 (79.3, 125.1)	21.2 (19.8, 23.5)
Fibre	19.2 (14.5, 24.9)	2.1 (1.7, 2.4)
Energy (kJ)	7298.4 (5890.1, 9234.2)	
P:C ratio	0.43 (0.39, 0.48)	
n-6:n-3 ratio	6.38 (5.22, 7.78)	
Energy-adjusted values	Grams	
Protein	121.9 (89.3, 128.6)	
Total fat	103.7 (97.4, 109.1)	
SFA	44.3 (39.6, 49.2)	
PUFA	13.5 (11.5, 16.2)	
n-3 Fatty acids	1.9 (1.7, 2.1)	
n-6 Fatty acids	11.1 (9.6, 13.9)	
MUFA	36.3 (34.4, 38.2)	
Total carbohydrate	250.0 (240.0, 264.3)	
Sugars	117.9 (106.1, 129.7)	
Starch	128.2 (116.4, 137.4)	
Fibre	26.7 (23.4, 30.0)	

P:C, protein-to-carbohydrate. n-6:n-3, omega-6-to-omega-3. [1] All values are medians; 25th and 75th percentiles in parentheses.

Table 4. Mixed-model regression analysis of the associations between diet during pregnancy and child systolic blood pressure up to age 4 years. Results presented for all dietary data (n = 129) [1].

	Systolic Blood Pressure (mmHg)								
	Crude model			**Adjusted model (a)**			**Adjusted model (b)**		
Maternal diet	β Coefficient	95% CI	P [2]	β Coefficient	95% CI	P [2]	β Coefficient	95% CI	P [2]
Protein (% E)	−0.36	−0.88, 0.16	0.17	−0.39	−0.90, 0.12	0.13	−0.48	−0.99, 0.03	0.07
Polyunsaturated fat (% E)	0.69	−0.02, 1.41	0.06	0.68	−0.04, 1.40	0.06	0.73	0.003, 1.45	0.05
Omega-6 fatty acids (% E)	**0.84**	**0.05, 1.64**	**0.04**	**0.86**	**0.06, 1.66**	**0.04**	**0.89**	**0.09, 1.69**	**0.03**
Fibre (g)	0.09	−0.06, 0.24	0.24	**0.26**	0.001, 0.53	0.05	0.27	0.002, 0.54	0.05
P:C ratio	−10.93	−24.53, 2.67	0.12	−12.23	−25.70, 1.24	0.07	**−14.14**	**−27.68, −0.60**	**0.04**
Energy adjusted values									
Protein (g)	−0.07	−0.16, 0.02	0.13	0.08	0.16, 0.01	0.09	0.09	0.17, 0.003	0.06
Polyunsaturated fat (g)	**0.43**	**0.06, 0.80**	**0.02**	**0.42**	**0.05, 0.80**	**0.03**	**0.44**	**0.06, 0.81**	**0.02**
Omega-6 fatty acids (g)	**0.50**	**0.10, 0.90**	**0.02**	**0.50**	**0.09, 0.90**	**0.02**	**0.51**	**0.10, 0.92**	**0.01**
Fibre (g)	0.20	−0.07, 0.46	0.14	0.27	0.01, 0.53	0.05	0.27	0.01, 0.54	0.05

P:C, protein to carbohydrate. % E, percentage of energy. [1] Analysis models: (a) adjusted for maternal energy intake and child birthweight; (b) adjusted for maternal energy intake, child birthweight and child BMI z-score. Energy-yielding dietary variables not presented in the table above did not return any significant results for any model.
[2] P-values were derived by linear mixed-model regression analyses.

The association between maternal P:C ratio during pregnancy and child mean systolic BP up to 4 years is presented in Figure 1. The surface plot highlighted that mean child systolic BP remained constant with changing proportions of dietary fat, but was influenced by the P:C ratio of maternal diet during pregnancy. A maternal diet with a P:C ratio of 0.29 corresponded with a child systolic BP of 104.5, compared with a systolic BP of 97.5 for a P:C ratio of 0.9. Child systolic BP was greatest at low proportions of dietary protein (<16% of energy) and high carbohydrate (>40% of energy) intakes.

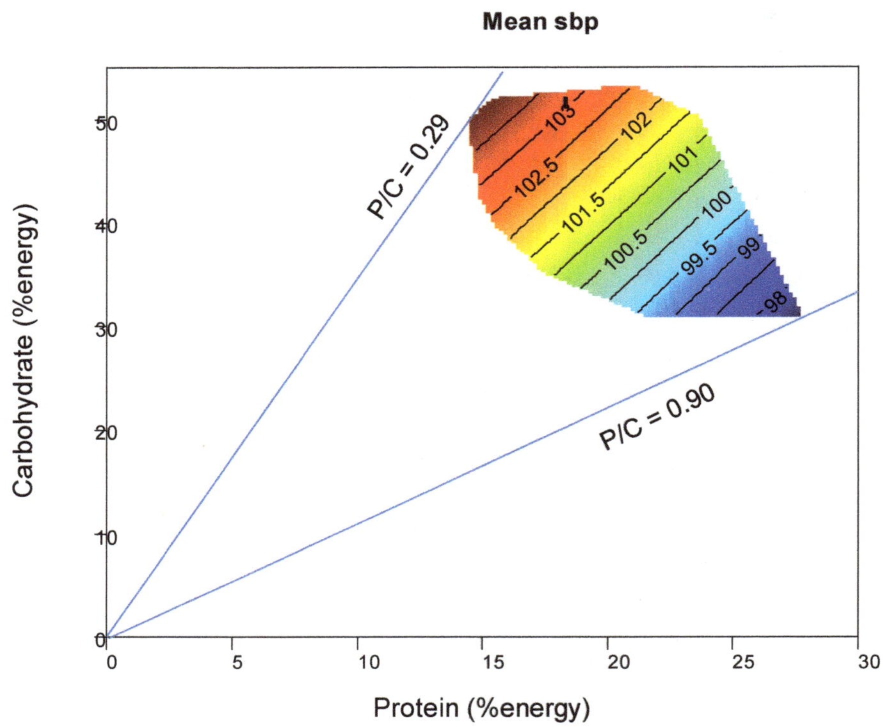

Figure 1. Effects of maternal macronutrient intake during pregnancy on child mean systolic blood pressure up to four years. Plotted onto arrays of maternal dietary macronutrient composition points are fitted surfaces for the response variable (child mean systolic blood pressure). The isolines for the child mean systolic blood pressure rise in elevation from dark blue to dark red. A maternal diet with a P:C ratio of 0.29 corresponded with a child systolic BP of 104.5, compared with a systolic BP of 97.5 for a P:C ratio of 0.9. Child systolic BP was greatest at low proportions of dietary protein (<16% of energy) and high carbohydrate (>40% of energy) intakes.

4. Discussion

This is the first prospective study to longitudinally examine the relationship between maternal diet during pregnancy and the trajectories of child BP up to four years. Results indicate that lower P:C ratios in maternal diet are associated with increased child systolic BP up to four years of age. Childhood systolic BP was also positively associated with maternal intake of PUFA and *n*-6 fatty acids, despite remaining constant with changing total fat intake.

Strong evidence supports the tracking of BP from childhood to adult life [4]. Women who gave birth during the Dutch famine in 1944–1945 illustrate that offspring BP as young adults was inversely associated with the P:C ratio of the average ration during the third trimester, but not associated with any absolute measure of intake [26]. This suggests that long-term health may be linked more strongly to the macronutrient ratio of maternal diet as opposed to absolute intakes. This study is the first to confirm similar findings in children. Mean childhood BP measures were within normal ranges (*i.e.*, below the 90th percentile) [27]. However, mean systolic BP and diastolic BP measures within this study were significantly higher than those reported by other contemporary birth cohorts [11,13]. The most likely explanation for these higher values is that BP was only measured on one occasion at each time point rather than an average of the two or three values used in other studies. The P:C ratio may further influence non-energy providing micronutrients that may affect childhood BP. Intervention studies have shown that a modest increase in dietary protein (5.3% of energy) with a corresponding reduction in carbohydrate subsequently decreased sodium intake (25mmol/day) in adults, in conjunction with a reduction in blood pressure [28]. Macronutrient ratios may influence offspring health and disease [16]. Future research is required to include the P:C ratio when evaluating the influence of maternal macronutrient composition during pregnancy on offspring health outcomes, and consider its impact on micronutrient intakes.

While potential molecular mechanisms related to our findings are poorly understood, animal models provide important mechanistic insights and suggest that nutritional deprivation or excess during pregnancy may stimulate epigenetic processes [5,13]. These events lead to both acute changes in offspring tissue structure and organ development, and permanent alterations in gene expression through DNA and histone methylation or histone acetylation [29,30], with subsequent cardio-metabolic consequences [5]. Rodent and sheep models support findings in the current study and provide strong evidence of a relationship between maternal protein intake during pregnancy and offspring cardiovascular function [6,8,31]. Offspring of nutritionally deprived animals commonly display elevated BP, while offspring exposed to protein or energy restriction during pregnancy show abnormal vascular function in isolated resistance arteries [32]. Additional consequences include increased sympathetic outflow [6], possibly due to altered interactions between the aberrant central signaling pathways in the renin-angiotensin system and sympathetic efferent activity [32]. While others have suggested mechanistic changes in renal sodium transport, including altered mRNA expression of α_1- and β_1- Na^+/K^+ ATPase and renal tubular bumetanide-sensitive and thiazidesensitive sodium co-transporters [5]. However, evidence for associations between maternal diet during pregnancy and offspring cardiovascular function in human cohorts, while valuable, is indirect. Causality cannot be inferred from this study because of its observational nature and the possibility of residual confounding cannot be excluded. Therefore, the effect of variations in maternal macronutrient composition requires further investigation using (i) animal model interventions; (ii) observational studies using statistical approaches such as propensity score analysis, to address residual confounding; or (iii) opportunistic examination within interventions targeting maternal nutrition to improve pregnancy dietary intake.

Compelling arguments have emerged from animal models of dietary balance (specifically the ratio of dietary P:C) regarding nutritional targets for optimal health and ageing [16]. The balance of macronutrients, rather than the absolute intake of a single nutrient, is a key determinant of lifespan [16]. In insect and mouse models, diets with decreased P:C were associated with increased lifespan and improved cardio-metabolic outcomes in later life [16]. These data are supported indirectly by a systematic review showing increased mortality in human studies associated with low carbohydrate diets [16], and a recent study showing increased mortality and cancer in humans on high protein diets [16]. Both high and low P:C diets have benefits and risks [33], which highlights an important role for macronutrient balance in optimizing the relationship between diet and disease risk. Recent evidence indicates that the interaction of a dominant protein appetite with weaker carbohydrate and fat appetites is a primary driver of total energy intake in mice and humans (termed "protein leverage") [15]. The findings suggest that pregnant women may be driven to achieve a "target" percentage protein intake, as the median percentage of energy from protein throughout pregnancy within our sample was stable at 19% [14]. This potentially dominant appetite for protein during pregnancy may significantly influence the development of offspring BP in early childhood and thus play an important role in the development of pediatric and adult hypertension. Coupled with a severe decrease in P:C ratio being related to a greater tendency to store excess body fat and increased risk of decreased longevity associated with obesity [15], maternal macronutrient ratio may further increase the risk of elevated blood pressure through its influence on offspring adiposity [14]. Research investigating protein leverage during pregnancy, including the role of macronutrient balance (maternal prenatal and offspring postnatal diet) in the development of offspring blood pressure up until adulthood, and secondary outcomes such as increased adiposity, are required before pregnancy dietary recommendation to optimize childhood blood pressure can be formulated.

The role of maternal pregnancy PUFA intakes with development and regulation of child BP remains unclear. It is known that dietary PUFA intakes play a role in BP regulation and have usually been associated with beneficial effects [34]. However, emerging evidence suggests that PUFA classes (*n*-3 and *n*-6) have differential health effects, with *n*-6 PUFAs and PUFA ratios generating scientific debate regarding their role in human physiological processes [34]. Both classes of fatty acids have been shown to reduce BP in adult rats and hypertensive subjects [35,36]. However, significant reductions in BP in normotensive subjects have not been shown, nor have beneficial effects of PUFA on CVD risk markers been reported universally [36]. Arguments for reduced *n*-6 intakes surround the notion that inflammation plays a key role in CVD mechanisms [36]. Recent evidence from the Sydney Diet Heart Study reported that in men aged 30 to 59 years, substituting dietary *n*-6 linoleic acid (LA) in place of SFA showed no cardiovascular benefit and actually increased the risk of death from all causes, coronary heart disease and CVD [37]. The proposed mechanistic model linking *n*-6 PUFAs to cardiovascular pathogenesis is based on a diet-induced increase in the production of bioactive oxidized LA metabolites [37]. Oxidized LA metabolites are the most abundant oxidized fatty acids in oxidized low-density lipoprotein molecules. Ramsden and colleagues hypothesize that oxidative stress combined with diets high in *n*-6 LA facilitate this oxidation, leading to oxidized LA metabolite mediated atherosclerotic progression and increased cardiovascular mortality [37]. Increased circulating oxidized low-density lipoprotein has been reported in hypertensive men [38] and women with pre-eclampsia [39]. Limited research has been conducted in pregnancy. There is a lack of population-based research examining the relationship between maternal pregnancy PUFA intake and offspring BP. Results in the current study support a positive relationship between trajectory of childhood systolic BP up to age four years and maternal PUFA and *n*-6 fatty acids intakes during pregnancy, despite BP remaining constant with changing maternal total fat intake and being altered with P:C ratio. The influence of maternal diet on child BP may also be secondary to its influence on maternal BP during pregnancy. A higher maternal BP during pregnancy could reflect the mother's own fetal experience, which consequently influences the intrauterine environment she provides for her children. Further research to elucidate the role of *n*-6 fatty acids in cardiovascular disease mechanisms, particularly maternal and child blood pressure, is warranted.

Limitations of the current study include the use of self-reported FFQ data to measure dietary intake. Dietary data is strengthened by the similarities between the daily mean energy intake reported in our study (8070 kJ/day) and that reported in a representative sample of pregnant women in the Australian Longitudinal Study on Women's Health (7795 kJ/day) in 2003 [40]. Macronutrient distributions were also similar to the population nation data in pregnancy [40]. Physical activity data for children were unable to be obtained for our sample. BP measurements should be interpreted with caution. Automated BP monitors overestimate systolic BP and underestimate diastolic BP [41], and thus are not recommended for use in children in clinical settings where the accuracy of the absolute measurement is required [41]. In epidemiological studies where differences in BP between groups are more important than absolute levels, automated BP monitors such as the Dinamap are appropriate to reduce observer bias and digit preference [41]. Lastly, the WATCH study contained a higher proportion of women with post-school qualifications, socio-economic advantage and in a married or de facto relationship, but had a similar proportion of overweight/obesity and indigenous ethnicity compared to the Australian population [14]. Therefore, care should be taken in extrapolating results at the population level.

5. Conclusions

This study provides some evidence for an optimal maternal macronutrient profile associated with a healthy child BP. The development of systolic BP up to four years was positively associated with higher maternal PUFA intakes and a lower P:C ratio. Future focus on the maternal protein-to-carbohydrate ratio during pregnancy will be an important research area and may offer strategy to optimize offspring cardiovascular health. Further research has the potential to elucidate the role of maternal diet in childhood BP and in refining dietary recommendations provided to pregnant women in order to optimize offspring health long-term.

Acknowledgments

The authors would like to thank all WATCH Study participants who have generously volunteered their time and personal information. We thank Kim Colyvas and Fran Baker of the University of Newcastle for their advice and guidance with the statistical analyses, and Trish Engel and Therese Finnegan (Midwives) for their involvement in the recruitment process.

Author Contributions

All authors helped design the study and directed its implementation, including quality assurance and control. M.B., S.J.S. and D.R. worked on the statistical analyses and M.B. was responsible for the preparation of the manuscript. All authors have made a significant contribution to the research and the development of the manuscript.

References

1. Muntner, P.; He, J.; Cutler, J.A.; Wildman, R.P.; Whelton, P.K. Trends in blood pressure among children and adolescents. *JAMA* **2004**, *291*, 2107–2113.
2. World Health Organisation. *Cardiovascular Diseases (CVDs)*; World Health Organisation: Geneva, Switzerland, 2013.
3. Sun, S.S.; Liang, R.; Huang, T.T.; Daniels, S.R.; Arslanian, S.; Liu, K.; Grave, G.D.; Siervogel, R.M. Childhood obesity predicts adult metabolic syndrome: The Fels longitudinal study. *J. Pediatr.* **2008**, *152*, 191–200.
4. Chen, X.; Wang, Y. Tracking of blood pressure from childhood to adulthood: A systematic review and meta-regression analysis. *Circulation* **2008**, *117*, 3171–3180.
5. Poston, L. Influence of maternal nutritional status on vascular function in the offspring. *Microcirculation* **2011**, *18*, 256–262.
6. Nuyt, A.M.; Alexander, B.T. Developmental programming and hypertension. *Curr. Opin. Nephrol. Hypertens.* **2009**, *18*, 144–152.
7. Ojeda, N.B.; Grigore, D.; Alexander, B.T. Developmental programming of hypertension: Insight from animal models of nutritional manipulation. *Hypertension* **2008**, *52*, 44–50.
8. Grigore, D.; Ojeda, N.B.; Alexander, B.T. Sex differences in the fetal programming of hypertension. *Gend. Med.* **2008**, *5*, S121–S132.
9. Langley-Evans, S.C.; Jackson, A.A. Increased systolic blood pressure in adult rats induced by fetal exposure to maternal low protein diets. *Clin. Sci. (Lond.)* **1994**, *86*, 217–222.
10. Symonds, M.E.; Stephenson, T.; Budge, H. Early determinants of cardiovascular disease: The role of early diet in later blood pressure control. *Am. J. Clin. Nutr.* **2009**, *89*, 1518S–1522S.
11. Normia, J.; Laitinen, K.; Isolauri, E.; Poussa, T.; Jaakkola, J.; Ojala, T. Impact of intrauterine and post-natal nutritional determinants on blood pressure at 4 years of age. *J. Hum. Nutr. Diet.* **2013**, *26*, 544–552.
12. Aaltonen, J.; Ojala, T.; Laitinen, K.; Piirainen, T.J.; Poussa, T.A.; Isolauri, E. Evidence of infant blood pressure programming by maternal nutrition during pregnancy: A prospective randomized controlled intervention study. *J. Pediatr.* **2008**, *152*, 79–84.
13. Brion, M.J.; Leary, S.D.; Lawlor, D.A.; Smith, G.D.; Ness, A.R. Modifiable maternal exposures and offspring blood pressure: A review of epidemiological studies of maternal age, diet, and smoking. *Pediatr. Res.* **2008**, *63*, 593–598.
14. Blumfield, M.L.; Hure, A.J.; MacDonald-Wicks, L.; Smith, R.; Simpson, S.J.; Giles, W.B.; Raubenheimer, D.; Collins, C.E. Dietary balance during pregnancy is associated with fetal adiposity and fat distribution. *Am. J. Clin. Nutr.* **2012**, *96*, 1032–1041.
15. Simpson, S.J.; Raubenheimer, D. Obesity: The protein leverage hypothesis. *Obes. Rev.* **2005**, *6*, 133–142.
16. Simpson, S.J.; Le Couteur, D.G.; Raubenheimer, D. Putting the balance back in diet. *Cell* **2015**, in press.
17. Hure, A.J.; Collins, C.E.; Giles, W.B.; Wright, I.M.R.; Smith, R. Protocol for the Women and their Children's Health (WATCH) Study: A cohort of pregnancy and beyond. *J. Epidemiol.* **2012**, *22*, 267–275.

18. Hure, A.J.; Smith, R.; Collins, C.E. A recruiting failure turned success. *BMC Health Serv. Res.* **2008**, *8*, 64, doi:10.1186/1472-6963-8-64.
19. Blumfield, M.L.; Hure, A.J.; MacDonald-Wicks, L.K.; Smith, R.; Simpson, S.J.; Raubenheimer, D.; Collins, C.E. The association between the macronutrient content of maternal diet and the adequacy of micronutrients during pregnancy. *Nutrients* **2012**, *4*, 1958–1976.
20. Hure, A.J.; Collins, C.E.; Giles, W.B.; Paul, J.W.; Smith, R. Greater maternal weight gain during pregnancy predicts a large but lean phenotype: A prospective cohort study. *Matern. Child Health J.* **2012**, *16*, 1374–1384.
21. Hodge, A.; Patterson, A.J.; Brown, W.J.; Ireland, P.; Giles, G. The Anti Cancer Council of Victoria FFQ: Relative validity of nutrient intakes compared with weighed food records in young to middle-aged women in a study of iron supplementation. *Aust. N. Z. J. Public Health* **2000**, *24*, 576–583.
22. Willett, W.C.; Howe, G.R.; Kushi, L.H. Adjustment for total energy intake in epidemiologic studies. *Am. J. Clin. Nutr.* **1997**, *65*, 1220S–1228S.
23. WHO; Multicentre Growth Reference Study Group. *WHO Child Growth Standards: Length/Height-for-Age, Weight-for-Age, Weight-for-Length, Weight-for-Height and Body Mass Index-for-Age: Methods and Development*; World Health Organisation: Geneva, Switzerland, 2006.
24. Meltzer, H.M.; Brantsaeter, A.L.; Ydersbond, T.A.; Alexander, J.; Haugen, M. Methodological challenges when monitoring the diet of pregnant women in a large study: Experiences from the Norwegian Mother and Child Cohort Study (MoBa). *Matern. Child Nutr.* **2008**, *4*, 14–27.
25. Pink, B. *An introduction to Socioeconomic Indexes for Areas*; Australian Bureau of Statistics; Commonwealth of Australia: Canberra, Australia, 2006.
26. Roseboom, T.J.; van der Meulen, J.H.; van Montfrans, G.A.; Ravelli, A.C.; Osmond, C.; Barker, D.J.; Bleker, O.P. Maternal nutrition during gestation and blood pressure in later life. *J. Hypertens.* **2001**, *19*, 29–34.
27. U.S. Department of Health and Human Services. The forth report on the diagnosis, evaluation, and treatment of high blood pressure in children and adolescents. *Pediatrics* **2004**, *114*, S555–S576.
28. Hodgson, J.M.; Burke, V.; Beilin, L.J.; Puddey, I.B. Partial substitution of carbohydrate intake with protein intake from lean red meat lowers blood pressure in hypertensive persons. *Am. J. Clin. Nutr.* **2006**, *83*, 780–788.
29. Gluckman, P.D.; Hanson, M.A.; Cooper, C.; Thornburg, K.L. Effect of in utero and early-life conditions on adult health and disease. *N. Engl. J. Med.* **2008**, *359*, 61–73.
30. Hanley, B.; Dijane, J.; Fewtrell, M.; Grynberg, A.; Hummel, S.; Junien, C.; Koletzko, B.; Lewis, S.; Renz, H.; Symonds, M.; *et al.* Metabolic imprinting, programming and epigenetics—A review of present priorities and future opportunities. *Br. J. Nutr.* **2010**, *104*, S1–S25.
31. Baum, M. Role of the kidney in the prenatal and early postnatal programming of hypertension. *Am. J. Physiol. Renal Physiol.* **2010**, *298*, F235–F247.
32. Van Abeelen, A.F.; Veenendaal, M.V.; Painter, R.C.; de Rooij, S.R.; Thangaratinam, S.; van der Post, J.A.; Bossuyt, P.M.; Elias, S.G.; Uiterwaal, C.S.; Grobbee, D.E.; *et al.* The fetal origins of hypertension: A systematic review and meta-analysis of the evidence from animal experiments of maternal undernutrition. *J. Hypertens.* **2012**, *30*, 2255–2267.

33. Blumfield, M.L.; Collins, C.E. High-protein diets during pregnancy: Healthful or harmful for offspring. *Am. J. Clin. Nutr.* **2014**, *100*, 993–995.
34. Khandelwal, S.; Kelly, L.; Malik, R.; Prabhakaran, D.; Reddy, S. Impact of omega-6 fatty acids on cardiovascular outcomes: A review. *J. Prev. Cardiol.* **2013**, *2*, 325–336.
35. Miura, K.; Stamler, J.; Nakagawa, H.; Elliott, P.; Ueshima, H.; Chan, Q.; Brown, I.J.; Tzoulaki, I.; Saitoh, S.; Dyer, A.R.; *et al.* Relationship of dietary linoleic acid to blood pressure. *Hypertension* **2008**, *52*, 408–414.
36. Harris, W.S.; Mozaffarian, D.; Rimm, E.; Kris-Etherton, P.; Rudel, L.R.; Appel, L.J.; Engler, M.M.; Engler, M.B.; Sacks, F. Omega-6 fatty acids and risk for cardiovascular disease: A science advisory from the American heart association nutrition subcommittee of the council on nutrition, physical activity, and metabolism; council on cardiovascular nursing; and council on epidemiology and prevention. *Circulation* **2009**, *119*, 902–907.
37. Ramsden, C.E.; Zamora, D.; Leelarthaepin, B.; Majchrzak-Hong, S.F.; Faurot, K.R.; Suchindran, C.M.; Ringel, A.; Davis, J.M.; Hibbeln, J.R. Use of dietary linoleic acid for secondary prevention of coronary heart disease and death: Evaluation of recovered data from the Sydney Diet Heart Study and updated meta-analysis. *BMJ* **2013**, *346*, e8707, doi:10.1136/bmj.e8707.
38. Frostegard, J.; Wu, R.; Lemne, C.; Thulin, T.; Witztum, J.L.; de Faire, U. Circulating oxidized low-density lipoprotein is increased in hypertension. *Clin. Sci. (Lond)* **2003**, *105*, 615–620.
39. Qiu, C.; Phung, T.; Vadachkoria, S.; Muy-Rivera, M.; Sanchez, S.E.; Williams, M.A. Oxidized low-density lipoprotein (Oxidized LDL) and the risk of preeclampsia. *Physiol. Res.* **2006**, *55*, 491.
40. Hure, A.; Young, A.; Smith, R.; Collins, C. Diet and pregnancy status in Australian women. *Public Health Nutr.* **2009**, *12*, 853–861.
41. Barker, M.E.; Shiell, A.W.; Law, C.M. Evaluation of the Dinamap 8100 and Omron M1 blood pressure monitors for use in children. *Paediatr. Perinat. Epidemiol.* **2000**, *14*, 179–186.

7

Placental Adaptations in Growth Restriction

Song Zhang [1], Timothy R.H. Regnault [2,3], Paige L. Barker [1], Kimberley J. Botting [1], Isabella C. McMillen [1], Christine M. McMillan [1], Claire T. Roberts [4] and Janna L. Morrison [1,*]

1. Early Origins of Adult Health Research Group, Sansom Institute for Health Research, University of South Australia, Adelaide, SA 5001, Australia; E-Mails: song.zhang@unisa.edu.au (S.Z.); barpl002@mymail.unisa.edu.au (P.L.B.); kb555@cam.ac.uk (K.J.B.); caroline.mcMillen@newcastle.edu.au (I.C.M); mcmcm003@mymail.unisa.edu.au (C.M.M.)
2. Departments of Obstetrics and Gynecology, University of Western Ontario, London, ON N6A 5C1, Canada; E-Mail: tim.regnault@uwo.ca
3. Departments of Physiology and Biochemistry, University of Western Ontario, London, ON N6A 5C1, Canada
4. The Robinson Research Institute, University of Adelaide, Adelaide, SA 5005, Australia; E-Mail: claire.roberts@adelaide.edu.au

* Author to whom correspondence should be addressed; E-Mail: janna.morrison@unisa.edu.au

---

Abstract: The placenta is the primary interface between the fetus and mother and plays an important role in maintaining fetal development and growth by facilitating the transfer of substrates and participating in modulating the maternal immune response to prevent immunological rejection of the conceptus. The major substrates required for fetal growth include oxygen, glucose, amino acids and fatty acids, and their transport processes depend on morphological characteristics of the placenta, such as placental size, morphology, blood flow and vascularity. Other factors including insulin-like growth factors, apoptosis, autophagy and glucocorticoid exposure also affect placental growth and substrate transport capacity. Intrauterine growth restriction (IUGR) is often a consequence of insufficiency, and is associated with a high incidence of perinatal morbidity and mortality, as well as increased risk of cardiovascular and metabolic diseases in later life. Several different experimental methods have been used to induce placental insufficiency and IUGR in animal models and a range of factors that regulate placental growth and substrate transport capacity have been demonstrated. While no model system completely recapitulates human IUGR, these animal models allow us to carefully dissect cellular and molecular mechanisms to improve our understanding and facilitate development of therapeutic interventions.

Keywords: placental morphology; vascularity; substrate transport; IUGR

1. Introduction

In eutherian mammals, the placenta is the primary interface between the fetus and mother. One of the main functions of the placenta is to deliver nutrients and oxygen to the fetus. Failure of the placenta to deliver an adequate supply of nutrients to the fetus is termed placental insufficiency and results in intrauterine growth restriction (IUGR), affecting up to 5%–10% of pregnancies in developed countries [1–3]. IUGR is also associated with a high incidence of perinatal morbidity and mortality and an increased risk of cardiovascular disease and type II diabetes in later life [4–7]. In this review, we will focus on placental structure and function, factors affecting placental nutrient transport capacity, animal models of IUGR and regulation of placental growth and substrate transport in the IUGR pregnancy.

2. Placental Structure and Function

In mammals, the placenta is the primary interface between the fetus and mother and plays an important role in maintaining fetal growth by performing several physiological functions, which, following birth, are controlled by the kidney, gastrointestinal tract, lungs and endocrine glands. The main functions of the placenta include modulation of the mother's immune response to prevent immunological rejection termed tolerance, facilitating the exchange of respiratory gases, water, ions, nutrients and wastes between the maternal and fetal circulations, and producing and secreting hormones, cytokines and other signalling molecules required to maintain pregnancy and to ensure placental and fetal development and growth [8].

Maternal blood supply to the placenta is established at the end of the first trimester of human pregnancy, with maternal blood entering the intervillous space of the placenta from the transformed spiral arterioles for substrate transport to the fetus [9–11]. The barrier between the maternal and the fetal circulations in the human hemochorial placenta consists of three fetal cellular layers: (i) the syncytiotrophoblast, a multinucleated epithelial layer formed following the fusion of the mononucleated villous cytotrophoblasts; (ii) villous stromal tissue and (iii) the fetal capillary endothelium (Table 1) [12]. The syncytiotrophoblast has two polarized plasma membranes: the maternal-facing microvillous plasma membrane (MVM) and the basal membrane (BM). The syncytiotrophoblast is the main regulator of substrate exchange and nutrient transporters are expressed on both plasma membranes [13].

Table 1. An across species comparison of placental shape and structure [14–16].

Species	Placental Shape	Placental Structure
Humans	Discoid	Hemochorial
Ruminants (Sheep, cattle, goats)	Cotyledonary	Epitheliochorial
Rodents (rats, mice)	Discoid	Hemochorial
Pigs	Diffuse	Epitheliochorial
Horses	Diffuse	Epitheliochorial
Carnivores (cats, dogs)	Zonary	Epitheliochorial
Primates	Discoid	Hemochorial

It is important to understand the role of placental function in the IUGR fetus from a clinical and scientific point of view. However, *in vivo* studies of the human placenta are difficult as the methodology presents risks to both the mother and fetus. Therefore, the majority of the body of knowledge about the placenta and its function is a result of ultrasound studies across gestation or those performed in placentas collected at delivery or in animal models. In terms of morphological similarities, the placenta of higher primates is the most comparable to that of the human, with a discoid hemomonochorial structure, where fetal trophoblast cells are in direct contact with the maternal blood supply [15]. However, primates that are suitable for experimental studies are small, have small fetuses, and often abort or deliver prematurely following intrauterine surgery, limiting their use in placental studies [17]. Therefore placental nutrient transport and exchange has been extensively studied in the rabbit, guinea pig, rat, mice and human [18–20]. However, one of the most widely used animal models for studies of fetal development and placental function is the sheep [21–23].

One of the advantages of working with sheep compared to other animal models of pregnancy is that the functional responses of the sheep fetus to short or long periods of placental insufficiency can be studied *in utero* [24–28]. Like the human, organogenesis in the sheep occurs during early gestation with the functional maturation of the renal and cardiovascular systems by late gestation [23]. In addition, pregnant ewes are comparable to humans in size with equally large fetuses that tolerate intrauterine surgery well and most organ systems develop before birth [29]. Therefore, vascular catheters can be surgically implanted in the fetus, exteriorized through the ewes' flank and maintained for several weeks, allowing for repetitive blood sampling from unanaesthetised pregnant ewes and their fetuses to measure blood gases, hormones and cardiovascular parameters in response to placental insufficiency during late gestation [23,30].

In sheep, implantation begins at ~14–16 days gestation (term = 150 ± 3 days gestation) and is complete by ~22 days gestation, marking the initiation of placentation [31], which is the process of placental growth and development, resulting in the maturation of functional units called placentomes. Sheep have a non-invasive, cotyledonary type of placentation in which specialized areas of the endometrium termed caruncles are attachment sites for trophoblasts of the chorion forming 50–90 placentomes during a normal singleton pregnancy (Table 1) [14,16]. Placentomes are divided into the maternal (caruncle) and fetal (cotyledon) portions and consist of interdigitated maternal crypts and fetal villi that develop through synchronised growth between the trophoblast and caruncular endometrium [16,32]. Morphologically, the maternal portion of the placentome is composed of maternal connective tissue, maternal capillaries and maternal epithelial cells; while the fetal portion of the placentome is composed of fetal trophoblasts, connective tissue and fetal capillaries. The placentomes grow rapidly following implantation and reach maximum weight at ~75–80 days gestation, from which point weight declines until term [33]. However, placentomes undergo progressive structural remodelling, with attenuation of all cell layers in both fetal and maternal tissues, bringing fetal and maternal capillaries in close proximity to allow increased capacity for substrate transfer during the second half of gestation when fetal demand for nutrients is high [16].

Placentomes are classified into four types (A–D) based on their gross morphology [34]. The fetal side of the placentome is defined as a thin hemophagous zone where maternal blood extravasates between the maternal crypts and fetal villi. Type A placentomes are rounder in shape and the hemophagous zone is inverted inside of the bulk of the placentome in which only a small area of the zone is visible externally. Type D placentomes are flatter in shape and the hemophagous zone is everted and covers the entire fetal surface of the placentome. Type B and C placentomes are intermediate in the degree of hemophagous zone eversion that is present. Throughout gestation, type A and B placentomes dominate, accounting for ~60% of the total number in a normal pregnancy. Type C and D placentomes are less common, occurring with greater frequency in multiple pregnancies and during late gestation. They are larger, heavier and more everted compared to type A placentomes. Although, the placentome types have different structures, it is not known if they have differential functions [32]. Previous studies have suggested that placentome eversion is an adaptation that occurs to increase the efficiency of placental nutrient transfer to the fetus [35]. In sheep, gross placentome morphology changes progressively throughout gestation with an increase in the number of everted placentomes, type C and D, in late gestation at 125–135 days [35,36]. Interestingly, it has been reported that early exposure to high plasma cortisol concentrations decreases the proportion of type C and D placentomes, which indicates that developmental shifts in placentome classification are not restricted to eversion [16].

3. Factors Affecting Placental Substrate Transport Capacity

Birth weight depends not only on maternal nutrition but also on the placenta's ability to transport substrates from the maternal to the fetal circulation [10]. Placental efficiency or fetal-placental weight ratio, defined as grams of fetus per gram of placenta, can vary between species and pregnancies [37]. At any gestational age, placental efficiency measurements provide an indication of the conditions experienced *in utero* and the extent to which placental adaptations during intrauterine development have occurred in order to meet fetal growth demands. These morphological and/or functional adaptations determine placental substrate transport capacity and efficiency to the fetus. The major substrates required for fetal growth include oxygen, glucose, amino acids and fatty acids [9,12,13].

While the placenta regulates the transport of nutrients to the fetus according to the mother's ability to deliver them, fetal demands as well as hormones and growth factors secreted by the placenta, the weight, size and shape of the placenta also affect its ability to transfer nutrients [38–40]. The transfer of highly permeable molecules, such as gases, oxygen and carbon dioxide, is influenced by blood flow and occurs via simple diffusion, whereas less permeable substrates are transferred through passive and active transport processes. Glucose is transported across the placenta via facilitated diffusion and is orchestrated by hormones secreted by the placenta [11]. Therefore, net glucose transfer is highly dependent on the maternal-fetal concentration gradient. Nutrients such as amino acids are transported via active transport using the charge provided by sodium ions and those that are transported via exchange for another amino acid [13]. Furthermore, these processes also depend on morphological characteristics of the placenta, such as placental size, surface area for exchange, vascularity as well as blood flow [15].

3.1. Fetal Oxygenation

Simple molecules such as oxygen and carbon dioxide are transported by diffusion and bulk flow. Oxygen (O_2) plays a critical role in the development and function of the placenta and fetal hypoxaemia is a common condition of complicated pregnancy. Oxygen diffuses from the maternal to the fetal circulation across a placental epithelial layer that consumes O_2. This O_2 consumption generates a transepithelial oxygen partial pressure (PO_2) difference whose magnitude depends upon the rate of umbilical and uterine blood flow, fetal and maternal blood oxygen carrying capacity, haemoglobin oxygen binding affinity, placental surface area and placental permeability [41]. Placental gas exchange occurs across cellular layers between the uterine and fetal circulations, once vascular beds have matured to allow adequate supply across the two circulations [14]. As a result, placental oxygen levels are low in the first trimester, increasing significantly by the second trimester. Therefore the fetus develops in a hypoxic environment during early pregnancy until the utero-placental vasculature can provide efficient gas exchange. Currently, much of the understanding of fetal and placental respiration is from the study of sheep in late gestation [42]. As the placenta is a highly metabolically active organ, it consumes a large quantity of the oxygen taken up from maternal circulation; some 80% in mid-gestation [42] and 40%–60% in late gestation [43]. Moreover, despite decreases in maternal oxygenation and uterine blood flow, the PO_2 gradient across the placenta remains constant in order to sustain fetal oxygen delivery at a normal rate [44].

3.2. Placental Size and Morphology

Placental size has a direct effect on the capacity for nutrient transfer via changes in surface area for transport. Placental weight is positively correlated with birth weight at term in many animal models [15]. In humans, placental weight progressively increases throughout pregnancy, while in rodents and sheep, placental weight increases before plateauing in mid to late gestation and then declines until term [45]. The small placenta increases nutrient transport capacity via morphological adaptations such as increased relative surface area for nutrient exchange, vascularity and decreased barrier thickness. These adaptations affect placental transport capacity and alter fetal to placental weight ratio.

3.3. Blood Flow and Vascularity

Blood flow is a major determinant of placental function and fetal growth. Vascularity of the sheep placenta increases in mid gestation, due to increases in the number and surface density of the placental capillaries, particularly those in the fetal side of the placentomes [46]. Vasculogenesis, formation of new blood vessels, and angiogenesis, formation of new branches from pre-existing vessels [47], are critical to form a vascular system needed for effective transport of nutrients, oxygen, and waste products. Several factors have been identified as important regulators of these processes, including the vascular endothelial growth factor (VEGF) family, basic fibroblast growth factor (bFGF), epidermal growth factor (EGF), platelet-derived growth factor (PDGF) and angiopoietin-1 and -2 [48]. The VEGF proteins and receptors

VEGFR1 (FLT-1) and VEGFR2 (FLK-1) are the most studied family of growth factors known to regulate the processes of vasculogenesis and angiogenesis. In pregnancy, VEGF is expressed by human villous and extravillous trophoblasts and also participates in the proliferation, migration, and metabolic activity of trophoblasts [49]; bFGF acts as a modulator of tissue differentiation and placental angiogenesis [48]. Angiopoietin-1 and its antagonist angiopoietin-2 act on the angiopoietin receptor (TIE-2) to regulate vascular integrity and remodeling [50]. Angiopoietin-1 and -2 have both been detected in decidual and placental tissues [51]. Vascular growth is necessary to increase placental-fetal blood flow across gestation [52–54]. Therefore fetal growth is linked to the capacity of the placenta to supply oxygen and nutrients for transfer to the fetus [55].

3.4. Insulin-Like Growth Factors

Insulin-like growth factors (IGFs), IGF-1 and IGF-2, are single chained polypeptides that promote fetal and neonatal growth, acting in response to fetal, maternal and placental signals such as nutrients, oxygen and hormones via the IGF receptors, IGF-1R and IGF-2R, and the insulin receptor (InsR). IGF-2 is the most abundant of the fetal IGFs, however, deletion of either *Igf* gene results in reduced birth weight [55]. IGF-1 regulates fetal growth in response to nutrient availability while IGF-2 stimulates placental growth and differentiation [56]. Furthermore IGFs regulate substrate transport and hormone secretion and influence fetal growth indirectly by influencing maternal substrate availability or directly by influencing placental nutrient uptake and transport [56]. In human trophoblasts, IGF-1 and IGF-2 stimulate glucose and amino acid uptake [57]. Elevated maternal plasma IGF-1 has been shown to increase fetal glucose and amino acid uptake in the guinea pig in early pregnancy [27,28]. In sheep, elevated plasma IGF-1 concentrations in early pregnancy are associated with increased maternal plasma glucose concentrations and enhanced fetal growth [56]. Furthermore in late pregnancy, acute treatment with IGF-1 alters placental metabolic function and increases glucose delivery to the sheep fetus [58]. IGF-1 stimulates system A amino acid uptake in cultured trophoblast cells and can act by both the IGF-1R and InsR [57]. Interestingly, in a knockout mouse model, deletion of the gene transcript for placenta specific expression of *Igf2* results in the reduction of placental growth while fetal growth is maintained in association with an up-regulation of glucose transporter (GLUT3) and amino acid transporter (SNAT2) during mid gestation, however IUGR still develops near term [59–61].

3.5. Placental Apoptosis, Autophagy and Glucocorticoid Actions

The role of the apoptosis cascade has been characterized in human villous trophoblast turnover and syncytium formation [62]. Apoptosis occurs in placentas of normal human pregnancies, and is regulated by the effector caspase pathway and the apoptosis inhibitor B-cell lymphoma 2 (BCL-2) in the trophoblast [62].

Autophagy is a highly regulated and dynamic process involving invagination and degradation of cytoplasmic components that maintain cellular homeostasis and promote cell survival in response to environmental stresses such as starvation and hypoxia [63]. Autophagy-related proteins such as beclin-1, light chain 3 isoform B (LC3B), and damage-regulated autophagy modulator (DRAM) are present in the trophoblast of human placenta during early, mid and late gestation [64,65]. Beclin-1 is part of an early complex that promotes synthesis and growth of pre-autophagosomal membranes [66]. LC3B is synthesized as proLC3B and converted to LC3B-I by autophagy-related proteases, which is further processed into LC3B-II and integrated into membranes of autophagosomes upon induction of autophagy [66]. DRAM is a lysosomal protein that regulates autophagy in a p53-dependent manner [67].

In utero, the placenta and embryo/fetus are each exposed to physiological glucocorticoids arising from either the maternal or fetal adrenal glands. Glucocorticoid actions are moderated by the glucocorticoid receptor and two isoforms of intracellular 11β-hydroxysteroid dehydrogenases (11βHSDs) [68]. 11βHSD1, which is a reduced nicotinamide adenine dinucleotide phosphate-dependent isoform, acts to convert biologically inert cortisone to the active cortisol, whereas 11βHSD2, which is a unidirectional nicotinamide adenine dinucleotide-dependent enzyme, catalyzes the conversion of the biologically active cortisol to the inert cortisone. In placenta, 11βHSD1 protein is expressed specifically in the placental villous endothelial cells, amnion, chorionic and extravillous trophoblasts, while 11βHSD2 protein is localized exclusively in the syncytiotrophoblast and invasive extravillous trophoblasts with no expression in the chorion or amnion [69]. 11βHSD1 expression increases throughout pregnancy in response to progesterone in human placenta [70]. In human pregnancy, placental 11βHSD2 activity increases markedly in the third trimester of pregnancy at a time when maternal circulating levels of glucocorticoid are rising [71]. In contrast, the placental inactivation of cortisol via placental 11βHSD2 activity decreases in the latter stages of gestation in sheep and is not present in term ovine placenta [72]. The fetus is normally protected from the high levels of maternal cortisol by placental 11βHSD2 [69].

3.6. Placental Transporter Abundance

The placenta's ability to transport substrates for fetal growth is also influenced by the abundance, activity and localization of transporters in the placental membranes [73]. Furthermore, transport of nutrients such as glucose and amino acids is also determined by the placental barrier and specifically the expression and activity of particular nutrient transport systems in the placental syncytiotrophoblast plasma membranes, MVM and BM [9]. Glucose and amino acid uptake into fetal circulation is dependent on three steps: (1) uptake from maternal circulation by transporters on the microvillous membrane of the syncytiotrophoblast; (2) transport across cytoplasm of the syncytiotrophoblast; and (3) transport across the fetal-facing basal membrane of the syncytiotrophoblast into fetal circulation [14]. Enhanced expression of nutrient transporters per unit of surface area is another key compensatory mechanism used to increase efficiency of the small placenta. Activity of placental glucose and amino acid transport systems is influenced by a wide range of environmental factors including heat stress, hypoxia, under- and overnutrition as well as exposure to placental hormones [55]. Placental glucose, amino acid and fatty acid transport systems are discussed in detail below.

3.6.1. Placental Glucose Transport Systems

Glucose is the primary nutrient required for the fetus and placenta [13,74]. However, the fetus and placenta have a limited ability for producing glucose, therefore glucose availability is dependent on supply from the maternal circulation [13,75–77]. Placental glucose uptake and transport to the fetus occurs down the concentration gradient from maternal to fetal circulation where it crosses the placental barrier via facilitated transport [14,78]. This is mediated by a family of sodium-independent transporter proteins, encoded by 14 different genes of the SCL2A family, called glucose transporters (GLUTs) [78]. GLUTs are present on both plasma membranes of the syncytiotrophoblast [13]. As glucose is transported down the concentration gradient, higher maternal glucose concentrations compared to fetal glucose concentrations drive net glucose transport toward the fetus. A high density of GLUTs in the MVM, together with a large surface area, allows for rapid glucose uptake into the syncytiotrophoblast. This provides adequate glucose supply for placental consumption while also maintaining a gradient between the syncytiotrophoblast and fetal circulation, ensuring fetal supply [13]. GLUT expression on the BM is much lower than the MVM and is associated with a smaller placental surface area, which suggests transport across the BM is the rate-limiting step of placental glucose metabolism [9,13]. The sheep and human placenta have two primary glucose transporters including GLUT1 (SLC2A1) and GLUT3 (SLC2A3) and less abundant glucose transporters including GLUT4 (SLC2A4) and GLUT8 (SLC2A8).

GLUT1 is insulin independent and ubiquitously expressed in a variety of human tissues including muscle, adipose, brain and endothelial cells [74]. GLUT1 is the main glucose transporter in the placenta and is highly expressed on both the microvillous and basal membranes of the syncytiotrophoblast [13,79]. In humans, GLUT1 expression is higher in the MVM compared to the BM, allowing for increased glucose uptake from maternal circulation [9,80]. In sheep, GLUT1 is localised to the base of the syncytial layer of the placenta, which is derived from the maternal epithelial cells and chorionic binucleated cells, and the baso-lateral surface of the trophoblast layer [81]. However, GLUT1 has not been found on the interdigitated microvilli of the trophoblast and syncytial layer [14]. In sheep, placental GLUT1 mRNA expression increases throughout gestation, peaking at 120 days in singleton pregnancies and 140 days in twins [79].

GLUT3 is insulin independent and its expression is cell-specific, depending on the stage of pregnancy [78]. In both humans and sheep, GLUT3 is expressed throughout gestation but decreases toward term, and therefore plays a greater role in the transport of glucose during early fetal development [74,78]. Furthermore, GLUT3 expression in the placenta has been detected in the cytotrophoblast but not the syncytiotrophoblast in the first trimester of human pregnancy [78]. However, in the third trimester placental GLUT3 expression is localised to the vascular endothelial cells of the fetal blood vessels and stromal cells [14,78,80]. In sheep, GLUT3 has been found on the microvillous junction between the syncytium and trophoblast layer [81]. Interestingly, GLUT3 is only expressed in one other tissue aside from the placenta, the brain [74,80]. The brain, like the fetus, depends on a constant supply of glucose in order to sustain energy production. Therefore, expression of GLUT3 in the placenta may maintain glucose supply to the fetus, even when maternal plasma glucose concentrations are low [14]. Furthermore, GLUT3 has a higher affinity for glucose than GLUT1 and is therefore more efficient in transporting glucose at low concentrations [81]. The high affinity of GLUT3 for glucose means that in conditions where maternal glucose concentrations are lower than normal, GLUT3 may be the key transporter in tissues where glucose is the primary metabolic substrate [74].

GLUT4 is insulin dependent and its immunostaining was detected in fibroblasts from amnion and chorion [82]. A strong GLUT4 signal was also observed in intravillous stromal cells, appearing to co-localize with InsR [83]. GLUT8 was localized to the chorionic epithelial layer and uterine epithelial cell from mid to late gestation and its expression in placenta increased during late gestation [84,85].

3.6.2. Placental Amino Acid Transport Systems

The human placenta expresses more than 20 different amino acid transporters [13]. Fetal amino acid concentrations are generally higher than maternal amino acid concentrations, reflecting an active transport mechanism across the placenta [13,86]. However, the placenta not only transports amino acids from mother to fetus but also produces and utilizes amino acids to meet its own metabolic need, and therefore plays a key role in determining the flux of amino acids into the fetal circulation [9]. Many types of placental amino acid transporters have been identified and are characterized into distinct systems [13,86]. There are several major classes of amino acid transporters present in the placenta, including neutral amino acid transporters, cationic amino acid transporters and anionic amino acid transporters [87,88].

System A amino acid transporters are an example of neutral amino acid transporters that facilitate the uptake of small non-essential neutral amino acids such as alanine, glycine and serine. Uptake occurs against their concentration gradient simultaneously with the transport of extracellular sodium into the cell. While system A transporters are present on both placental membranes, expression is greater on the MVM. System A activity contributes to the high intracellular concentration of amino acids such as glycine, which is exchanged for extracellular essential amino acids by system L transporters [9]. Therefore, system A transporters are important for the placental transport of both non-essential and essential amino acids [13]. System A consists of three sodium-coupled neutral amino acid transporter (SNAT) proteins, each encoded by independently regulated genes: SNAT1 (SLC38A1), SNAT2 (SLC38A2) and SNAT4 (SLC38A4) [59,89]. SNAT2 is ubiquitously expressed in mammalian tissues, while SNAT1 is predominately expressed in the brain, heart and placenta and SNAT4 expressed in the liver and placenta [89]. Throughout gestation, the activity of system A transporter increases, although the individual contributions of the three SNATs to total system A activity varies [13]. SNAT1 and 4 are found on both the MVM and the BM of the placenta [90]. SNAT1 has been shown to play a significant role in the human term placenta [91]. SNAT4, which has a lower substrate affinity for neutral amino acids, has a higher contribution in the first trimester placenta than the term placenta [89].

System L transporters are sodium independent exchangers of neutral amino acids. Non-essential amino acids are exchanged for essential amino acids with aromatic or branched side chains such as leucine or phenylalanine to allow for transport against their concentration gradient [92]. System L transporters consist of a heterodimer formed from a light chain protein, large neutral amino acid transporter (LAT)1 (SLC7A5) or LAT2 (SLC7A8), and a heavy chain transmembrane protein: 4F2hc/CD98 (SLC3A2) [92,93]. 4F2hc and LAT1 expression is higher in term than mid gestation placentas [93]. Localization of the LAT isoforms are polarized, with LAT1 predominately found on the MVM and LAT2 on the BM [94], although LAT2 has also been shown to have functional activity in the MVM [95]. However, localization of LAT2 on the BM allows for the exchange of amino acids between non-essential amino acids in the fetal circulation and essential amino acids in the syncytiotrophoblast cytoplasm [96]. Two additional system L light chains, LAT3 and LAT4 have recently been reported in placental tissues [97,98]. They are localized to the BM and may play an important role in the net efflux of amino acids to the fetus [99]. While transporting a restricted group of system L substrates (leucine, isoleucine and phenylalanine), LAT3 and LAT4 also appear to differ from the traditional system L transport in that they do not require the co-expression of 4F2hc and function as facilitative diffusion transporters [99,100].

It is well established that the cationic amino acid transporter (CAT) is the main transporter for cationic amino acids in MVM [101]. Kamath *et al.* also found that CAT1 (SLC7A1), CAT2 (SLC7A2), and CAT4 (SLC7A4) are expressed in cultured trophoblast cells and in BeWo choriocarcinoma cells [102], supporting the possibility that multiple members of the CAT family are present in BM of the placenta. CAT is a sodium independent electrogenic transporter, which interacts only weakly with neutral amino acids and therefore is specific for cationic amino acids.

Anionic or system X_{AG} amino acid transporters are capable of sodium dependent and D-aspartate-inhibitable glutamate/aspartate transport activity. A family of five anionic amino acid transporters (excitatory amino acid transporters EAAT1-5) have been cloned and, of these, EAAT1-4 are expressed in the human and rat placenta [103–105]. EAAT1-4 are present in both plasma membranes of the syncytiotrophoblast and increase over the last trimester [105,106].

3.6.3. Placental Fatty Acid Transporter Systems

Fatty acids are important precursors of bioactive molecules, which are structural components of cells and provide a major source of energy [13]. Two sources of fatty acids are taken up by the placenta from the maternal circulation, the esterified fatty acids that are present in triglycerides (TG) and the nonesterified fatty acids (NEFA) [13]. The primary source of fatty acids taken up by the placenta is maternal TG because their uptake increases in the last trimester compared with NEFAs [107].

Fatty acid transfer from the mother to the fetus can be accomplished via simple diffusion, as with NEFAs [107]. However, in late gestation the rate of simple diffusion may not be adequate to supply the fetus [13,108]. Kazantzis and Stahl stated that the cellular membrane fatty acid transport proteins (FATPs) are important for the cellular uptake of long chain fatty acids [108]. There are five transport proteins in humans, including FATP1-4 and FATP6 [109]. FATP1 is present on both the MVM and the BM, but the exact cellular location of the others remains unknown [110]. Fatty acid translocase (CD36) is the membrane-associated protein expressed in placenta with the ability to transport fatty acids [110]. Upon entering the syncytiotrophoblast the hydrophobic fatty acids are transported across the cytosol to the BM or to other sites within the cell where they undergo esterification or beta oxidation. To accomplish this they bind with fatty acid binding proteins (FABPs) [13]. There are four forms of the fatty acid binding proteins in the human placenta, including FABP1 and FABP3-5 [111].

We have summarized the major placental changes in morphology and substrate transport capacity that regulate placental efficiency and fetal growth in normal pregnancies. As we know, placental insufficiency results in a failure of the placenta to deliver an adequate supply of substrates to the fetus and IUGR develops. Therefore, several different experimental methods used to produce placental insufficiency and induce IUGR in animal models and a range of factors that regulate placental growth and substrate transport capacity have been discussed in human and animal IUGR studies below.

4. The Placenta and Development of Intrauterine Growth Restriction

Intrauterine growth restriction is clinically defined as a birth weight below the tenth centile for gestational age where the fetus does not meet its growth potential [23,112]. IUGR affects 6% of

Australian pregnancies [1] and is associated with a high incidence of perinatal morbidity and mortality [7]. IUGR neonates have a greater risk of hypoxic-ischaemic encephalopathy, intraventicular haemorrhage and necrotizing enterocolitis with longer hospital stays and higher health care costs [23]. Furthermore, epidemiological, clinical and experimental studies from around the world highlight an association between a poor intrauterine environment and poor health outcomes in adulthood [7,113–115]. In particular, these studies have demonstrated a significant relationship between small size at birth and the risk of developing coronary heart disease, hypertension and type 2 diabetes in adulthood [4–6]. Causes of IUGR can be of maternal, fetal or placental origin, including maternal smoking, alcohol and drug abuse, genetic defects, chromosomal abnormalities or placental pathologies [116]. In the developing world, IUGR is likely to be a consequence of poor maternal nutritional status prior to or during pregnancy whereas, in the developed world IUGR is commonly a consequence of placental insufficiency [117].

Several different experimental methods have been used to produce placental insufficiency and induce IUGR in both small and large animal models, and previously discussed in detail [23]. For example, methodologies include reduction of uterine blood flow by vascular occlusion or ligation in rats, guinea pigs and sheep, hyperthermia, placental infarction by repetitive embolization in pregnant ewes or uterine caruncletomy of non-pregnant ewes [23]. As sheep are used in all of these methodologies to induce IUGR, the sheep models of placental insufficiency are summarized below (Table 2).

Table 2. Summary of experimental models of placental insufficiency and their impact on the placenta and the fetus.

Experimental Intervention		Impact on the Placenta	Impact on the Fetus
Surgical Umbilical Artery Ligation (SUAL)	Isolation and ligation of one umbilical artery close to the fetal abdomen	placental infarction causing ↓ umbilical blood flow and ↓ placental substrate transfer [118,119]	Hypoxemia IUGR
Maternal Hyperthermia	Exposure of pregnant ewes to an environment with an increased ambient temperature	↓ uterine artery flow and ↓ placental weight due to ↑ maternal temperature [2,30]	IUGR
Placental Embolism	Repeated injection of microspheres (15μm) into the placenta via the umbilical artery through a catheter implanted in the descending aorta or fetal umbilical vein	block placental capillaries causing ↓ placental surface area [120]	Hypoxemia Hypoglycemia IUGR
Uterine Carunclectomy	Surgical removal of the majority of the endometrial caruncles from the uterus of non-pregnant ewes prior to conception	↓ placental weight due to ↓ placentomes [116]	Hypoxemia Hypoglycemia IUGR

5. Animal Models of Placental Insufficiency

5.1. Single Umbilical Artery Ligation (SUAL)

Single umbilical artery ligation (SUAL) involves the isolation and ligation of one umbilical artery close to the fetal abdomen [118]. SUAL causes a partial infarction of the placenta, which reduces umbilical blood flow and causes a reduction in the capacity of the placenta to transfer substrates and induces IUGR in the sheep fetus [118,119]. Furthermore, SUAL fetuses are significantly smaller than control fetuses from 117 days gestation and are chronically hypoxaemic (PO_2 < 17 mmHg), but not acidotic in late gestation [121].

5.2. Maternal Hyperthermia

The hyperthermia-induced model of placental insufficiency induces fetal growth restriction by exposing pregnant ewes to an environment with an increased ambient temperature with a diurnal cycle of 40 °C for 12 h and 35 °C for 12 h, from ~38 days gestation until ewes are sacrificed at post mortem [2,122]. Ewes can be exposed to this treatment for ~17 days (early gestation), ~52 days (mid gestation) or ~96 ± 5 days (late gestation). This hyperthermia treatment results in an increase in maternal core body temperature from ~39 °C to 40 °C in hyperthermia pregnant ewes [53,123]. It also results in a redistribution of blood flow toward the peripheral vascular system, leading to a reduction in uterine and umbilical artery blood flow and a decrease in placental weight and IUGR [2,30].

5.3. Placental Embolism

Placental embolism of the placental vasculature aims to mimic the onset of IUGR in late gestation. This procedure involves repeated injection of microspheres (15 μm) into the placenta via the umbilical artery through a catheter implanted in the descending aorta or fetal umbilical vein [124–126]. The microspheres block the placental capillaries resulting in reduced surface area for the transfer of substrates from mother to fetus [120]. Placental embolism in late gestation causes acute decreases in placental substrate supply after each daily injection over a period of 10–20 days, which leads to chronic fetal hypoxemia, hypoglycemia and IUGR.

5.4. Endometrial Carunclectomy

Uterine carunclectomy limits the number of placentomes after surgical removal of the majority of the endometrial caruncles from the uterus of nonpregnant ewes prior to conception. This restricts the number of placentomes that form during pregnancy, consequently limiting placental and fetal growth [116]. Experimental restriction of placental growth results in fetuses that are chronically hypoxaemic and hypoglycemic [127]. Furthermore, the changes to nutrient supply and fetal blood gases in placentally restricted (PR) sheep fetuses are similar to those measured in cordocentesis studies of human infants who are born small for gestational age [116,121]. PR fetuses also have reduced placental and fetal weights at term [128].

6. Regulation of Placental Growth and Substrate Transport in IUGR Pregnancy

Fetal growth is dependent on substrate supply, which is dependent on substrate transport and its regulation. These processes also depend on morphological characteristics of the placenta, such as placental size, morphology, blood flow and vascularity. Therefore placental nutrient transfer capacity is specifically regulated by signals of fetal, maternal and placental origin in an effort to control fetal growth. However, in late gestation, when fetal nutrient demand is at its greatest, the compensatory upregulation is no longer sufficient to meet fetal demand and thus IUGR develops [129,130]. Here, we focus on the morphological and functional changes in the regulation of placental growth and substrate transport capacity in human pregnancy complicated with IUGR and animals models of placental insufficiency.

6.1. Placental Size and Morphology

In human pregnancies, Chen and coworkers have found a significant decrease in villi vascular density and cell proliferation in both trophoblast and stromal cell compartments within the IUGR placentas compared with control placentas at 25 to 41 weeks of gestation [131]. Other reports have shown a decrease in surface area, volume, and number of terminal villi, a reduced number of capillaries as well as an increased thickness of the exchange barrier in the stroma of IUGR placentas as compared with placentas from normal pregnancies [132,133]. Undernutrition in guinea pigs during pregnancy increases barrier thickness and reduces placental weight and placental area involved in nutrient exchange during late gestation [134]. In contrast, hypoxia during pregnancy cause a reduction in the barrier thickness between maternal and fetal circulation in the human and guinea pig placenta that has a direct effect on diffusional exchange [135,136]. In pregnant sheep, the total surface of the cotyledons and surface occupied by vasculature were greater at high altitude, whereas the number of cotyledons was smaller at high altitude [137]. These placental morphological changes may improve maternal and fetal exchange and display an efficient mechanism of adaptation to hypobaric hypoxia.

Experimental restriction of placental size by surgical removal of implantation sites prior to conception, multiple pregnancy or adverse conditions in early gestation restricts fetal growth, but increases fetal to placental weight ratio and placental efficiency in late pregnancy [15,53]. Conversely, an increased fetal to placental weight ratio may suggest fetal adaptations in response to the small placenta, which maximizes transplacental concentration gradients and/or partitioning of placentally derived nutrients to support and maintain fetal growth during suboptimal intrauterine conditions [55]. Adverse conditions, such as maternal undernutrition and hypoxemia resulted in increased eversion of placentomes and an increased proportion of type C and D placentomes in late gestation sheep fetuses [138,139]. In contrast, adverse intrauterine conditions induced by umbilical cord compression is associated with an increased proportion of type A and B, and fewer type C- and D placentomes during late gestation in sheep [140]. Therefore, adverse conditions in the intrauterine environment determine placental morphology during late gestation depending on the type and duration of the insult.

6.2. Oxygen Supply/Uptake, Blood Flow and Vascularity

In situations of placental insufficiency and IUGR, there appears to be an underdevelopment of the placental epithelial sites, with low hindrance to transplacental O_2 diffusion reducing the surface area of exchange between the uterine and umbilical circulations, and resulting in decreased fetal umbilical oxygen supply [30,132]. Under hypoxic conditions, hypoxia inducible factor (HIF)-1, which consists of two subunits HIF-1α and HIF-1β, acts on the cell nucleus and regulates the expression of genes with hypoxia response element (HRE). HIFs recruit mechanisms to increase oxygen supply (erythropoiesis, angiogenesis, and vasodilation), decrease oxygen demand (increased glycolysis coupled with decreased oxidative metabolism), and regulate the cell cycle, apoptosis, and autophagy [141]. *In vitro* studies have demonstrated that hypoxia can affect the proliferation, differentiation, and invasion of cytotrophoblast cells [142]. Following a three day exposure to low oxygen, there was decreased HIF-1α and unchanged HIF-2α mRNA expression in cultured murine ectoplacental cones [143]. Hypoxia resulted in an increase in the transcription and translation of VEGF in cultured placental fibroblasts [144]. Low oxygen levels also resulted in a shift of the angiopoietin-1: angiopoietin-2 ratio in favor of angiopoietin-2, leading to vessel instability, angiogenesis and vessel remodeling [145].

Morphological studies show that physiological remodelling of the maternal uterine vasculature into spiral arteries is deficient in IUGR pregnancies due to inadequate trophoblast invasion [146,147]. This results in maternal blood entering the placenta at an abnormally high rate, which causes damage to the placental villi and may harm endocrine and transport functions of the placenta. The intensity of VEGF-A immunostaining in syncytiotrophoblast was significantly reduced in placental villous tissue from pregnancies complicated by IUGR and preeclampsia compared with the control group [148]. However, it has been shown that the expression of VEGF-A and bFGF was significantly higher in cytotrophoblasts, syncytiotrophoblasts, extravillous trophoblasts, vascular smooth muscle cells, chorionic villous stromal cells and villous vascular endothelial cells of the IUGR placenta when compared with those collected from normal-term pregnancies using semi-quantitative immunohistochemistry [149]. This suggests that these factors play a role in promoting increased endothelial cell proliferation, migration and pathological angiogenesis. Similarly in sheep, hyperthermia-induced placental restriction resulted in increased uterine blood flow and increased VEGF, angiopoietin-1, angiopoietin-2 and TIE-2 expression in the fetal portion (cotyledon) of the placentome in early gestation as well as reduced expression in FLT-1 and FLK-1 in the cotyledonary tissue in mid gestation, suggesting a disorganized fetal capillarisation and angiogenesis as well as compensatory transport capacity for the fetal circulation to uptake nutrients from the maternal circulation, which fails to maintain placental and fetal growth [53,54,123]. These alterations in angiogenic growth factors could impair normal placental vascular development and may contribute to the development of placental insufficiency, and ultimately intrauterine growth restriction.

6.3. IGFs

In knockout mice with a deletion of the placental-specific transcript (P0) of the *Igf2* gene, placental surface area is reduced and placental thickness increased, leading to reduced placental growth and fetal growth restriction [60,61]. Placental IGF-I mRNA expression was lower in the growth-restricted groups compared with normal pregnancies [150]. Similarly, the mRNA expression of IGF1, IGFBP1 and human placental growth hormone was significantly lower in placentas from human IUGR pregnancies compared with that in placentas of fetuses with normal growth [151]. However in sheep, caruncle IGF1 mRNA expression was increased at 90 days gestation in the placentas of hyperthermia-induced IUGR compared with the control group [152]. Cotyledon IGF2 and caruncle IGFBP4 mRNA expression were also elevated at 55 days gestation in these placentas [152]. In contrast, maternal hypoxia in mice from mid to late gestation resulted in a decrease in placental mRNA expression of IGF2, IGF1R and IGF2R [153].

6.4. Apoptosis, Autophagy and Glucocorticoid Action

Placentas from women with IUGR pregnancies show enhanced apoptosis when compared with those from normal pregnancy [154,155]. Cultured trophoblasts exposed to hypoxia alone show an upregulation of p53 activity and BCL-2-like protein 4 (BAX) expression and decreased expression of the anti-apoptotic BCL-2, all of which promote apoptosis [156]. Hypoxia/re-oxygenation results in even more marked apoptosis regulated by increased expression of the pro-apoptotic BAX and BCL-2 homologous antagonist (BAK) mRNA and protein and reduced expression of BCL-2 mRNA in human placental villous tissues [157]. Expression of p53 and the active form of caspase-3 is upregulated in villi from IUGR compared to control pregnancies, and the increase is predominantly in the villous trophoblast in humans [158,159]. The association between altered trophoblast cell turnover in IUGR and increased p53 expression was also shown to be reminiscent of that following exposure to hypoxia [160].

Compared with normal pregnant women, women with IUGR had increased placental levels of autophagy-related proteins including LC3B-II, beclin-1, DRAM, and p53 [161]. Furthermore, hypoxia induces apoptotic and autophagic changes in primary human cytotrophoblasts [162].

Placental 11βHSD2 activity was significantly reduced in deliveries complicated by IUGR compared with the term deliveries and with appropriately grown preterm deliveries, suggesting that glucocorticoids may, in part, contribute to impaired fetal growth closely controlled through placental 11βHSD2 expression [71]. There is evidence that exposure of the pregnant sheep to maternal undernutrition for a period extending beyond the preimplantation period, from 60 days before and the first 30 days after conception or from early to mid gestation (between 28 and 78 days gestation), results in a decrease in placental 11βHSD2 expression or activity [72,163]. In mice, maternal hypoxia during mid to late gestation resulted in a decrease in placental glucocorticoid receptor (GR) mRNA expression as well as placental 11βHSD2 mRNA and protein expression [153]. A previous study by Mericq *et al* found a lower expression and activity of 11βHSD1 in both chorionic and basal plates of the placentas from full term small for gestation age newborns compared with those in the placentas from appropriate for gestational age newborns, suggesting a possible compensatory mechanism to diminish the higher cortisol concentrations in fetuses with IUGR [164].

6.5. Glucose Transport Systems

Alterations in placental glucose transport have been implicated in adverse perinatal conditions such as IUGR and fetal hypoxia [165]. As glucose transport is dependent on the glucose concentration gradient from mother to fetus, the IUGR pregnancy has increased the transplacental glucose gradient and glucose uptake across the placenta [10] and this represents an example of how the IUGR fetus adapts to restricted placental size. In carunclectomized ewes with smaller placentas and a larger proportions of type D placentomes, the rate of glucose transfer to the fetus per gram of placenta is greater than that in controls [166,167]. Exposure to hypoxic conditions resulted in an upregulation in GLUT1 protein abundance and trans-epithelial glucose transport in BeWo choriocarcinoma cells [168]. GLUT3 mRNA expression and protein abundance in the trophoblast on the maternal aspect of the placenta was increased in the full-term IUGR placenta compared with normal placenta [169]. Increased placental GLUT3 expression was associated with increased activation of placental HIF-1α, suggesting that hypoxia may play a role in the upregulation of GLUT3. However, placental GLUT1 mRNA expression was decreased in the maternal aspect of the IUGR placenta and GLUT4 mRNA expression was increased in the fetal aspect of the IUGR placenta when compared with the control pregnancies, although there was no difference in placental GLUT1 or GLUT4 protein abundance between the treatment groups [169] (Table 3). Similarly, placental GLUT1, but not GLUT3 immunostaining in the terminal villi of severe preeclampsia cases (both with and without IUGR) was significantly lower compared with the control group [170]. Chronic hypoxia *in vivo* with high altitude pregnancies also resulted in a decrease in GLUT1 expression in the BM but not MVM of the placenta, leading to reduced nutrient supply and fetal growth [171]. In mice, maternal hypoxia during mid to late gestation resulted in a decrease in placental GLUT1 mRNA and protein expression in female fetuses, but no change in placental GLUT3 mRNA expression in both female and male fetuses [153]. Another study demonstrated that GLUT1 protein abundance is not altered in IUGR babies when compared to those that are appropriate for gestational age (AGA) [172]. Placental GLUT8 mRNA expression and protein abundance was decreased in late gestation in a sheep model of IUGR caused by placental insufficiency, which may contribute in part to the placental glucose transport deficit that occurs in this model [84]. Taken together, these data along with amino acid and fatty acid transport systems mentioned below suggest that the regulation of nutrient transport in the IUGR pregnancies may depend on the timing and type of the insult, and be species-specific and different from *in vivo* and *in vitro* studies.

Table 3. Summary of human and sheep models of IUGR and their impact on oxygen transfer, placental glucose, amino acid and fatty acid transporters.

Models of IUGR	Impact on Glucose Transporters	Impact on Amino Acid Transporters	Impact on Fatty Acid Transporters
Human IUGR	↓ GLUT1 mRNA, ↔ GLUT1 protein [169] ↑ GLUT4 mRNA, ↔ GLUT1 protein [169] ↑ GLUT3 mRNA & protein [169] ↓ GLUT1 protein [171] ↓ GLUT1 protein ↔ GLUT3 protein [170] ↔ GLUT1 protein [172]	↓ System A transporter activity [173,174] ↓ SNAT2 mRNA & protein [175]	NS
Sheep			
Surgical Umbilical Artery Ligation (SUAL)	NS	NS	NS
Maternal Hyperthermia	↓ GLUT8 mRNA & protein	↑ LAT-1 & LAT-2 mRNA [19]	NS
Placental Embolism	NS	NS	NS
Uterine Caruncleectomy	NS	NS	NS

NS, not studied.

6.6. Amino Acid Transport Systems

In the IUGR placenta the different amino acid transport systems are affected. Tracer studies of placental amino acid transport have demonstrated that there is a significant reduction in the transplacental flux/fetal turnover ratios of essential amino acids [176–178]. For example, reduced uptake of leucine and lysine was found in vesicles from human IUGR placenta compared with the controls, suggesting decreased activity of placental transporters for cationic and neutral amino acids [176]. Similarly, there was a reduction of maternal leucine flux into the placenta and fetus in the hyperthermia sheep model of IUGR [178]. However, studies of fetal plasma amino acid concentrations have produced inconclusive results. Although earlier reports showed decreased fetal plasma amino acid concentrations [178], subsequent human and animal studies showed maintained or increased amino acid concentrations [22,177,179]. In severely growth restricted sheep fetuses, where placental and fetal weights are reduced by 40%–60%, umbilical uptake of oxygen, glucose and essential amino acids is significantly reduced, whereas the fetal/maternal ratio of the amino acids that are transported from the placenta to fetus showed normal or elevated fetal concentrations compared to control fetuses [22,30]. A previous study has shown that transplacental and total placental clearance of a branched-chain amino acid analogue, the non-metabolisable neutral amino acid aminocyclopentane-l-carboxylic acid per 100 g placenta, were significantly reduced in a sheep model of hyperthermia-induced IUGR, suggesting impaired placental non-essential amino acid transport in the IUGR placenta [180].

In normal pregnancy, system A transporter activity was shown to be the highest in the smallest babies per milligram of microvillous protein [181]. In contrast, placental system A transporter activity was not only reduced in IUGR compared with normal pregnancies but also related to the severity of IUGR [173,174]. Placental SNAT2 mRNA expression and syncytiotrophoblast immunostaining were significantly decreased in IUGR placentas with reduced umbilical blood flows compared with those in control placentas [175]. Hypoxia also decreases placental system A transport and activity in full-term human trophoblasts [182]. In mice, maternal hypoxia during mid to late gestation resulted in an increase in placental GLUT1 mRNA expression in female fetuses, but no change in placental SNAT4 mRNA expression. There was also a decrease in placental SNAT2 mRNA expression in both female and male fetuses [153]. Interestingly, placental LAT-1 and LAT-2 mRNA expression was elevated in the moderately growth restricted sheep fetuses where placental and fetal weight was reduced by 25% compared with the control placenta [19].

6.7. Fatty Acid Transport Systems

Hypoxia enhances the expression of FABP1, -3, and -4 in term human trophoblasts, suggesting that FABPs play a role in fat accumulation in the hypoxic placenta [111]. Similarly, hypoxia also resulted in increased FATP2 expression and reduced FATP4 expression in cultured primary term human trophoblasts [183]. However, placental CD36 mRNA expression was unaltered in human pregnancy complicated with IUGR [184].

7. Conclusions

The placenta is the main interface between the fetus and mother. Placental insufficiency results in a failure of the placenta to deliver an adequate supply of substrates to the fetus and IUGR develops. A range of human and animal studies in IUGR pregnancies have suggested that placental restriction and insufficiency may result in a series of placental changes such as altered placental growth and placental substrate transport capacity, increased apoptosis and autophagy and increased glucocorticoid action (Figure 1). Such placental morphological and functional changes may consequently lead to decreased fetal growth and IUGR, which is modified by compensatory changes in placental efficiency. We have also noted that there are different patterns of placental changes associated with the human IUGR pregnancy and animal models of placental insufficiency induced IUGR. These differences may be dependent on the nature of the causes of IUGR, the time, duration and severity of insult exposure, species and *in vivo* or *in vitro* studies. While no model system completely encapsulates complete human IUGR, these model systems do allow us to carefully dissect aspects of the issue so as to further expand our understanding of the cellular and molecular mechanisms involved, and promote the development of therapeutic interventions.

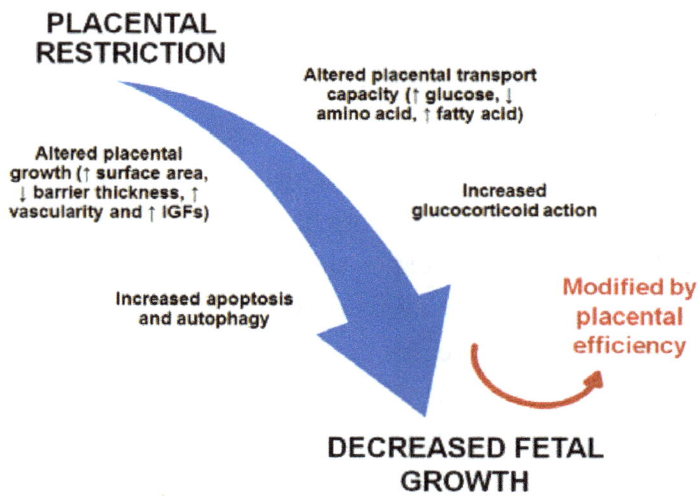

Figure 1. Summary of the placental adaptations that occur in the placental insufficiency-induced IUGR fetus and contribute to decreased fetal growth.

Acknowledgments

Janna L. Morrison was supported by a Career Development Award from the National Health and Medical Research Council (NHMRC) (APP1066916) and a South Australian Cardiovascular Research Network Fellowship (CR10A4988). Claire T. Roberts was supported by a Senior Research Fellowship from the NHMRC (APP1020749).

Author Contributions

Song Zhang compiled the review and wrote the manuscript. Timothy R.H. Regnault and Janna L. Morrison participated in the writing and critical review of the manuscript. Paige L. Barker participated in the writing. All authors commented, edited and approved the paper.

References

1. Li, Z.; Zeki, R.; Hilder, L.; Sullivan, E.A. *Australia's Mothers and Babies 2010*, Ca. no. PER 57 ed.; AIHW National Perinatal Epidemiology and Statistics: Canberra, Australia, 2012.
2. Limesand, S.W.; Rozance, P.J.; Zerbe, G.O.; Hutton, J.C.; Hay, W.W., Jr. Attenuated insulin release and storage in fetal sheep pancreatic islets with intrauterine growth restriction. *Endocrinology* **2006**, *147*, 1488–1497.
3. Bamfo, J.E.; Odibo, A.O. Diagnosis and management of fetal growth restriction. *J. Pregnancy* **2011**, *2011*, doi:10.1155/2011/640715.
4. Barker, D.J. Developmental origins or chronic disease. *Public Healh* **2012**, *126*, 185–189.
5. Barker, D.J.; Gluckman, P.D.; Godfrey, K.M.; Harding, J.E.; Owens, J.A.; Robinson, J.S. Fetal nutrition and cardiovascular disease in adult life. *Lancet* **1993**, *341*, 938–941.
6. Li, C.C.Y.; Maloney, C.A.; Cropley, J.E.; Suter, C.M. Epigenetic programming by maternal nutritions: Shaping future generations. *Epigenomics* **2010**, *2*, 539–549.
7. Barker, D.J.; Gelow, J.; Thornburg, K.; Osmond, C.; Kajantie, E.; Eriksson, J.G. The early origins of chronic heart failure: Impaired placental growth and initiation of insulin resistance in childhood. *Eur. J. Heart Fail.* **2010**, *12*, 819–825.
8. Jansson, T.; Powell, T.L. Role of the placenta in fetal programming: Underlying mechanisms and potential interventional approaches. *Clin. Sci. (Lond.)* **2007**, *113*, 1–13.
9. Jones, H.N.; Powell, T.L.; Jansson, T. Regulation of placental nutrient transport—A review. *Placenta* **2007**, *28*, 763–774.
10. Marconi, A.M.; Paolini, C.L. Nutrient transport across the intrauterine growth-restricted placenta. *Semin. Perinatol.* **2008**, *32*, 178–181.
11. Gude, N.M.; Roberts, C.T.; Kalionis, B.; King, R.G. Growth and function of the normal human placenta. *Thromb. Res.* **2004**, *114*, 397–407.
12. Sibley, C.P.; Brownbill, P.; Dilworth, M.; Glazier, J.D. Review: Adaption in placental nutrient supply to meet fetal growth demand: Implications for programmings. *Placenta* **2010**, *24*, 70–74.
13. Lager, S.; Powell, T.L. Regulation of nutrient transport across the placenta. *J. Pregnancy* **2012**, *2012*, 1–14.
14. Barry, J.S.; Anthony, R.V. The pregnant sheep as a model for human pregnancy. *Theriogenology* **2008**, *69*, 55–67.
15. Fowden, A.L.; Ward, J.W.; Wooding, F.P.B.; Forhead, A.J.; Constancia, M. Programming placental nutrient transfer capacity. *J. Physiol.* **2006**, *572*, 5–15.
16. Ward, J.W.; Forhead, A.J.; Wooding, F.P.B.; Fowden, A.L. Functional significance and cortisol dependence of the gross morphology of ovine placentomes during late gestation. *Biol. Reprod.* **2006**, *74*, 137–145.
17. Ahokas, R.A.; McKinney, E.T. *Development and Physiology of the Placenta and Membrane*; The Global Library of Women's Medicine: London, UK, 2008.
18. Fowden, A.L.; Sferruzzi-Perri, A.N.; Coan, P.M.; Burton, G. Placental efficiency and adaptation: Endocrine regulation. *J. Physiol.* **2009**, *587*, 3459–3472.

19. Regnault, T.R.; Marconi, A.M.; Smith, C.H.; Glazier, J.D.; Novak, D.A.; Sibley, C.P.; Jansson, T. Placental amino acid transport systems and fetal growth restriction—A workshop report. *Placenta* **2005**, *26*, 76–80.
20. Roberts, C.T.; Sohlstrom, A.; Kind, K.L.; Grant, P.A.; Earl, R.A.; Robinson, J.S.; Khong, T.Y.; Owens, P.C.; Owens, J.A. Altered placental structure induced by maternal food restriction in guinea pigs: A role for circulating IGF-II and IGFBP-2 in the mother? *Placenta* **2001**, *22*, 77–82.
21. Anthony, R.V.; Scheaffer, A.N.; Wright, C.D.; Regnault, T.R. Ruminant models of prenatal growth restriction. *Reprod. Suppl.* **2003**, *61*, 183–194.
22. Regnault, T.R.; de Vrijer, B.; Galan, H.L.; Wilkening, R.B.; Battaglia, F.C.; Meschia, G. Umbilical uptakes and transplacental concentration ratios of amino acids in severe fetal growth restriction. *Pediatr. Res.* **2013**, *73*, 602–611.
23. Morrison, J.L. Sheep models of intrauterine growth restriction: Fetal adaptations and consequences. *Clin. Exp. Pharmacol. Physiol.* **2008**, *35*, 730–743.
24. Gagnon, R.; Langridge, J.; Inchley, K.; Murotsuki, J.; Possmayer, F. Changes in surfactant-associated protein mRNA profile in growth-restricted fetal sheep. *Am. J. Physiol.* **1999**, *276*, 459–465.
25. Jones, C.T.; Roebuck, M.M.; Walker, D.W.; Lagercrantz, H.; Johnston, B.M. Cardiovascular, metabolic and endocrine effects of chemical sympathectomy and of adrenal demedullation in fetal sheep. *J. Dev. Physiol.* **1987**, *9*, 347–367.
26. Miller, S.L.; Chai, M.; Loose, J.; Castillo-Melendez, M.; Walker, D.W.; Jenkin, G.; Wallace, E.M. The effects of maternal betamethasone administration on the intrauterine growth-restricted fetus. *Endocrinology* **2007**, *148*, 1288–1295.
27. Mallard, E.C.; Rees, S.; Stringer, M.; Cock, M.L.; Harding, R. Effects of chronic placental insufficiency on brain development in fetal sheep. *Pediatr. Res.* **1998**, *43*, 262–270.
28. Robinson, J.S.; Hart, I.C.; Kingston, E.J.; Jones, C.T.; Thorburn, G.D. Studies on the growth of the fetal sheep. The effects of reduction of placental size on hormone concentration in fetal plasma. *J. Dev. Physiol.* **1980**, *2*, 239–248.
29. Dobbing, J.; Sands, J. Comparative aspects of the brain growth spurt. *Early Hum. Dev.* **1979**, *3*, 79–83.
30. Regnault, T.R.H.; de Vrijer, B.; Galan, H.L.; Wilkening, R.B.; Battaglia, F.C.; Meschia, G. Development and mechanisms of fetal hypoxia in severe fetal growth restriction. *Placenta* **2007**, *28*, 714–723.
31. Wilson, M.E. Role of placental function in mediating conceptus growth and survival. *J. Anim. Sci.* **2002**, *80*, 195–201.
32. Vonnahme, K.A.; Arndt, W.J.; Johnson, M.L.; Borowicz, P.P.; Reynolds, L.P. Effect of morphology on placentome size, vascularity and vasoreactivity in late pregnant sheep. *Biol. Reprod.* **2008**, *79*, 976–982.
33. Ehrhardt, R.A.; Bell, A.W. Growth and metabolism of the ovine placenta during mid-gestation. *Placenta* **1995**, *16*, 727–741.
34. Vatnick, I.; Schoknecht, P.A.; Darrigrand, R.; Bell, A.W. Growth and metabolism of the placenta after unilateral fetectomy in twin pregnant ewes. *J. Dev. Physiol.* **1991**, *15*, 351–356.

35. Robinson, J.S.; Hartwich, K.M.; Walker, S.K.; Erwich, J.J.; Owens, J.A. Early influences on embryonic and placental growth. *Acta Paediatr. Suppl.* **1997**, *423*, 159–164.
36. Alexander, G. Studies on the placenta of the sheep (*Ovis aries* L.). Effect of surgical reduction in the number of caruncles. *J. Reprod. Fertil.* **1964**, *30*, 307–322.
37. Wilson, M.E.; Ford, S.P. Comparative aspects of placental efficiency. *Reprod. Suppl.* **2001**, *58*, 223–232.
38. Barker, D.J.P.; Thornburg, K.L. Placental programming of chronic diseases, cancer and lifespan: A review. *Placenta* **2013**, *34*, 841–845.
39. Barker, D.J.; Bull, A.R.; Osmond, C.; Simmonds, S.J. Fetal and placental size and risk of hypertension in adult life. *BMJ* **1990**, *301*, 259–262.
40. Sibai, B.M.; Frangieh, A. Maternal adaptation to pregnancy. *Curr. Opin. Obstet. Gynecol.* **1995**, *7*, 420–426.
41. Carter, A.M. Factors affecting gas transfer across the placenta and the oxygen supply to the fetus. *J. Dev. Physiol.* **1989**, *12*, 305–322.
42. Bell, A.W.; Kennaugh, J.M.; Battaglia, F.C.; Makowski, E.L.; Meschia, G. Metabolic and circulatory studies of fetal lamb at midgestation. *Am. J. Physiol.* **1986**, *250*, 538–544.
43. Bonds, D.R.; Crosby, L.O.; Cheek, T.G.; Hagerdal, M.; Gutsche, B.B.; Gabbe, S.G. Estimation of human fetal-placental unit metabolic rate by application of the bohr principle. *J. Dev. Physiol.* **1986**, *8*, 49–54.
44. Campbell, A.G.; Dawes, G.S.; Fishman, A.P.; Hyman, A.I.; James, G.B. The oxygen consumption of the placenta and foetal membranes in the sheep. *J. Physiol.* **1966**, *182*, 439–464.
45. Coan, P.M.; Ferguson-Smith, A.C.; Burton, G. Developmental dynamics of the definitive mouse placenta assessed by stereology. *Biol. Reprod.* **2004**, *70*, 1806–1813.
46. Reynolds, L.P.; Borawicz, P.P.; Vonnahme, K.A.; Johnson, M.L.; Grazul-Bilska, A.T.; Wallace, J.M.; Caton, J.S.; Redmer, D.A. Animal models of placental angiogenesis. *Placenta* **2005**, *26*, 689–708.
47. Demir, R.; Seval, Y.; Huppertz, B. Vasculogenesis and angiogenesis in the early human placenta. *Acta Histochem.* **2007**, *109*, 257–265.
48. Charnock-Jones, D.S.; Kaufmann, P.; Mayhew, T.M. Aspects of human fetoplacental vasculogenesis and angiogenesis. I. Molecular regulation. *Placenta* **2004**, *25*, 103–113.
49. Ahmed, A.; Perkins, J. Angiogenesis and intrauterine growth restriction. *Baillieres Best Pract. Res. Clin. Obstet. Gynaecol.* **2000**, *14*, 981–998.
50. Maisonpierre, P.C.; Suri, C.; Jones, P.F.; Bartunkova, S.; Wiegand, S.J.; Radziejewski, C.; Compton, D.; McClain, J.; Aldrich, T.H.; Papadopoulos, N.; *et al.* Angiopoietin-2, a natural antagonist for tie2 that disrupts *in vivo* angiogenesis. *Science* **1997**, *277*, 55–60.
51. Plaisier, M.; Rodrigues, S.; Willems, F.; Koolwijk, P.; van Hinsbergh, V.W.; Helmerhorst, F.M. Different degrees of vascularization and their relationship to the expression of vascular endothelial growth factor, placental growth factor, angiopoietins, and their receptors in first-trimester decidual tissues. *Fertil. Steril.* **2007**, *88*, 176–187.
52. Cross, J.C.; Hemberger, M.; Lu, Y.; Nozaki, T.; Whiteley, K.; Masutani, M.; Adamson, S.L. Trophoblast functions, angiogenesis and remodeling of the maternal vasculature in the placenta. *Mol. Cell. Endocrinol* **2002**, *187*, 207–212.

53. Regnault, T.R.; de Vrijer, B.; Galan, H.L.; Davidsen, M.L.; Trembler, K.A.; Battaglia, F.C.; Wilkening, R.B.; Anthony, R.V. The relationship between transplacental O2 diffusion and placental expression of PLGF, VEGF and their receptors in a placental insufficiency model of fetal growth restriction. *J. Physiol.* **2003**, *550*, 641–656.
54. Hagen, A.S.; Orbus, R.J.; Wilkening, R.B.; Regnault, T.R.; Anthony, R.V. Placental expression of angiopoietin-1, angiopoietin-2 and tie-2 during placental development in an ovine model of placental insufficiency-fetal growth restriction. *Pediatr. Res.* **2005**, *58*, 1228–1232.
55. Fowden, A.L.; Forhead, A.J.; Coan, P.M.; Burton, G. The placenta and intrauterine programming. *J. Neuroendocrinol.* **2008**, *20*, 439–450.
56. Sferruzzi-Perri, A.N.; Owens, J.A.; Pringle, K.G.; Roberts, C.T. The neglected role of insulin-like growth factors in the maternal circulation regulating fetal growth. *J. Physiol.* **2011**, *589*, 7–20.
57. Roos, S.; Lagerlöf, O.; Wennergren, M.; Powell, T.L.; Jansson, T. Regulation of amino acid transporters by glucose and growth factors in cultured primary human trophoblast cells is mediated by mtor signalling. *Am. J. Physiol. Cell Physiol.* **2009**, *297*, 723–731.
58. Harding, J.E.; Liu, L.; Evans, P.C.; Gluckman, P.D. Insulin-like growth factor 1 alters feto-placental protein and carbohydrate metabolism in fetal sheep. *Endocrinology.* **1994**, *134,* 1509–1514.
59. Constancia, M.; Angiolini, E.; Sandovic, I.; Smith, P.; Smith, R.; Kelsey, G.; Dean, W.; Ferguson-Smith, A.C.; Sibley, C.P.; Reik, W.; *et al.* Adaption of nutrient supply to fetal demand in the mouse involves interaction between the Igf2 gene and placental transporter proteins. *Proc. Natl. Acad. Sci. USA* **2005**, *102*, 19219–19224.
60. Sibley, C.P.; Coan, P.M.; Ferguson-Smith, A.C.; Dean, W.; Hughes, J.; Smith, P.; Reik, W.; Burton, G.J.; Fowden, A.L.; Constancia, M. Placental-specific insulin-like growth factor 2 (Igf2) regulates the diffusional exchange characteristics of the mouse placenta. *Proc. Natl. Acad. Sci. USA* **2004**, *101*, 8204–8208.
61. Constancia, M.; Hemberger, M.; Hughes, J.; Dean, W.; Ferguson-Smith, A.; Fundele, R.; Stewart, F.; Kelsey, G.; Fowden, A.; Sibley, C.; *et al.* Placental-specific IGF-II is a major modulator of placental and fetal growth. *Nature* **2002**, *417*, 945–948.
62. Huppertz, B.; Kadyrov, M.; Kingdom, J.C. Apoptosis and its role in the trophoblast. *Am. J. Obstet. Gynecol.* **2006**, *195*, 29–39.
63. Klionsky, D.J.; Emr, S.D. Autophagy as a regulated pathway of cellular degradation. *Science* **2000**, *290*, 1717–1721.
64. Signorelli, P.; Avagliano, L.; Virgili, E.; Gagliostro, V.; Doi, P.; Braidotti, P.; Bulfamante, G.P.; Ghidoni, R.; Marconi, A.M. Autophagy in term normal human placentas. *Placenta* **2011**, *32*, 482–485.
65. Hung, T.H.; Hsieh, T.T.; Chen, S.F.; Li, M.J.; Yeh, Y.L. Autophagy in the human placenta throughout gestation. *PLoS One* **2013**, *8*, doi:10.1371/journal.pone.0083475.
66. Klionsky, D.J.; Abdalla, F.C.; Abeliovich, H.; Abraham, R.T.; Acevedo-Arozena, A.; Adeli, K.; Agholme, L.; Agnello, M.; Agostinis, P.; Aguirre-Ghiso, J.A.; *et al.* Guidelines for the use and interpretation of assays for monitoring autophagy. *Autophagy* **2012**, *8*, 445–544.
67. Crighton, D.; Wilkinson, S.; Ryan, K.M. Dram links autophagy to p53 and programmed cell death. *Autophagy* **2007**, *3*, 72–74.

68. Michael, A.E.; Thurston, L.M.; Rae, M.T. Glucocorticoid metabolism and reproduction: A tale of two enzymes. *Reproduction* **2003**, *126*, 425–441.
69. Korgun, E.T.; Ozmen, A.; Unek, G.; Mendilcioglu, I. *The Effects of Glucocorticoids on Fetal and Placental Development*; InTech: Rijeka, Croatia, 2012.
70. Alfaidy, N.; Li, W.; MacIntosh, T.; Yang, K.; Challis, J. Late gestation increase in 11beta-hydroxysteroid dehydrogenase 1 expression in human fetal membranes: A novel intrauterine source of cortisol. *J. Clin. Endocrinol. Metab.* **2003**, *88*, 5033–5038.
71. Shams, M.; Kilby, M.D.; Somerset, D.A.; Howie, A.J.; Gupta, A.; Wood, P.J.; Afnan, M.; Stewart, P.M. 11beta-hydroxysteroid dehydrogenase type 2 in human pregnancy and reduced expression in intrauterine growth restriction. *Hum. Reprod.* **1998**, *13*, 799–804.
72. Whorwood, C.B.; Firth, K.M.; Budge, H.; Symonds, M.E. Maternal undernutrition during early to midgestation programs tissue-specific alterations in the expression of the glucocorticoid receptor, 11beta-hydroxysteroid dehydrogenase isoforms, and type 1 angiotensin ii receptor in neonatal sheep. *Endocrinology* **2001**, *142*, 2854–2864.
73. Sibley, C.P.; Turner, M.A.; Cetin, I.; Ayuk, P.; Boyd, R.; D'Souza, S.W.; Glazier, J.D.; Greenwood, S.L.; Jansson, T.; Powell, T.L. Placental phenotypes of intrauterine growth. *Pediatr. Res.* **2005**, *58*, 827–832.
74. Brown, K.; Heller, D.S.; Zamudio, S.; Illsley, N.P. Glucose transporter 3 (GLUT3) protein expression in human placenta across gestation. *Placenta* **2011**, *32*, 1041–1049.
75. Magnusson, A.L.; Powell, T.L.; Wennergren, M.; Jansson, T. Glucose metabolism in the the human preterm and term placenta of IUGR fetuses. *Placenta* **2004**, *25*, 337–346.
76. DiGiacomo, J.E.; Hay, W.W., Jr. Placental-fetal glucose exchange and placental glucose consumption in pregnant sheep. *Am. J. Physiol.* **1990**, *258*, 360–367.
77. Hay, W.W., Jr. Placental-fetal glucose exchange and fetal glucose metabolism. *Trans. Am. Clin. Climatol. Assoc.* **2006**, *117*, 321–340.
78. Novakovic, B.; Gordon, L.; Robinson, W.P.; Desoye, G.; Saffery, R. Glucose as a fetal nutrients: Dynamic regulation of several glucose transporter genes by DNA methylation in the human placenta across gestation. *J. Nutr. Biochem.* **2013**, *24*, 282–288.
79. Dandrea, J.; Wilson, V.; Gopalakrishnan, G.; Heasman, L.; Budge, H.; Stephenson, T.; Symonds, M.E. Maternal nutritional manipulation of placental growth and glucose transporter 1 (GLUT-1) abundance in sheep. *Reproduction* **2001**, *122*, 793–800.
80. Larqué, E.; Ruiz-Palacios, M.R.; Koletzko, B. Placental regulation of fetal nutrient supply. *Curr. Opin. Clin. Nutr. Metab. Care* **2013**, *16*, 292–297.
81. Wooding, F.B.; Fowden, A.L.; Bell, A.W.; Ehrhardt, R.A.; Limesand, S.W.; Hay, W.W., Jr. Localisation of glucose transport in the ruminant placenta: Implications for sequential use of transporter isoforms. *Placenta* **2005**, *26*, 626–640.
82. Wolf, H.J.; Desoye, G. Immunohistochemical localization of glucose transporters and insulin receptors in human fetal membranes at term. *Histochemistry* **1993**, *100*, 379–385.
83. Xing, A.Y.; Challier, J.C.; Lepercq, J.; Cauzac, M.; Charron, M.J.; Girard, J.; Hauguel-de Mouzon, S. Unexpected expression of glucose transporter 4 in villous stromal cells of human placenta. *J. Clin. Endocrinol. Metab.* **1998**, *83*, 4097–4101.

84. Limesand, S.W.; Regnault, T.R.; Hay, W.W., Jr. Characterization of glucose transporter 8 (GLUT8) in the ovine placenta of normal and growth restricted fetuses. *Placenta* **2004**, *25*, 70–77.
85. Carayannopoulos, M.O.; Chi, M.M.; Cui, Y.; Pingsterhaus, J.M.; McKnight, R.A.; Mueckler, M.; Devaskar, S.U.; Moley, K.H. GLUT8 is a glucose transporter responsible for insulin-stimulated glucose uptake in the blastocyst. *Proc. Natl. Acad. Sci. USA* **2000**, *97*, 7313–7318.
86. Regnault, T.R.H.; Friedman, J.E.; Wilkening, R.B.; Anthony, R.V.; Hay, W.W., Jr. Fetoplacental transport and utilization of amino acids in IUGR. A review. *Placenta* **2005**, *26*, 52–62.
87. Grillo, M.A.; Lanza, A.; Colombatto, S. Transport of amino acids through the placenta and their role. *Amino Acids* **2008**, *34*, 517–523.
88. Desforges, M.; Sibley, C.P. Placental nutrient supply and fetal growth. *Int. J. Dev. Biol.* **2010**, *54*, 377–390.
89. Desforges, M.; Lacey, H.A.; Glazier, J.D.; Greenwood, S.L.; Mynett, K.J.; Speake, P.F.; Sibley, C.P. Snat4 isoform of system A amino acid transporter is expressed in human placenta. *Am. J. Physiol. Cell Physiol.* **2006**, *290*, 305–312.
90. Regnault, T.R.H.; de Vrijer, B.; Battaglia, F.C. Transport and metabolism of amino acids in placenta. *Endocrine* **2002**, *19*, 23–41.
91. Desforges, M.; Greenwood, S.L.; Glazier, J.D.; Westwood, M.; Sibley, C.P. The contribution of snat1 to system A amino acid transporter activity in human placental trophoblast. *Biochem. Biophys. Res. Commun.* **2010**, *398*, 130–134.
92. Verrey, F. System l: Heteromeric exchangers of large, neutral amino acids involved in directional transport. *Pflugers Arch.* **2003**, *445*, 529–533.
93. Okamoto, Y.; Sakata, M.; Ogura, K.; Yamamoto, T.; Yamaguchi, M.; Tasaka, K.; Kurachi, H.; Tsurudome, M.; Murata, Y. Expression and regulation of 4f2hc and hlat1 in human trophoblasts. *Am. J. Physiol.* **2002**, *282*, 196–204.
94. Gaccioli, F.; Roos, S.; Powell, T.L.; Jansson, T. Isoforms of the system L-amino acid transporter are differentially polarised to the syncytiotrophoblast plasma membrane in human placenta. *Reprod. Sci.* **2011**, *18*, 200.
95. Lewis, R.M.; Glazier, J.D.; Greenwood, S.L.; Bennett, E.J.; Godfrey, K.M.; Jackson, A.A.; Sibley, C.P.; Cameron, I.T.; Hanson, M.A. L-serine uptake by human placental microvillous membrane vesicles. *Placenta* **2007**, *28*, 445–452.
96. Kudo, Y.; Boyd, C.A.R. Characterisation of L-tryptophan transporters in human placenta: A comparison of brush border and basal membrane vesicles. *J. Physiol.* **2001**, *531*, 405–416.
97. Bodoy, S.; Martin, L.; Zorzano, A.; Palacin, M.; Estevez, R.; Bertran, J. Identification of lat4, a novel amino acid transporter with system l activity. *J. Biol. Chem.* **2005**, *280*, 12002–12011.
98. Babu, E.; Kanai, Y.; Chairoungdua, A.; Kim, D.K.; Iribe, Y.; Tangtrongsup, S.; Jutabha, P.; Li, Y.; Ahmed, N.; Sakamoto, S.; *et al*. Identification of a novel system l amino acid transporter structurally distinct from heterodimeric amino acid transporters. *J. Biol. Chem.* **2003**, *278*, 43838–43845.
99. Cleal, J.K.; Glazier, J.D.; Ntani, G.; Crozier, S.R.; Day, P.E.; Harvey, N.C.; Robinson, S.M.; Cooper, C.; Godfrey, K.M.; Hanson, M.A.; *et al*. Facilitated transporters mediate net efflux of amino acids to the fetus across the basal membrane of the placental syncytiotrophoblast. *J. Physiol.* **2011**, *589*, 987–997.

100. Cleal, J.K.; Brownbill, P.; Godfrey, K.M.; Jackson, J.M.; Jackson, A.A.; Sibley, C.P.; Hanson, M.A.; Lewis, R.M. Modification of fetal plasma amino acid composition by placental amino acid exchangers *in vitro*. *J. Physiol.* **2007**, *582*, 871–882.
101. Ayuk, P.T.; Sibley, C.P.; Donnai, P.; D'Souza, S.; Glazier, J.D. Development and polarization of cationic amino acid transporters and regulators in the human placenta. *Am. J. Physiol. Cell Physiol.* **2000**, *278*, 1162–1171.
102. Kamath, S.G.; Furesz, T.C.; Way, B.A.; Smith, C.H. Identification of three cationic amino acid transporters in placental trophoblast: Cloning, expression, and characterization of hcat-1. *J. Membr. Biol.* **1999**, *171*, 55–62.
103. Arriza, J.L.; Fairman, W.A.; Wadiche, J.I.; Murdoch, G.H.; Kavanaugh, M.P.; Amara, S.G. Functional comparisons of three glutamate transporter subtypes cloned from human motor cortex. *J. Neurosci.* **1994**, *14*, 5559–5569.
104. Fairman, W.A.; Vandenberg, R.J.; Arriza, J.L.; Kavanaugh, M.P.; Amara, S.G. An excitatory amino-acid transporter with properties of a ligand-gated chloride channel. *Nature* **1995**, *375*, 599–603.
105. Matthews, J.C.; Beveridge, M.J.; Malandro, M.S.; Rothstein, J.D.; Campbell-Thompson, M.; Verlander, J.W.; Kilberg, M.S.; Novak, D.A. Activity and protein localization of multiple glutamate transporters in gestation day 14 *vs.* Day 20 rat placenta. *Am. J. Physiol.* **1998**, *274*, 603–614.
106. Jansson, T. Amino acid transporters in the human placenta. *Pediatr. Res.* **2001**, *49*, 141–147.
107. Haggarty, P. Fatty acid supply to the human fetus. *Annu. Rev. Nutr.* **2010**, *30*, 237–255.
108. Kazantzis, M.; Stahl, A. Fatty acid transport proteins, implications in physiology and disease. *Biochim. Biophys. Acta* **2012**, *1821*, 852–857.
109. Schaiff, W.T.; Bildirici, I.; Cheong, M.; Chern, P.L.; Nelson, D.M.; Sadovsky, Y. Peroxisome proliferator-activated receptor-γ and retinoid X receptor signaling regulate fatty acid uptake by primary human placental trophoblasts. *J. Clin. Endocrinol. Metab.* **2005**, *90*, 4267–4275.
110. Campbell, F.M.; Bush, P.G.; Veerkamp, J.H.; Dutta-Roy, A.K. Detection and cellular localization of plasma membrane-associated and cytoplasmic fatty acid-binding proteins in human placenta. *Placenta* **1998**, *19*, 409–415.
111. Biron-Shental, T.; Schaiff, W.T.; Ratajczak, C.K.; Bildirici, I.; Nelson, D.M.; Sadovsky, Y. Hypoxia regulates the expression of fatty acid-binding proteins in primary term human trophoblasts. *Am. J. Obstet. Gynecol.* **2007**, *197*, 1–6.
112. McMillen, I.C.; Robinson, J.S. Developmental origins of the metabolic syndrome: Prediction, plasticity, and programming. *Physiol. Rev.* **2005**, *85*, 571–633.
113. Barker, D.J. Fetal programming of coronary heart disease. *Trends Endocrinol. Metab.* **2002**, *13*, 364–368.
114. Barker, D.J.; Osmond, C.; Forsen, T.J.; Kajantie, E.; Eriksson, J.G. Trajectories of growth among children who have coronary events as adults. *N. Engl. J. Med.* **2005**, *353*, 1802–1809.
115. Moore, V.M.; Miller, A.G.; Boulton, T.J.C.; Cockington, R.A.; Craig, I.H.; Magarey, A.M.; Robinson, J.S. Placental weight, birth measurements and blood pressure at age 8 years. *Arch. Dis. Child.* **1996**, *74*, 538–541.

116. McMillen, I.C.; Adams, M.B.; Ross, J.T.; Coulter, C.L.; Simonetta, G.; Owens, J.A.; Robinson, J.S.; Edwards, L.J. Fetal growth restriction: Adaptations and consequences. *Reproduction* **2001**, *122*, 195–204.
117. Morrison, J.L.; Duffield, J.A.; Muhulhausler, B.S.; Gentili, S.; McMillen, I.C. Fetal growth restriction, catch-up growth and the early origins of insulin resistance and visceral obesity. *Pediatr. Nephrol.* **2009**, *25*, 669–677.
118. Emmanouilides, G.C.; Townsend, D.E.; Bauer, R.A. Effects of single umbilical artery ligation in the lamb fetus. *Pediatrics* **1968**, *42*, 919–927.
119. Oh, W.; Omori, K.; Erenberg, A.; Emmanouilides, G.C. Umbilical blood flow and glucose uptake in lamb fetus following single umbilical artery ligation. *Biol. Neonate* **1975**, *26*, 291–299.
120. Cheung, C.Y.; Bogic, L.; Gagnon, R.; Harding, R.; Brace, R.A. Morphologic alterations in ovine placenta and fetal liver following induced severe placental insufficiency. *J. Soc. Gynecol. Investig.* **2004**, *11*, 521–528.
121. Sutherland, A.E.; Crossley, K.J.; Allison, B.J.; Jenkin, G.; Wallace, E.M.; Miller, S.L. The effects of intrauterine growth restriction and antenatal glucocorticoids on ovine fetal lung development. *Pediatr. Res.* **2012,** *76*, 689–696.
122. Early, R.J.; McBride, B.W.; Vatnick, I.; Bell, A.W. Chronic heat stress and prenatal development in sheep: Ii. Placental cellularity and metabolism. *J. Anim. Sci.* **1991**, *69*, 3610–3616.
123. Regnault, T.R.; Orbus, R.J.; de Vrijer, B.; Davidsen, M.L.; Galan, H.L.; Wilkening, R.B.; Anthony, R.V. Placental expression of VEGF, PLGF and their receptors in a model of placental insufficiency-intrauterine growth restriction (PI-IUGR). *Placenta* **2002**, *23*, 132–144.
124. Clapp, J.F., 3rd; Szeto, H.H.; Larrow, R.; Hewitt, J.; Mann, L.I. Umbilical blood flow response to embolization of the uterine circulation. *Am. J. Obstet. Gynecol.* **1980**, *138*, 60–67.
125. Gagnon, R.; Johnston, L.; Murotsuki, J. Fetal placental embolization in the late-gestation ovine fetus: Alterations in umbilical blood FLW and fetal heart rate patterns. *Am. J. Obstet. Gynecol.* **1996**, *175*, 63–72.
126. Louey, S.; Cock, M.L.; Stevenson, K.M.; Harding, R. Placental insufficiency and fetal growth restriction lead to postnatal hypotension and alterd postnatal growth in sheep. *Pediatr. Res.* **2000**, *48*, 808–814.
127. Owens, J.A.; Kind, K.L.; Carbone, F.; Robinson, J.S.; Owens, P.C. Circulating insulin-like growth factors-I and -II and substrates in fetal sheep following restriction of placental growth. *J. Endocrinol.* **1994**, *140*, 5–13.
128. Danielson, L.; IMcMillen, I.C.; Dyer, J.L.; Morrison, J.L. Restriction of placental growth results in greater hypotensive response to α-adrenergic blockade in sheep during late gestation. *J. Physiol.* **2005**, *563*, 611–620.
129. Soo, P.S.; Hiscock, J.; Botting, K.J.; Roberts, C.T.; Davey, A.K.; Morrison, J.L. Maternal undernutrition reduces P-glycoprotein in guinea pigs placenta and developing brain in late gestation. *Reprod. Toxicol.* **2012**, *33*, 374–381.
130. Robinson, J.S.; Kingston, E.J.; Jones, C.T.; Thornburn, G.D. Studies on experimental growth retardation in sheep. The effect of removal of endometrial caruncles on fetal size and metabolism. *J. Dev. Physiol.* **1979**, *1*, 379–398.

131. Chen, C.P.; Bajoria, R.; Aplin, J.D. Decreased vascularization and cell proliferation in placentas of intrauterine growth-restricted fetuses with abnormal umbilical artery flow velocity waveforms. *Am. J. Obstet. Gynecol.* **2002**, *187*, 764–769.
132. Mayhew, T.M.; Ohadike, C.; Baker, P.N.; Crocker, I.P.; Mitchell, C.; Ong, S.S. Stereological investigation of placental morphology in pregnancies complicated by pre-eclampsia with and without intrauterine growth restriction. *Placenta* **2003**, *24*, 219–226.
133. Krebs, C.; Macara, L.M.; Leiser, R.; Bowman, A.W.; Greer, I.A.; Kingdom, J.C. Intrauterine growth restriction with absent end-diastolic flow velocity in the umbilical artery is associated with maldevelopment of the placental terminal villous tree. *Am. J. Obstet. Gynecol.* **1996**, *175*, 1534–1542.
134. Roberts, C.T.; Owens, P.C.; Owens, J.A. Maternal food restriction reduces the exchange surface area and increases the barrier thickness of the placenta in the guinea pig. *Placenta* **2001**, *22*, 177–185.
135. Bacon, B.J.; Gilbert, R.D.; Kaufmann, P.; Smith, A.D.; Trevino, F.T.; Longo, L.D. Placental anatomy and diffusing capacity in guinea pigs following long-term maternal hypoxia. *Placenta* **1984**, *5*, 475–487.
136. Reshetnikova, O.S.; Burton, G.J.; Milovanov, A.P. Effects of hypobaric hypoxia on the fetoplacental unit: The morphometric diffusing capacity of the villous membrane at high altitude. *Am. J. Obstet. Gynecol.* **1994**, *171*, 1560–1565.
137. Parraguez, V.H.; Atlagich, M.; Diaz, R.; Cepeda, R.; Gonzalez, C.; de los Reyes, M.; Bruzzone, M.E.; Behn, C.; Raggi, L.A. Ovine placenta at high altitudes: Comparison of animals with different times of adaptation to hypoxic environment. *Anim. Reprod. Sci.* **2006**, *95*, 151–157.
138. Penninga, L.; Longo, L.D. Ovine placentome morphology: Effect of high altitude, long-term hypoxia. *Placenta* **1998**, *19*, 187–193.
139. Steyn, C.; Hawkins, P.; Saito, T.; Noakes, D.E.; Kingdom, J.C.P.; Hanson, M.A. Undernutrition during the first half of gestation increases the predominance of fetal tissue in late-gestation ovine placentomes. *Eur. J. Obstet. Gynecol. Reprod. Biol.* **2001**, *98*, 165–170.
140. Gardner, D.S.; Ward, J.W.; Giussani, D.A.; Fowden, A.L. The effect of a reversible period of adverse intrauterine conditions during late gestation on fetal and placental weight and placentome distribution in sheep. *Placenta* **2002**, *23*, 459–466.
141. Semenza, G.L. Hif-1: Mediator of physiological and pathophysiological responses to hypoxia. *J. Appl. Physiol.* **2000**, *88*, 1474–1480.
142. Caniggia, I.; Winter, J.L. Adriana and Luisa Castellucci award lecture 2001. Hypoxia inducible factor-1: Oxygen regulation of trophoblast differentiation in normal and pre-eclamptic pregnancies—A review. *Placenta* **2002**, *23*, 47–57.
143. Pringle, K.G.; Kind, K.L.; Thompson, J.G.; Roberts, C.T. Complex interactions between hypoxia inducible factors, insulin-like growth factor-ii and oxygen in early murine trophoblasts. *Placenta* **2007**, *28*, 1147–1157.
144. Wheeler, T.; Elcock, C.L.; Anthony, F.W. Angiogenesis and the placental environment. *Placenta* **1995**, *16*, 289–296.
145. Zhang, E.G.; Smith, S.K.; Baker, P.N.; Charnock-Jones, D.S. The regulation and localization of angiopoietin-1, -2, and their receptor tie2 in normal and pathologic human placentae. *Mol. Med.* **2001**, *7*, 624–635.

146. Toal, M.; Chan, C.; Fallah, S.; Alkazalen, F.; Chaddha, V.; Winderm, R.C.; Kingdom, J.C. Usefulness of a placental profile in high-risk pregnancies. *Am. J. Obstet. Gynecol.* **2007**, *196*, 363–371.
147. Pijnenborg, R.; Vercruysse, L.; Hanssens, M. The uterine spiral arteries in human pregnancy: Facts and controversies. *Placenta* **2006**, *27*, 939–958.
148. Lyall, F.; Young, A.; Boswell, F.; Kingdom, J.C.; Greer, I.A. Placental expression of vascular endothelial growth factor in placentae from pregnancies complicated by pre-eclampsia and intrauterine growth restriction does not support placental hypoxia at delivery. *Placenta* **1997**, *18*, 269–276.
149. Barut, F.; Barut, A.; Gun, B.D.; Kandemir, N.O.; Harma, M.I.; Harma, M.; Aktunc, E.; Ozdamar, S.O. Intrauterine growth restriction and placental angiogenesis. *Diagn. Pathol.* **2010**, *5*, doi:10.1186/1746-1596-5-24.
150. Akram, S.K.; Sahlin, L.; Ostlund, E.; Hagenas, L.; Fried, G.; Soder, O. Placental IGF-I, estrogen receptor, and progesterone receptor expression, and maternal anthropometry in growth-restricted pregnancies in the swedish population. *Horm. Res. Paediatr.* **2011**, *75*, 131–137.
151. Koutsaki, M.; Sifakis, S.; Zaravinos, A.; Koutroulakis, D.; Koukoura, O.; Spandidos, D.A. Decreased placental expression of hPGH, IGF-I and IGFBP-1 in pregnancies complicated by fetal growth restriction. *Growth Horm. IGF Res.* **2011**, *21*, 31–36.
152. De Vrijer, B.; Davidsen, M.L.; Wilkening, R.B.; Anthony, R.V.; Regnault, T.R. Altered placental and fetal expression of IGFS and IGF-binding proteins associated with intrauterine growth restriction in fetal sheep during early and mid-pregnancy. *Pediatr. Res.* **2006**, *60*, 507–512.
153. Cuffe, J.S.; Walton, S.L.; Singh, R.R.; Spiers, J.G.; Bielefeldt-Ohmann, H.; Wilkinson, L.; Little, M.H.; Moritz, K.M. Mid- to late term hypoxia in the mouse alters placental morphology, glucocorticoid regulatory pathways and nutrient transporters in a sex-specific manner. *J. Physiol.* **2014**, *592*, 3127–3141.
154. Erel, C.T.; Dane, B.; Calay, Z.; Kaleli, S.; Aydinli, K. Apoptosis in the placenta of pregnancies complicated with iugr. *Int. J. Gynaecol. Obstet.* **2001**, *73*, 229–235.
155. Smith, S.C.; Baker, P.N.; Symonds, E.M. Increased placental apoptosis in intrauterine growth restriction. *Am. J. Obstet. Gynecol.* **1997**, *177*, 1395–1401.
156. Levy, R.; Smith, S.D.; Chandler, K.; Sadovsky, Y.; Nelson, D.M. Apoptosis in human cultured trophoblasts is enhanced by hypoxia and diminished by epidermal growth factor. *Am. J. Physiol. Cell Physiol.* **2000**, *278*, 982–988.
157. Hung, T.H.; Chen, S.F.; Liou, J.D.; Hsu, J.J.; Li, M.J.; Yeh, Y.L.; Hsieh, T.T. Bax, Bak and mitochondrial oxidants are involved in hypoxia-reoxygenation-induced apoptosis in human placenta. *Placenta* **2008**, *29*, 565–583.
158. Levy, R.; Smith, S.D.; Yusuf, K.; Huettner, P.C.; Kraus, F.T.; Sadovsky, Y.; Nelson, D.M. Trophoblast apoptosis from pregnancies complicated by fetal growth restriction is associated with enhanced p53 expression. *Am. J. Obstet. Gynecol.* **2002**, *186*, 1056–1061.
159. Endo, H.; Okamoto, A.; Yamada, K.; Nikaido, T.; Tanaka, T. Frequent apoptosis in placental villi from pregnancies complicated with intrauterine growth restriction and without maternal symptoms. *Int. J. Mol. Med.* **2005**, *16*, 79–84.

160. Heazell, A.E.; Sharp, A.N.; Baker, P.N.; Crocker, I.P. Intra-uterine growth restriction is associated with increased apoptosis and altered expression of proteins in the p53 pathway in villous trophoblast. *Apoptosis* **2011**, *16*, 135–144.

161. Hung, T.H.; Chen, S.F.; Lo, L.M.; Li, M.J.; Yeh, Y.L.; Hsieh, T.T. Increased autophagy in placentas of intrauterine growth-restricted pregnancies. *PLoS One* **2012**, *7*, doi:10.1371/journal.pone.0040957.

162. Chen, B.; Longtine, M.S.; Nelson, D.M. Hypoxia induces autophagy in primary human trophoblasts. *Endocrinology* **2012**, *153*, 4946–4954.

163. Jaquiery, A.L.; Oliver, M.H.; Bloomfield, F.H.; Connor, K.L.; Challis, J.R.; Harding, J.E. Fetal exposure to excess glucocorticoid is unlikely to explain the effects of periconceptional undernutrition in sheep. *J. Physiol.* **2006**, *572*, 109–118.

164. Mericq, V.; Medina, P.; Kakarieka, E.; Marquez, L.; Johnson, M.C.; Iniguez, G. Differences in expression and activity of 11beta-hydroxysteroid dehydrogenase type 1 and 2 in human placentas of term pregnancies according to birth weight and gender. *Eur. J. Endocrinol.* **2009**, *161*, 419–425.

165. Zamudio, S.; Torricos, T.; Fik, E.; Oyala, M.; Echalar, L.; Pullockaran, J.; Tutino, E.; Martin, B.; Belliappa, S.; Balanza, E.; *et al.* Hypoglycemia and the origin of hypoxia-induced reduction in human fetal growth. *PLoS One* **2010**, *5*, doi:10.1371/journal.pone.0008551.

166. Owens, J.A.; Falconer, J.; Robinson, J.S. Restriction of placental size in sheep enhances efficiency of placental transfer of antipyrine, 3-o-methyl-d-glucose but not of urea. *J. Dev. Physiol.* **1987**, *9*, 457–464.

167. Owens, J.A.; Falconer, J.; Robinson, J.S. Effect of restriction of placental growth on fetal and utero-placental metabolism. *J. Dev. Physiol.* **1987**, *9*, 225–238.

168. Baumann, M.U.; Zamudio, S.; Illsley, N.P. Hypoxic upregulation of glucose transporters in BeWo choriocarcinoma cells is mediated by hypoxia-inducible factor-1. *Am. J. Physiol. Cell Physiol.* **2007**, *293*, 477–485.

169. Janzen, C.; Lei, M.Y.; Cho, J.; Sullivan, P.; Shin, B.C.; Devaskar, S.U. Placental glucose transporter 3 (GLUT3) is up-regulated in human pregnancies complicated by late-onset intrauterine growth restriction. *Placenta* **2013**, *34*, 1072–1078.

170. Dubova, E.A.; Pavlov, K.A.; Kulikova, G.V.; Shchegolev, A.I.; Sukhikh, G.T. Glucose transporters expression in the placental terminal villi of preeclampsia and intrauterine growth retardation complicated pregnancies. *Health* **2013**, *5*, 100–104.

171. Zamudio, S.; Baumann, M.U.; Illsley, N.P. Effects of chronic hypoxia *in vivo* on the expression of human placental glucose transporter. *Placenta* **2006**, *27*, 49–55.

172. Jansson, T.; Wennergren, M.; Illsley, N.P. Glucose transporter protein expression in human placenta throughout gestation and in intrauterine growth retardation. *J. Clin. Endocrinol. Metab.* **1993**, *77*, 1554–1562.

173. Jansson, T.; Ylven, K.; Wennergren, M.; Powell, T.L. Glucose transport and system A activity in syncytiotrophoblast microvillous and basal plasma membranes in intrauterine growth restriction. *Placenta* **2002**, *23*, 392–399.

174. Glazier, J.D.; Cetin, I.; Perugino, G.; Ronzoni, S.; Grey, A.M.; Mahendran, D.; Marconi, A.M.; Pardi, G.; Sibley, C.P. Association between the activity of the system A amino acid transporter in the microvillous plasma membrane of the human placenta and severity of fetal compromise in intrauterine growth restriction. *Pediatr. Res.* **1997**, *42*, 514–519.

175. Mando, C.; Tabano, S.; Pileri, P.; Colapietro, P.; Marino, M.A.; Avagliano, L.; Doi, P.; Bulfamante, G.; Miozzo, M.; Cetin, I. Snat2 expression and regulation in human growth-restricted placentas. *Pediatr. Res.* **2013**, *74*, 104–110.

176. Jansson, T.; Scholtbach, V.; Powell, T.L. Placental transport of leucine and lysine is reduced in intrauterine growth restriction. *Pediatr. Res.* **1998**, *44*, 532–537.

177. Paolini, C.L.; Marconi, A.M.; Ronzoni, S.; di Noio, M.; Fennessey, P.V.; Pardi, G.; Battaglia, F.C. Placental transport of leucine, phenylalanine, glycine, and proline in intrauterine growth-restricted pregnancies. *J. Clin. Endocrinol. Metab.* **2001**, *86*, 5427–5432.

178. Ross, J.C.; Fennessey, P.V.; Wilkening, R.B.; Battaglia, F.C.; Meschia, G. Placental transport and fetal utilization of leucine in a model of fetal growth retardation. *Am. J. Physiol.* **1996**, *270*, 491–503.

179. Anderson, A.H.; Fennessey, P.V.; Meschia, G.; Wilkening, R.B.; Battaglia, F.C. Placental transport of threonine and its utilization in the normal and growth-restricted fetus. *Am. J. Physiol.* **1997**, *272*, 892–900.

180. De Vrijer, B.; Regnault, T.R.; Wilkening, R.B.; Meschia, G.; Battaglia, F.C. Placental uptake and transport of ACP, a neutral nonmetabolizable amino acid, in an ovine model of fetal growth restriction. *Am. J. Physiol. Endocrinol. Metab.* **2004**, *287*, 1114–1124.

181. Godfrey, K.M.; Matthews, N.; Glazier, J.; Jackson, A.; Wilman, C.; Sibley, C.P. Neutral amino acid uptake by the microvillous plasma membrane of the human placenta is inversely related to fetal size at birth in normal pregnancy. *J. Clin. Endocrinol. Metab.* **1998**, *83*, 3320–3326.

182. Nelson, D.M.; Smith, S.D.; Furesz, T.C.; Sadovsky, Y.; Ganapathy, V.; Parvin, C.A.; Smith, C.H. Hypoxia reduces expression and function of system A amino acid transporters in cultured term human trophoblasts. *Am. J. Physiol. Cell Physiol.* **2003**, *284*, 310–315.

183. Mishima, T.; Miner, J.H.; Morizane, M.; Stahl, A.; Sadovsky, Y. The expression and function of fatty acid transport protein-2 and -4 in the murine placenta. *PLoS One* **2011**, *6*, doi:10.1371/journal.pone.0025865.

184. Laivuori, H.; Gallaher, M.J.; Collura, L.; Crombleholme, W.R.; Markovic, N.; Rajakumar, A.; Hubel, C.A.; Roberts, J.M.; Powers, R.W. Relationships between maternal plasma leptin, placental leptin mRNA and protein in normal pregnancy, pre-eclampsia and intrauterine growth restriction without pre-eclampsia. *Mol. Hum. Reprod.* **2006**, *12*, 551–556.

8

Developmental Programming of Cardiovascular Disease Following Intrauterine Growth Restriction: Findings Utilising a Rat Model of Maternal Protein Restriction

Vladislava Zohdi [1,†], Kyungjoon Lim [2,†], James T. Pearson [3,4,*] and M. Jane Black [1]

1 Department of Anatomy and Developmental Biology, Monash University, Melbourne, VIC 3800, Australia; E-Mails: vladislava.zohdi@monash.edu (V.Z.); jane.black@monash.edu (M.J.B.)
2 Neuropharmacology Laboratory, Baker IDI Heart and Diabetes Institute, P.O. Box 6492 St Kilda Rd Central, Melbourne 8008, Australia; E-Mail: joon.lim@bakeridi.edu.au
3 Department of Physiology, Monash University, Melbourne, VIC 3800, Australia
4 Monash Biomedical Imaging, Monash University, Melbourne, VIC 3800, Australia

† These authors contributed equally to this work.

* Author to whom correspondence should be addressed; E-Mail: james.pearson@monash.edu

---

Abstract: Over recent years, studies have demonstrated links between risk of cardiovascular disease in adulthood and adverse events that occurred very early in life during fetal development. The concept that there are embryonic and fetal adaptive responses to a sub-optimal intrauterine environment often brought about by poor maternal diet that result in permanent adverse consequences to life-long health is consistent with the definition of "programming". The purpose of this review is to provide an overview of the current knowledge of the effects of intrauterine growth restriction (IUGR) on long-term cardiac structure and function, with particular emphasis on the effects of maternal protein restriction. Much of our recent knowledge has been derived from animal models. We review the current literature of one of the most commonly used models of IUGR (maternal protein restriction in rats), in relation to birth weight and postnatal growth, blood pressure and cardiac structure and function. In doing so, we highlight the complexity of developmental programming, with regards to timing, degree of severity of the insult, genotype and the subsequent postnatal phenotype.

Keywords: diabetes; heart; IUGR; hypertension; maternal diet

1. Introduction

The importance of maternal nutrition to growth of the foetus has long been recognised with inadequate maternal nutrition, as a result of undernutrition and/or malnutrition, linked to induction of intrauterine growth restriction (IUGR) and potential adverse impacts on lifelong health of the offspring. Importantly, over recent decades both epidemiological and experimental studies have shown an association between IUGR and an increased risk of cardiovascular disease later in life [1–6]. This association has been linked to "developmental programming" whereby sub-optimal growth during pregnancy results in fetal adaptations, including altered organogenesis, which can then render the offspring vulnerable to disease processes later in life [7]. The purpose of this review is to provide an overview of the current knowledge relating to IUGR and the long-term effects of IUGR on the heart. There is particular emphasis on maternal protein restriction which is a popular animal model used to induce IUGR and the subsequent effects on long-term cardiac health.

2. Low Birth Weight is Linked to Long-Term Cardiovascular Disease

It is now well established that events occurring during early life can also impact on long term levels of blood pressure and cardiovascular health [8–11], with impaired growth in early life leading to long term vulnerability to cardiovascular disease. Over recent decades many epidemiological studies have linked low birth weight with long term heart disease [12–17] and with other disease processes that are directly associated with an increased propensity for cardiovascular disease, such as metabolic disease [18,19], insulin resistance [20,21], non-insulin dependent diabetes [22,23], renal disease [24] and hypertension [25,26].

In 1977, Forsdahl was the first to report a close correlation between increased rates of death from ischaemic heart disease and poverty in childhood and adolescent years in Norway [27]. Similar relationships were reported in early studies from England and Wales [28]. In the 1980s Barker and colleagues reported in a cohort of 10,141 men from Hertfordshire, England, born between 1911 and 1930 that the incidence of death from ischaemic heart disease was highest in the men with lowest birth weights and weights at one year of age, compared to individuals of normal birth weight; this was independent of lifestyle factors [29]. This is when the importance of maternal diet during pregnancy to the long-term health of her offspring was first recognised.

Since then, there have been many epidemiological studies in many populations worldwide that have confirmed these observations [3,11,15,30–35]. Of particular interest are the findings of the Nurses' Health Study in which the health of 121,700 women in the USA was retrospectively followed up from 1976 and interestingly, the strong associations between low birth weight and coronary heart disease remained after adjustments were made for adult smoking, physical activity, dietary habits and socio-economic status [3]. This association is strongest when there is accelerated body growth after birth [4,15,36–40] and collectively, these studies suggest that it is the accelerated postnatal growth that characteristically occurs in small-for-gestational age infants, rather than low birth weight per se, that leads to the increased risk of cardiovascular disease later in life.

Negative correlations between birth weight and levels of blood pressure in adult life are also now well established [41–44]. The first studies indicating that high blood pressure might have its origins in utero were population-based studies in the UK and other parts of Europe [8,9,31,45–47]. These studies have pointed out that an increase in birth weight was associated with a fall in blood pressure in adulthood. These correlations are reported to remain regardless of common risk factors such as alcohol consumption and body mass index in adulthood [48–50]. The results from a longitudinal study by Uiterwaal and colleagues following up 252 males and 231 females for 14 years demonstrated a strong and consistent inverse association between birth weight and systolic blood pressure after adjustment for body weight and height. This association persisted from adolescence into adulthood [49]. The links between IUGR and increased risk of disease in adulthood appear to be strongest when there is an accelerated postnatal catch up in growth [51,52].

3. Catch-Up Growth

The "catch-up" growth or "postnatal accelerated growth" hypothesis was proposed approximately fifteen years ago by Alan Lucas and Atul Singhal [53,54]. This hypothesis proposes deleterious consequences to offspring when postnatal growth rate exceeds otherwise normal linear growth, predisposing subjects to increased risk of developing metabolic and cardiovascular disease.

It is well established that postnatal weight gain is an important indicator for the programming of adult disease [55]. Accelerated weight gain in childhood is itself a risk factor for elevated blood pressure later in life [56,57] and this is likely to be compounded by low birth weight. Findings from a number of clinical studies have revealed that postnatal catch-up in growth in low birth weight subjects can lead to adverse effects on cognitive function [58], blood pressure [37], cardiac function [59–61], insulin sensitivity and secretion [62], development of type 2 diabetes [63] and obesity [64] both in childhood and in early adulthood. For example, in a study from Helsinki, low birth weight children who had not only caught-up in body weight with their age matched counterparts, but were heavier by the seventh year of life were shown to develop hypertension in adulthood [65] and coronary heart disease [15]. In another study metabolic syndrome has also been reported in men at 58 years of age [66] who were born of low birth weight and experienced accelerated catch-up growth in early adulthood, up to 18 years of age. In a prospective Australian study, where a longitudinal pregnancy cohort was followed up from birth until 13 years of age, it was reported that growth trajectory in childhood predicted cardiovascular risk; cardiovascular risk was high in adolescents with restricted prenatal growth followed by accelerated postnatal growth [38]. In addition, a prospective US study where data were collected from a large biracial cohort of pregnant women and their offspring concluded that increasing growth percentiles during any period of early childhood increases the risk for high blood pressure [37].

4. Low Birth Weight and IUGR

Low birth weight is defined as birth weight below 2.5 kg [67], irrespective of gestational age and is universal to all ethnic groups/populations (according to the World Health Organisation) and can result from inappropriate growth in utero [68], preterm birth [69] or a combination of both. This review focuses on the effect of IUGR rather than preterm birth.

In clinical practice IUGR is generally assigned to small for gestational age infants with a birth weight and/or birth length below the 10th percentile for gestational age [70]. It occurs as an abnormal restriction of foetal growth due to adverse genetic or environmental influences [71].

In general, growth restriction commencing from early pregnancy leads to proportional or symmetrical growth restriction, whereas in infants where there is mid-trimester or third trimester growth restriction there is disproportionate or asymmetrical growth restriction [72]. When there is symmetrical growth restriction the growth of the head, femur and abdomen is equally affected [71], whereas in asymmetric growth restriction there is disproportional growth of the foetus, with preferential blood flow to the brain, termed brain sparing, resulting in a baby with a relatively normal head size but a below normal body size [73]. This asymmetric type of growth restriction develops when oxygen or substrate supply to the foetus is reduced during the last trimester of pregnancy, often due to a reduced functional capacity of the placenta [74]. There are a number of studies suggesting that asymmetrical growth restriction in foetuses results in a worse outcome later in life than symmetrical growth restriction [75].

IUGR is not a specific disease per se but a manifestation of many maternal and foetal factors leading to poor foetal growth. There are many causes of IUGR including environmental and genetic factors. In general, IUGR usually results from nutrient and/or oxygen deprivation to the foetus, often due to both maternal and foetal factors [76]. Experimental evidence indicates that the primary environmental factor that regulates foetal growth in animals and humans is nutrient delivery to the foetus [70,77]. Nutrient delivery is dependent on maternal nutritional intake and adequate maternal blood flow, which is essential for normal placental function [78]. In developed countries placental insufficiency is the leading cause of IUGR [76], whereas in developing countries maternal malnutrition is the major cause of IUGR resulting from long-term nutrient deprivation to the growing foetus [79]. As a result of the early observations of the link between IUGR and long term disease the developmental programming hypothesis evolved.

5. Early Life Programming for Long-Term Disease

The concept that there are embryonic and foetal adaptive responses to a suboptimal intrauterine environment that result in permanent adverse consequences is consistent with the definition of "programming" [80,81]. "Programming" refers to the idea that an insult or stimulus applied during a critical or sensitive period of development can have long lasting or persistent effects on the structure or function of an organism [53]; the "programming" can be either beneficial or detrimental to long term health. Both prenatal life and early postnatal life are "critical periods" that are characterised by a high degree of plasticity [82–84] and a high cell proliferation rate in the developing tissues [85,86]. Therefore, exposure to an adverse stimulus during these "critical periods" can lead to detrimental consequences in the growth of tissues and organs [55,87], which in turn, can cause persistent alterations in body function. In addition, adaptive programming of the foetus to IUGR can lead to modifications of biochemical and hormonal pathways within the foetus, again rendering the individual susceptible to disease later in life [88].

Potential programming effects on tissue structure and on the number of functional units formed in vital organs.

Adverse environmental factors acting during the developmental period have the potential to disturb the processes of cell proliferation and differentiation [89]. The vulnerability of particular organs and organ systems to exposure to insults during gestation usually coincides with the periods in development when the organs are first forming and/or during "critical periods" of cellular proliferation and differentiation [85,90]. Indeed, a reduction in cell number, or a change in the balance of cell types within tissues, has been observed in a number of animal models in response to an altered intrauterine environment [91,92]. Such changes may account for subsequent alterations in gene expression and physiological function. Certainly, a reduction in the complement of the functional units within vital organs has the potential to adversely impact on the functional capacity and adaptive capabilities in adulthood. This is especially important given that the proliferative capacity of the functional units in many vital organs usually ceases prior to birth, or soon after birth, hence reduced foetal growth can lead to a lifelong deficit in the functional capacity of vital organs (Figure 1).

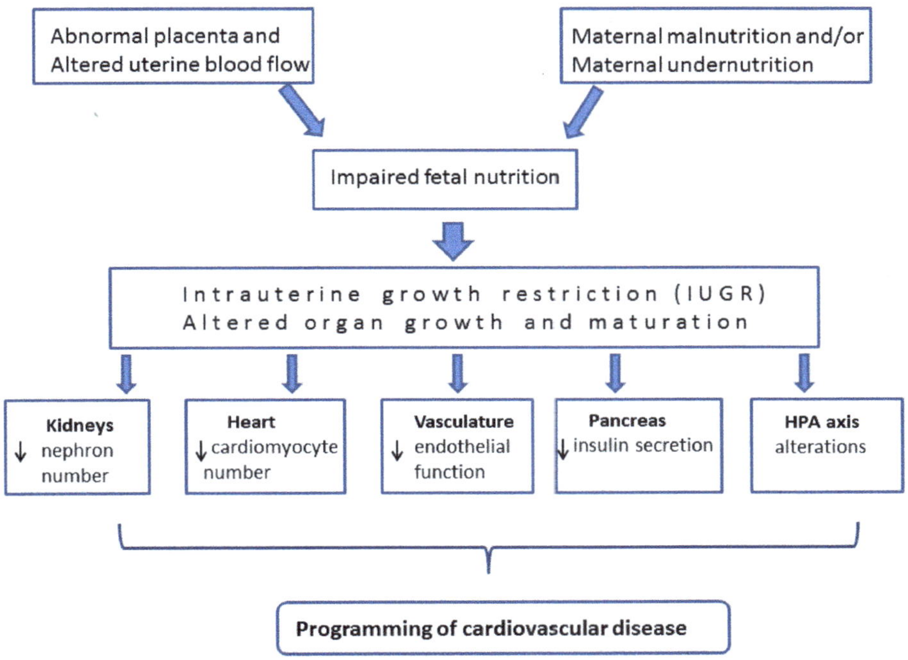

Figure 1. Diagram showing how impaired maternal nutrition and/or abnormal placental function leads to intrauterine growth restriction (IUGR) and subsequent changes to organs that play a key role in cardiovascular function. These changes have the potential to program for long-term cardiovascular disease.

For example, a reduction in:

(1) Nephron number has been observed in offspring in response to a maternal prenatal low-protein diet in the rat [93,94], mouse [95], and following uterine artery ligation in the guinea pig [96] and rabbit [97] and following placental embolization in sheep [98].
(2) Total cardiomyocyte number in the offspring of rats exposed to maternal protein restriction or placental insufficiency during pregnancy [99] and in lambs exposed to placental insufficiency the total complement of cardiomyocytes has been shown to be directly related to heart size [100].
(3) The numbers of secondary muscle fibres has been reported in the young offspring of a variety of species, including rats [101], pigs [102] and sheep [103] following maternal undernutrition during the critical proliferative period for muscle fibre development.

(4) Total pancreatic weight, islet cell mass and the relative proportion of β-cells within the islets [104] has been reported to be lower in IUGR rat offspring.

Furthermore, it has been shown that the vasculature undergoes permanent changes in reactivity as a result of maternal nutrient restriction [105]. In addition, there are reports of persistent alterations of the hypothalamic-pituitary-adrenal (HPA) axis of IUGR rat offspring [106,107] and this is postulated to play a critical role in the observed association between foetal growth restriction and subsequent cardiovascular and metabolic diseases.

Figure 1 collectively shows the sequence of events that can potentially lead to the programming for increased risk of cardiovascular disease in IUGR offspring.

6. Animal Model of IUGR—Maternal Protein Restriction in Rats

Much of our knowledge relating to the short term and long-term effects of IUGR has been derived from animal studies. A number of animal models of poor maternal nutrition and/or placental insufficiency have been developed over recent years to investigate the causes and consequences of IUGR. A variety of species have been studied, including: rodents, sheep and primates; and both, maternal dietary manipulations or surgical interventional techniques have been employed [108–114]. One of the most extensively studied and well-characterised animal models is maternal protein restriction in rats. Regardless of how severe the protein restriction is (mild- 9% diet or severe- 5% diet) the end result is reduction in body weight of the offspring [115–119].

In our laboratory over the past decade we have comprehensively examined the cardiovascular phenotype of rat offspring following maternal protein restriction. However, as our studies have progressed, it has become clearly apparent, that the cardiovascular and metabolic phenotype of the offspring using this model differs between different laboratories, which likely relates to subtle differences in study design. This in turn, makes comparison of the findings between studies difficult. For example, there are differences in the strain of rats studied, levels of maternal protein restriction in the diet, timing of administration of the diet to the dams and postnatal differences in body growth and levels of blood pressure of the offspring. These differences are highlighted in Table 1.

In our studies, Wistar-Kyoto (WKY) female breeder rats are fed a low protein diet for two weeks prior to birth to get the dams accustomed to the diet, then during pregnancy and for two weeks during lactation as the rodent organ systems are still developing in the early postnatal period. To avoid a high mortality rate in the offspring [120] we have chosen moderate protein restriction (8.7% casein in the diet) for the dams [121–128], rather than a more severe protein deprivation (6% casein) that is sometimes used by other investigators [129–131].

In the following sections we compare our findings with others; in doing so, we highlight differences in the maternal protein restriction model, which may account for conflicting findings between laboratories (Table 1).

Table 1. Studies investigating the effects of administration of a maternal low protein diet (LPD) in rats on the phenotype of the offspring—highlighting differences in the rat strains studied, severity of the dietary protein restriction and the timing of the diet administration. The table is organized according to the severity of maternal protein restriction. Studies conducted in our laboratory are highlighted in grey.

Author and Year of the Study	Rat Strain and Age of Offspring at Investigation	Diets	Timing of the Diet	Major Findings in the LPD Group
Woods *et al.* 2004 [93]	Sprague-Dawley 22 weeks	NPD: 19.0% casein LPD: 5.0% casein	During pregnancy	↓ birth wt ↓ body wt at 22 weeks ↓ nephron number ↑ MAP at 22 weeks
Dagan *et al.* 2009 [132]	Sprague-Dawley 6 weeks	NPD: 20.0% casein LPD: 6.0% casein	During pregnancy	↑ SBP at 6 weeks birth wt and body wt were not reported
Habib *et al.* 2011 [133]	Sprague-Dawley 9 and 12 weeks	NPD: 20.0% casein LPD: 6.0% casein	During pregnancy	↓ birth wt ↓ body wt at 12 weeks ↑SBP at 9 and 12 weeks ↓ nephron number
Langley and Jackson, 1994 [134]	Wistar 9 and 21 weeks	NPD: 18.0% casein LPD: 12.0% , 9%, and 6% casein	2 weeks prior to and during pregnancy	↓ body wt in 6%LPD group at 21 weeks ↔ body wt in 9% and 12% LPD group at 21 weeks ↑ SBP in all three LPD groups at 9 weeks ↑ SBP in 9% and 6% LPD groups at 21 weeks
Manning *et al.* 2002 [130]	Sprague-Dawley 4 and 8 weeks	NPD: 20.0% casein LPD: 6.0% casein	During pregnancy	↓ birth wt ↔ body wt at 4 weeks ↔ SBP at 4 weeks ↑ SBP at 8 weeks

Table 1. *Cont.*

Manning and Vehaskari, 2001 [135]	Sprague-Dawley 4, 8 and 45 weeks	NPD: 20.0% casein LPD: 6.0% casein	During pregnancy	↓birth wt ↔ body wt at 4 weeks ↑ SBP at 8 until 40 weeks ↓ survival rate at 45 weeks
Sathishkumar *et al.* 2009 [131]	Sprague-Dawley 52 weeks	NPD: 18.0% casein LPD: 6.0% casein	During pregnancy	↓ birth wt ↓ body weight at 52 weeks ↑ MAP at 52 weeks ↑ vascular contraction ↓ vascular relaxation
Tonkiss *et al.* 1998 [136]	Sprague-Dawley 14 weeks	NPD: 25.0% casein LPD: 6.0% casein	5 weeks prior to and during pregnancy	↓ birth wt ↔ body wt at 14 weeks ↑ DBP at 14 weeks ↔ SBP at 14 weeks
Vehaskari *et al.* 2001 [137]	Sprague-Dawley 8 weeks and 78 weeks	NPD: 20.0% casein LPD: 6.0% casein	During pregnancy	↓birth wt ↔ body wt at 2 weeks ↔ SBP at 4 weeks ↑ SBP at 8 weeks ↓ survival at 78 weeks
Coupe *et al.* 2009 [138]	Sprague-Dawley 36 weeks	NPD: 20.0% casein LPD: 8.0% casein	During pregnancy	↓ birth wt ↔ body wt at 36 weeks ↓ triglycerides, glucose
Hoppe *et al.* 2007 [95]	Sprague-Dawley 4 and 19 weeks	NPD: 20.0% casein LPD: 8.0% casein	2 weeks prior to and during pregnancy and 3 weeks postnatally	↓ body wt at 4 and 19 weeks ↓ organ weights (except brain) ↓ MAP at 19 weeks ↓ nephron number
Ozanne *et al.* 1996 [121]	Wistar 12 weeks	NPD: 20.0% casein LPD: 8.0% casein	During pregnancy and 3weeks postnatally	↓ body wt at 12 weeks ↓ size of tibialis anterior muscle ↑ insulin sensitivity

Table 1. *Cont.*

Plank *et al.* 2006 [124]	Wistar 10 weeks	NPD: 17.0% casein LPD: 8.0% casein	During pregnancy	↓ birth wt ↓ body length at birth ↔ body wt at 8 weeks ↔ MAP at 10 weeks ↑ inflammatory markers
Plank *et al.* 2008 [139]	Wistar 17 weeks	NPD: 17.0% casein LPD: 8.0% casein	During pregnancy	↓ birth wt ↓ body length at birth ↓ body wt at 3weeks ↔ body length at 3 weeks ↔ body wt at 17 weeks ↑ MAP at 17 weeks
Zeng *et al.* 2013 [140]	Sprague-Dawley 1 to 78 weeks	NPD: 20.0% casein LPD: 8.0% casein	During pregnancy	↓ birth weight ↔ body wt at 4 and 8 weeks ↑ body wt at 12, 52 and 78 weeks ↑ insulin secretion
Menendez-Castro *et al.* 2011 [141]	Wistar 10 weeks	NPD: 17.2% casein LPD: 8.4% casein	During pregnancy	↓ birth wt ↓ body wt at 10 weeks ↔ relative heart wt ↔ MAP at 10 weeks ↔ SBP at 10 weeks ↑ myocardial collagen I and collagen IV at 10 weeks
Menendez-Castro *et al.* 2014 [6]	Wistar 10 weeks	NPD: 17.2% casein LPD: 8.4% casein	During pregnancy	↓ ejection fraction ↓ fractional shortening ↑ LV diameters at systole and diastole at 10 weeks

Table 1. *Cont.*

Woods *et al.* 2001 [122]	Sprague-Dawley 21 weeks	NPD: 19.0% casein LPD: 8.5% casein	During pregnancy	↓ birth wt ↔ body wt at 3 and 21 weeks ↓ nephron number at 21 weeks ↑ MAP at 21 weeks
Woods *et al.* 2005 [142]	Sprague-Dawley 22 and 50 weeks	NPD: 19.0% casein LPD: 8.5% casein	During pregnancy	↓ birth wt ↔ body wt at 4 and 22 weeks ↓ body wt at 50 weeks ↔ MAP at 22 and 50 weeks ↔ nephron number
Corstius *et al.* 2005 [99]	WKY at birth	NPD: 20.0% casein LPD: 8.7% casein	2 weeks prior to and during pregnancy and 2 weeks postnatally	↓ birth wt ↓ heart wt ↓ cardiomyocyte number
Lim *et al.* 2006 [143]	WKY 24 weeks	NPD: 20.0% casein LPD: 8.7% casein	2 weeks prior to and during pregnancy and 2 weeks postnatally	↓ body wt at 2 and 24 weeks ↔ heart wt at 24 weeks ↑ LV + S interstitial fibrosis
Lim *et al.* 2010 [144]	WKY 4 weeks	NPD: 20.0% casein LPD: 8.7% casein	2 weeks prior to and during pregnancy and 2 weeks postnatally	↓ body wt at 4 weeks ↑ relative heart volume at 4weeks ↔ cardiomyocyte number
Lim *et al.* 2011a [145]	WKY 32 weeks	NPD: 20.0% casein LPD: 8.7% casein	2 weeks prior to and during pregnancy and 2 weeks postnatally	↓ birth wt ↓ body wt at 32 weeks ↑ insulin sensitivity ↔ SBP at 32 weeks ↔ body composition ↔ locomotor activity
Lim *et al.* 2011b [146]	WKY 32 weeks	NPD: 20.0% casein LPD: 8.7% casein	2 weeks prior to and during pregnancy and 2 weeks postnatally	↓ birth wt ↓ body wt at 32 weeks ↓ kidney wt at 32 weeks ↔ MAP at 32 weeks

Table 1. *Cont.*

Lim *et al.* 2012 [147]	WKY 32 weeks	NPD: 20.0% casein LPD: 8.7% casein	2 weeks prior to and during pregnancy and 2 weeks postnatally	↓ body wt at 32 ↑ relative heart wt ↑ LV + S interstitial fibrosis ↔ SBP at 32 weeks
Zimanyi *et al.* 2004 [117]	WKY 4 and 40 weeks	NPD: 20.0% casein LPD: 8.7% casein	2 weeks prior to and during pregnancy and 2 weeks postnatally	↓ birth wt ↓ body wt at 40 weeks ↓ kidney volume, nephron number at 4 weeks ↔ SBP at 40 weeks
Zimanyi *et al.* 2006 [94]	WKY 4 and 24 weeks	NPD: 20.0% casein LPD: 8.7% casein	2 weeks prior to and during pregnancy and 2 weeks postnatally	↓ birth wt ↓ body wt at 24 weeks ↓ nephron number at 4 weeks ↔ MAP at 24 weeks
Zohdi *et al.* 2011 [148]	WKY 14 weeks	NPD: 20.0% casein LPD: 8.7% casein	2 weeks prior to and during pregnancy and 2 weeks postnatally	↓ birth wt ↓ body wt at 14 weeks ↓ heart wt at 14 weeks ↔ MAP at 14 weeks ↑ arterial elastance, total peripheral resistance
Zohdi *et al.* 2013 [149]	WKY 18 weeks	NPD: 20.0% casein LPD: 8.7% casein	2 weeks prior to and during pregnancy and 2 weeks postnatally	↓ birth wt ↓ body wt at 18 weeks ↔ heart weight at 18 weeks ↔ cardiac fibrosis ↑ biochemical composition in the heart

Table 1. *Cont.*

Zohdi *et al.* 2014 [150]	WKY 18 weeks	NPD: 20.0% casein LPD: 8.7% casein	2 weeks prior to and during pregnancy and 2 weeks postnatally	↓ birth wt ↓ body wt at 18 weeks ↓ aortic peak systolic velocity at 18 weeks ↔ SBP at 18 weeks ↔ basal cardiac function at 18 weeks
Alwasel and Ashton, 2009 [125]	Wistar 4 weeks	NPD: 18.0% casein LPD: 9.0% casein	During pregnancy	↔ body wt at 4 weeks ↑ MAP
Bellinger *et al.* 2006 [123]	Wistar 36 weeks and 72 weeks	NPD: 18.0% casein LPD: 9.0% casein	During pregnancy	↔ birth wt ↔ body wt at 36 weeks ↓ body wt at 72 weeks
Boubred *et al.* 2009 [126]	Sprague-Dawley 4, 8, 16, 52 and 100 weeks	NPD: 22.0% casein LPD: 9.0% casein	During pregnancy	↓ birth wt ↔ SBP at 4 and 52 weeks ↑ SBP at 8 and 16 weeks ↔ body wt at 100 weeks
Brawley *et al.* 2003 [151]	Wistar 18 weeks	NPD: 18.0% casein LPD: 9.0% casein	During pregnancy	↔ birth wt ↓ body wt at 9 weeks ↔ body wt at 18 weeks ↑ SBP at 18 weeks
Cheema *et al.* 2005 [118]	Wistar 1–40 weeks	NPD: 18.0% casein LPD: 9.0% casein	2 weeks prior and during pregnancy	↓ birth wt ↓ body wt at 40 weeks LV hypertrophy at 40 weeks
Elmes *et al.* 2007 [152]	Wistar 4, 8 and 24 weeks	NPD: 18.0% casein LPD: 9.0% casein	During pregnancy	↑ SBP at 4 and 8 weeks ↔ baseline cardiac function ↓ recovery to myocardial ischemia at 24 weeks

Table 1. *Cont.*

Gardner *et al.* 1997 [153]	Wistar 6 weeks	NPD: 18.0% casein LPD: 9.0% casein	2 weeks prior to and during pregnancy	↔ body wt at 6 weeks ↑ SBP at 6 weeks
Harrison and Langley-Evans, 2009 [154]	Wistar, 8 and 10 weeks F_1, F_2, F_3 generational study	NPD: 18.0% casein LPD: 9.0% casein	During pregnancy	↔ body wt at 10 weeks in all generations ↑ SBP at 8 weeks in F_1 and F_2 ↓ nephron number in F_1 and F_2
Langley-Evans *et al.* 1994 [155]	Wistar 4 weeks	NPD: 18.0% casein LPD: 9.0% casein	2 weeks prior to and during pregnancy	↓ birth wt ↑ SBP at 4 weeks
Langley-Evans *et al.* 1996 [156]	Wistar 7 weeks	NPD: 18.0% casein LPD: 9.0% casein	During pregnancy	↓ birth wt ↔ body wt at 7 weeks ↑ SBP at 7 weeks
Langley-Evans *et al.* 1999 [116]	Wistar 4 and 19 weeks	NPD: 18.0% casein LPD: 9.0% casein	2 weeks prior to and during pregnancy	↔ body wt at 4 and 19 weeks ↑ SBP at 4 and 19 weeks
McMullen and Langley-Evans, 2005 [157]	Wistar 4 weeks	NPD: 18.0% casein LPD: 9.0% casein	During pregnancy	↔ birth wt ↔ body wt at 4 weeks ↑ SBP at 4 weeks
McMullen *et al.* 2004 [158]	Wistar 4 weeks	NPD: 18.0% casein LPD: 9.0% casein	2 weeks prior to and during pregnancy	↑ SBP at 4 weeks ↓ nephron number birth wt and body wt were not reported
Mehta *et al.* 2002 [159]	Wistar 52 weeks	NPD: 18.0% casein LPD: 9.0% casein	During pregnancy	↔ birth wt ↔ body wt at 52 weeks ↓ bone mineral content ↓ bone mineral density

Table 1. *Cont.*

Nwagwu *et al.* 2000 [160]	Wistar 4, 12 and 20 weeks	NPD: 18.0% casein LPD: 9.0% casein	During pregnancy	↔ birth wt ↑ SBP at all three ages ↓ kidney: body wt at 4weeks ↔ kidney morphometry at 12 weeks
Pladys *et al.* 2005 [161]	Wistar 9 to12 weeks	NPD: 18.0% casein LPD: 9.0% casein	During pregnancy	↔ birth wt ↔ body wt at 12 weeks ↑ MAP at 9 to 12 weeks ↔ adult arterial structure
Sherman and Langley-Evans, 2000 [127]	Wistar 4 and 12 weeks	NPD: 18.0% casein LPD: 9.0% casein	During pregnancy	↑ body wt at 4 weeks ↔ body wt at 12 weeks ↑ SBP at 4 and 12 weeks
Swali *et al.* 2010 [128]	Wistar 4, 8 and 12 weeks	NPD: 18.0% casein LPD: 9.0% casein	During pregnancy	↔ birth wt ↔ body wt between 4 and 12 weeks ↔ SBP at 4 weeks ↑ SBP at 8 weeks ↓ SBP at 12 weeks
Tappia *et al.* 2005 [162]	Wistar 3 weeks	NPD: 18.0% casein LPD: 9.0% casein	2 weeks prior to and during pregnancy	↓ birth wt ↓ saturated cardiac fatty acids ↑ unsaturated cardiac fatty acids
Tappia *et al.* 2011 [163]	Wistar 1, 4 and 8 weeks	NPD: 18.0% casein LPD: 9.0% casein	2 weeks prior to and during pregnancy	↑ LV internal diameter at all ages ↑ LV wall thickness at 4 weeks
Torrens *et al.* 2006 [164]	Wistar 15 weeks	NPD: 18.0% casein LPD: 9.0% casein	2 weeks prior to and during pregnancy	↔ birth weights ↑ SBP at 15 weeks
Ohishi *et al.* 2012 [165]	Sprague-Dawley 10 weeks	NPD: 20.0% casein LPD: 10.0% casein	During pregnancy and 3 weeks postnatally	↓ body wt at 10 weeks ↓ grip strength at 10 weeks ↑ motor activity at 10 weeks

Table 1. *Cont.*

Reyes-Castro *et al.* 2011 [166]	Wistar 17 and 21 weeks	NPD: 20.0% casein LPD: 10.0% casein	During pregnancy and 3 weeks postnatally	↓ birth wt ↔ body length at birth ↓ body wt at 17 and 21 weeks ↓ cognitive function at 21 weeks
Zambrano *et al.* 2006 [167]	Wistar 16 and 18 weeks	NPD: 20.0% casein LPD: 10.0% casein	During pregnancy and 3 weeks postnatally	↓ birth wt in females ↔ birth wt in males ↓ body wt at 3 and 18 weeks for both sexes ↑ insulin sensitivity

MAP: mean arterial pressure; NPD: normal protein diet; LV: left ventricle; LV + S: left ventricle plus interventricular septum; SBP: systolic blood pressure; wt: weight; WKY: Wistar-Kyoto; ↑: increased; ↓: decreased; ↔: unchanged.

7. Low Birth Weight and Postnatal Body Growth

In accordance with our findings, many laboratories worldwide have shown that administration of a protein restricted diet to rat dams during pregnancy leads to growth restriction in the offspring (Table 1). Given the relative consistency of these findings, maternal protein restriction in rats has now become one of the most commonly used animal models of IUGR (Table 1). To the contrary, however, the long-term effects on body weight are not always the same; in some laboratories the offspring undergo postnatal catch up in body growth, whereas in others the body weight of the offspring remains attenuated throughout life (Table 1). It is a consistent finding in our laboratory that the low protein diet (LPD) offspring are born small and they then remain significantly smaller throughout life when compared to normal protein diet (NPD) control offspring [99,117,143–145,147–149]; this is also reported in some other research groups [95,141]. In contrast, catch-up in body growth in the IUGR rat offspring is often reported following maternal protein restriction [51,137,140].

Why there are differences in postnatal growth in the offspring between studies is unknown. It is conceivable that it may be the prolonged maternal protein restriction after birth for two weeks during lactation in our studies that leads to the persistent attenuation of body growth in the LPD offspring. In our studies, we have chosen to feed the rat dams the specialized diets (LPD and NPD) for the first two weeks of lactation as rats are an altricial species and are born at a time when their organs are very immature. For instance, in the heart maturation of cardiomyocytes, which occurs late in gestation in humans, occurs in the first two weeks after birth in the rat [168]. Likewise, in the kidney nephrogenesis is complete by term birth in the human but continues in the first two weeks after birth in the rat. Hence, in order to more closely mimic the effect of IUGR on organ development, we have considered it appropriate to continue the maternal protein restriction until two weeks after birth.

In addition, there is another important difference in relation to the dietary feeding regime to the rat dams in our studies, compared to many other studies. In our studies, the dams commence the diet 2 weeks prior to mating, in order to get the dams accustomed to the specialised diets. In contrast, in the majority of studies utilising the maternal protein restriction model, they have commenced feeding the diet to the dams at the beginning of pregnancy. Hence, it may be the feeding of the low protein diet to the dams during the periconceptional period that has led to the long-term attenuation of postnatal growth and to some of the other differences in findings, compared to other studies using the maternal protein restriction model. Indeed, there have been a number of recent studies demonstrating long-term effects on the offspring, as a result of insults; including impaired nutrition, experienced by the mothers at around the time of conception [92,169–172], thus highlighting the importance of the periconceptional period in long-term programming [129,173,174]. Hence, in future studies, it would certainly be beneficial to explore the effects of the timing of the low protein diet to the dams on the long-term outcomes in the offspring, in order to differentiate the importance of the periconceptional, pregnancy and lactation periods in mediating the long-term effects.

8. Elevated Blood Pressure in Adulthood is not a Direct Corollary of IUGR

Over recent decades there have been many epidemiological studies that describe a direct link between being born small with an elevation of blood pressure in adulthood [8,31,48,175–177]. Interestingly, however, our studies using the maternal protein restriction model in rats do not support this concept. The blood pressure measurements in our studies have been performed using various methods; (tail cuff plethysmography, intra-arterial and high fidelity pressure sensor; and the outcome is always the same. The IUGR LPD offspring remain normotensive through to adulthood and their levels of blood pressure are not different to the non-IUGR NPD offspring, thus demonstrating that an elevation in blood pressure is not a direct corollary of IUGR.

The findings in relation to the effects of IUGR on blood pressure later in life using animal models differs widely amongst studies; some studies report no effects on blood pressure, whereas others report an elevation in blood pressure in adulthood (Table 1). In our studies the absence of an elevation in blood pressure in the adult IUGR offspring is in agreement with other previously reported studies [95,142,178] yet contrary to others [93,116,132–134,139,151,155,156]. Collectively, the findings clearly indicate that induction of hypertension in adulthood is not a direct corollary of being born small. The question thus arises why do the IUGR offspring in some studies develop high blood pressure in adulthood and in other studies blood pressure in adult IUGR offspring is not affected? There are a number of potential explanations for the discrepancies in findings. It may be that when body growth remains attenuated throughout life that blood pressure is not affected. It is likely that the cardiovascular system is programmed in utero and hence, cardiovascular function may only be adversely affected when there is a mismatch in prenatal and postnatal growth. Certainly, there are a number of experimental studies supporting this concept in the programming of metabolic disease. Importantly in this regard, using our model of maternal protein restriction in rats there is improved insulin sensitivity supporting the concept that it is the "mismatch" in prenatal and postnatal growth that leads to impaired glucose metabolism [179–183], the majority of studies shown in Table 1 support this concept in relation to the programming of hypertension [122,126,130,135,156]. Hence, when the IUGR LPD offspring experience accelerated postnatal growth, such that body weight is no longer different to the non-IUGR NPD offspring, these offspring generally exhibit a significant elevation in blood pressure. However, it is important to point out, that there are a few studies shown in Table 1, where body weights in the LPD offspring, at the time of examination, were still less than controls but blood pressure was significantly elevated [93,131,133].

An alternative explanation for the differences observed in levels of adult blood pressure may relate to whether the protocols used to measure blood pressure leads to stress in the animals. Indeed, there have been a number of studies suggesting that it is an elevated stress response in IUGR offspring that subsequently leads to the elevation in blood pressure rather than a direct etiological effect [39,128,136,178,184,185]. Hence, when rats are stressed during some procedures used to measure blood pressure, there will be an elevated stress response in the IUGR offspring, and hence, a concomitant elevated blood pressure response. This is similar to the "white coat hypertension" often experienced by human subjects when their blood pressure is measured in a clinical setting (and they have become stressed during the procedure) [186–190]. Certainly measurements of tail-cuff blood pressure can lead to stress in the animals, especially if they have not been well conditioned to the procedure. In early studies in the field, "one off" measurements were performed using tail-cuffs [155,156] and it is highly likely, that the rats were stressed during these procedures. In such studies, blood pressure would have been elevated in both IUGR and non-IUGR offspring during these procedures; however, if there was an elevated stress response in IUGR offspring this would lead to a greater elevation of blood pressure in these offspring. Van Abeelen and colleagues addressed this issue in a recent systemic review where they included 101 experimental studies from sheep, guinea pigs, rats and mice looking at the effects of maternal undernutrition (34 studies of maternal general undernutrition and 67 studies of low protein undernutrition) on the blood pressure in the offspring [185]. They pointed out that the values of blood pressure reported from tail-cuff measurements overestimate the "true value" of blood pressure when taken by a direct method using intra-arterial catheters. Furthermore, they have indicated that a direct comparison between tail-cuff and radiotelemetry would be beneficial when conducting studies [185]. In this regard, Swali and colleagues have reported simultaneous measurements of blood pressure, using tail-cuffs and telemetry, in IUGR and control offspring during baseline and under various stress conditions [128]. They found a good correlation between tail-cuff and radiotelemetry derived blood pressure data in control rats; however, in the IUGR group the tail-cuff method revealed hypertension at eight weeks of age but the telemetry method indicated significantly lower blood pressure at twelve weeks of age compared to controls [128]. Hence, their interpretation of these findings was that the increase in systolic blood pressure in LPD offspring reflects an increase in peripheral vascular resistance as well as change in the degree of amplification of blood pressure between central and peripheral regions.

9. Cardiac Remodelling in the Adult IUGR Heart with Normal Basal Function

In our analyses of the adult hearts of the IUGR LPD offspring we have no evidence of overt structural abnormalities in the myocardium of LPD offspring compared to NPD offspring in early adulthood (18 weeks of age) as assessed by echocardiography [150] and there is no significant difference in the amount of interstitial collagen deposition within the myocardium between the LPD and NPD groups [149]. Interestingly, however, when the biochemical composition of the left ventricle was assessed using FTIR micro-spectroscopy [149] there were marked differences detected in the biochemical spectra of the growth-restricted myocardium. In particular, there was a significant increase in the intensity of lipids, proteoglycans and carbohydrates as indicated by the increased absorbance of the 1455 and 1388 cm^{-1}, 1228 cm^{-1}, 1038 cm^{-1} bands, respectively. However, the protein, lipid and proteoglycan spatial distribution was similar within the myocardium of the left ventricular free wall and interventricular septum of the LPD and NPD adult offspring [149]. Interestingly, the spatial distribution of carbohydrates was different in the IUGR and non-IUGR hearts at 18 weeks of age with the most striking difference between the NPD and LPD myocardium observed in the absorbance band at 1228 cm^{-1}, which is due to the presence of proteoglycans. Importantly, in this regard it has been shown that an increase in proteoglycan deposition can ultimately affect cardiac performance [191,192]. The increase in carbohydrate content in the myocardium of IUGR offspring may be indicative of altered glucose metabolism within the LPD offspring. Certainly, experimental studies link IUGR with programming of altered glucose metabolism [193,194]. We have not directly assessed glucose metabolism in the IUGR offspring in our model of maternal protein restriction. However, in a previous study in our laboratory we have shown that maternal protein restriction leads to the programming of improved postnatal whole body insulin sensitivity when postnatal growth is similar to that in utero [145], which does not support the concept that glucose metabolism is impaired. Future studies are required to further investigate the cause of the increased carbohydrate content in the LV myocardium and determine whether it relates to altered glucose metabolism. It is conceivable that the biochemical changes that we have observed in the heart of the adult IUGR LPD offspring may have developed during foetal life. In support of our findings, Tappia and colleagues showed an altered phospholipid profile and fatty acid content in IUGR offspring at birth [162].

Although no differences in myocardial collagen were observed between LPD and NPD offspring at 18 weeks of age we have detected an increase in interstitial fibrosis in LPD offspring at 24 weeks of age [143] and at 32 weeks of age [147]; hence, it is conceivable that there may be an exacerbated deposition of collagen within the myocardium as the LPD offspring age. Interestingly, at 18 weeks of age we found minimal evidence of overt cardiac dysfunction under basal conditions in the IUGR offspring as assessed using both echocardiography and P-V catheterization techniques; fractional shortening a measure of myocardial contractility was normal [150]. Likewise, in another study from our laboratory there was preserved fractional shortening of the cardiac muscle in the IUGR offspring at 32 weeks of age [147]. Given our findings in relation to blood pressure and body weight, it is not really surprising that basal cardiac function was normal in the IUGR offspring; with normal blood pressure and attenuated postnatal body growth of the IUGR offspring the hemodynamic demands on the cardiovascular system are not likely to have increased in the IUGR offspring in adulthood. However, it is important to note, that when the hearts were challenged with dobutamine that the increase in both stroke volume and cardiac output were attenuated and the arterial elastance remained significantly elevated in the IUGR offspring, indicative of increased afterload on the heart [148]. In addition, echocardiographic analysis demonstrated a significant increase in end systolic dimensions and a significant reduction in aortic peak systolic velocity; which may indicate direct adverse effects on aortic compliance or mild impairment of systolic function. Others have shown in a rat model of maternal protein restriction that ejection fraction is significantly depressed in IUGR offspring very early in life at two weeks of age but subsequently normalised with no difference in ejection fraction between the IUGR and control offspring at 40 weeks of age as assessed by echocardiography [118]. Contrary to our findings, however, Menendez-Castro and colleagues have reported a significantly reduced ejection fraction as evaluated by echocardiography early in life at 10 weeks of age in IUGR offspring exposed to maternal protein restriction even though blood pressure was normal [6].

10. Challenging the Adaptive Capabilities of the IUGR Heart

Over recent years we have tested the hypothesis that IUGR acts as a primary insult to the heart, rendering the heart susceptible to secondary postnatal insults, such as hypertension, high salt diet and hyperglycaemia. It is well known that hypertension leads to left ventricular hypertrophy [195–199] and hence, it was considered likely that when the adaptive capabilities of the IUGR heart are challenged by hypertension, the pathological changes that ensue in the heart would be exacerbated in the heart of offspring that were born IUGR. In our studies, hypertension was induced by continuous infusion, at a pressor dose, of the potent vasopressor hormone angiotensin II (Ang II) [200]. Importantly, given that the IUGR LPD offspring in our studies do not normally develop high blood pressure in adulthood, we were able to look at the secondary effects of induction of hypertension, independent of an underlying primary hypertension.

Contrary to our initial hypothesis, when hypertension was induced as a secondary cardiac insult, the response to hypertension was not exacerbated in the IUGR offspring. The cardiac hypertrophic growth response to Ang II infusion, as assessed using echocardiography, was not different between the IUGR and non-IUGR offspring; however, there were differences in cardiac tissue structure. Unexpectedly, in the Ang II infused IUGR adult offspring the levels of interstitial collagen in the left ventricle myocardium was markedly reduced when compared to the non-IUGR offspring (unpublished observations from our laboratory). Hence, our findings do not support the concept that the IUGR heart is necessarily more vulnerable to hypertension in adulthood and importantly, our findings suggest that in some circumstances the IUGR heart may be somewhat protected from adverse remodelling. Further studies are required to elucidate the mechanisms for the reduced deposition of collagen.

In other studies in our laboratory we have examined the effects of induction of diabetes in adulthood, as a secondary postnatal insult, on the growth of the IUGR and non-IUGR heart [147]. Similar to that seen with induction of hypertension, the overall cardiac growth response to induction of diabetes, assessed by echocardiography, was not different between the IUGR and non-IUGR hearts. Importantly, however, the level of fibrosis was significantly greater in the IUGR diabetic hearts compared to non-IUGR diabetic hearts [147]. Collectively, our findings suggest that the IUGR heart may be better able to structurally adapt to a haemodynamic challenge, but not to the challenge of hyperglycaemia. However, this may be a somewhat simplistic interpretation of findings given that the mechanisms of the induction of cardiac hypertrophy are complex and both secondary insults are likely to involve haemodynamic and endocrine mechanisms.

There have been a number of studies that have examined the effect of a high salt diet administered postnatally, as a secondary lifestyle insult, on blood pressure in IUGR offspring [95,117,201–203]. Interestingly, several studies have shown that the increase in blood pressure in response to a high salt diet is similar between IUGR offspring and non-IUGR offspring [117,204], whereas some report salt-sensitive hypertension [93] and others report a reduction in blood pressure [95]. In our maternal protein restriction model it was previously shown that there was no difference in the elevation of blood pressure response to a high salt diet between LPD and NPD offspring [117]. Given that a high salt diet, is linked to induction of cardiac fibrosis [205,206] it would be interesting in future studies to compare the structural remodelling in the LPD IUGR offspring relative to NPD controls following the feeding of a high salt diet in adolescence/adulthood.

11. Conclusions

In summary, the findings of this review highlight the importance of maternal diet on the long-term cardiovascular outcomes of the offspring. Upon comparison of the findings between different laboratories using rat models of maternal protein restriction we highlight the many differences in the cardiovascular phenotype of the offspring between studies, which may relate to the rat strains studied, severity of the dietary protein restriction and the timing of the diet administration. In addition, this review emphasizes the complexity of the mechanisms relating to the developmental programming of heart disease and highlights directions for future research that are required to establish the importance of the periconceptional, pregnancy, lactational and post-weaning windows in life-long developmental programming.

Acknowledgments

Vladislava Zohdi was supported by an Australian Postgraduate Research Award and Kyungjoon Lim was supported by National Health and Medical Research Council scholarship whilst conducting this study.

Author Contributions

Vladislava Zohdi and Kyungjoon Lim wrote the manuscript, Vladislava Zohdi made the table, made Kyungjoon Lim the figure. James T. Pearson and Mary Jane Black critically revised the manuscript.

References

1. Barker, D.J.; Gluckman, P.D.; Godfrey, K.M.; Harding, J.E.; Owens, J.A.; Robinson, J.S. Fetal nutrition and cardiovascular disease in adult life. *Lancet* **1993**, *341*, 938–941.
2. Barker, D.J. Intra-uterine programming of the adult cardiovascular system. *Curr. Opin. Nephrol. Hypertens.* **1997**, *6*, 106–110.
3. Rich-Edwards, J.W.; Stampfer, M.J.; Manson, J.E.; Rosner, B.; Hankinson, S.E.; Colditz, G.A.; Willett, W.C.; Hennekens, C.H. Birth weight and risk of cardiovascular disease in a cohort of women followed up since 1976. *BMJ* **1997**, *315*, 396–400.
4. Forsen, T.; Eriksson, J.G.; Tuomilehto, J.; Osmond, C.; Barker, D.J. Growth in utero and during childhood among women who develop coronary heart disease: Longitudinal study. *BMJ* **1999**, *319*, 1403–1407.
5. Tappia, P.S.; Guzman, C.; Dunn, L.; Aroutiounova, N. Adverse cardiac remodeling due to maternal low protein diet is associated with alterations in expression of genes regulating glucose metabolism. *Nutr. Metab. Cardiovasc. Dis.* **2013**, *23*, 130–135.
6. Menendez-Castro, C.; Toka, O.; Fahlbusch, F.; Cordasic, N.; Wachtveitl, R.; Hilgers, K.F.; Rascher, W.; Hartner, A. Impaired myocardial performance in a normotensive rat model of intrauterine growth restriction. *Pediatr. Res.* **2014**, *75*, 697–706.
7. Hales, C.N.; Barker, D.J. The thrifty phenotype hypothesis. *Br. Med. Bull.* **2001**, *60*, 5–20.
8. Barker, D.J.; Osmond, C.; Golding, J.; Kuh, D.; Wadsworth, M.E. Growth in utero, blood pressure in childhood and adult life, and mortality from cardiovascular disease. *BMJ* **1989**, *298*, 564–567.
9. Barker, D.J.; Bull, A.R.; Osmond, C.; Simmonds, S.J. Fetal and placental size and risk of hypertension in adult life. *BMJ* **1990**, *301*, 259–262.
10. Barker, D.J.; Martyn, C.N. The fetal origins of hypertension. *Adv. Nephrol. Necker Hosp.* **1997**, *26*, 65–72.
11. Eriksson, J.G.; Forsen, T.J.; Kajantie, E.; Osmond, C.; Barker, D.J. Childhood growth and hypertension in later life. *Hypertension* **2007**, *49*, 1415–1421.
12. Barker, D.J. Fetal origins of coronary heart disease. *BMJ* **1995**, *311*, 171–174.
13. Fall, C.H.; Vijayakumar, M.; Barker, D.J.; Osmond, C.; Duggleby, S. Weight in infancy and prevalence of coronary heart disease in adult life. *BMJ* **1995**, *310*, 17–19.

14. Leon, D.A.; Lithell, H.O.; Vagero, D.; Koupilova, I.; Mohsen, R.; Berglund, L.; Lithell, U.B.; McKeigue, P.M. Reduced fetal growth rate and increased risk of death from ischaemic heart disease: Cohort study of 15,000 swedish men and women born 1915–29. *BMJ* **1998**, *317*, 241–245.
15. Eriksson, J.G.; Forsen, T.; Tuomilehto, J.; Winter, P.D.; Osmond, C.; Barker, D.J. Catch-up growth in childhood and death from coronary heart disease: Longitudinal study. *BMJ* **1999**, *318*, 427–431.
16. Eriksson, J.G.; Forsen, T.; Tuomilehto, J.; Osmond, C.; Barker, D.J. Early growth and coronary heart disease in later life: Longitudinal study. *BMJ* **2001**, *322*, 949–953.
17. Barker, D.J.; Osmond, C.; Forsen, T.J.; Kajantie, E.; Eriksson, J.G. Trajectories of growth among children who have coronary events as adults. *N. Engl. J. Med.* **2005**, *353*, 1802–1809.
18. Boney, C.M.; Verma, A.; Tucker, R.; Vohr, B.R. Metabolic syndrome in childhood: Association with birth weight, maternal obesity, and gestational diabetes mellitus. *Pediatrics* **2005**, *115*, 290–296.
19. Harville, E.W.; Srinivasan, S.; Chen, W.; Berenson, G.S. Is the metabolic syndrome a "small baby" syndrome?: The bogalusa heart study. *Metab. Syndr. Relat. Disord.* **2012**, *10*, 413–421.
20. Goh, K.L.; Shore, A.C.; Quinn, M.; Tooke, J.E. Impaired microvascular vasodilatory function in 3-month-old infants of low birth weight. *Diabetes Care* **2001**, *24*, 1102–1107.
21. Barker, D.J. The developmental origins of insulin resistance. *Horm. Res.* **2005**, *64* (Suppl. 3), 2–7.
22. Lopes, A.A.; Port, F.K. The low birth weight hypothesis as a plausible explanation for the black/white differences in hypertension, non-insulin-dependent diabetes, and end-stage renal disease. *Am. J. Kidney Dis.* **1995**, *25*, 350–356.
23. Vaag, A.A.; Poulsen, P.; Feinberg, M.R. Is low birth weight a risk factor for development of non-insulin-dependent diabetes mellitus? *Ugeskr. Laeger* **1998**, *160*, 2377–2381.
24. White, S.L.; Perkovic, V.; Cass, A.; Chang, C.L.; Poulter, N.; Spector, T.; Haysom, L.; Craig, J.C.; Salmi, I.A.; Chadban, S.J.; *et al.* Is low birth weight an antecedent of ckd in later life? A systemic review of observational studies. *Am. J. Kidney Dis.* **2009**, *54*, 248–261.
25. Mackenzie, H.S.; Lawler, E.V.; Brenner, B.M. Congenital oligonephropathy: The fetal flaw in essential hypertension? *Kidney Int. Suppl.* **1996**, *55*, 30–34.
26. Keller, G.; Zimmer, G.; Mall, G.; Ritz, E.; Amann, K. Nephron number in patients with primary hypertension. *N. Engl. J. Med.* **2003**, *348*, 101–108.
27. Forsdahl, A. Are poor living conditions in childhood and adolescence an important risk factor for arteriosclerotic heart disease? *Br. J. Prev. Soc. Med.* **1977**, *31*, 91–95.
28. Williams, D.R.; Roberts, S.J.; Davies, T.W. Deaths from ischaemic heart disease and infant mortality in england and wales. *J. Epidemiol. Community Health* **1979**, *33*, 199–202.
29. Barker, D.J.; Winter, P.D.; Osmond, C.; Margetts, B.; Simmonds, S.J. Weight in infancy and death from ischaemic heart disease. *Lancet* **1989**, *2*, 577–580.
30. Valdez, R.; Athens, M.A.; Thompson, G.H.; Bradshaw, B.S.; Stern, M.P. Birthweight and adult health outcomes in a biethnic population in the USA. *Diabetologia* **1994**, *37*, 624–631.
31. Law, C.M.; Shiell, A.W. Is blood pressure inversely related to birth weight? The strength of evidence from a systemic review of the literature. *J. Hypertens.* **1996**, *14*, 935–941.

32. Stein, C.E.; Fall, C.H.; Kumaran, K.; Osmond, C.; Cox, V.; Barker, D.J. Fetal growth and coronary heart disease in south india. *Lancet* **1996**, *348*, 1269–1273.
33. Jones, S.E.; Nyengaard, J.R. Low birth weight and cardiovascular disease: Myth or reality? *Curr. Opin. Lipidol.* **1998**, *9*, 309–312.
34. Frontini, M.G.; Srinivasan, S.R.; Xu, J.; Berenson, G.S. Low birth weight and longitudinal trends of cardiovascular risk factor variables from childhood to adolescence: The bogalusa heart study. *BMC Pediatr.* **2004**, *4*, doi:10.1186/1471-2431-4-22.
35. Banci, M.; Saccucci, P.; Dofcaci, A.; Sansoni, I.; Magrini, A.; Bottini, E.; Gloria-Bottini, F. Birth weight and coronary artery disease. The effect of gender and diabetes. *Int. J. Biol. Sci.* **2009**, *5*, 244–248.
36. Yajnik, C. Interactions of perturbations in intrauterine growth and growth during childhood on the risk of adult-onset disease. *Proc. Nutr. Soc.* **2000**, *59*, 257–265.
37. Hemachandra, A.H.; Howards, P.P.; Furth, S.L.; Klebanoff, M.A. Birth weight, postnatal growth, and risk for high blood pressure at 7 years of age: Results from the collaborative perinatal project. *Pediatrics* **2007**, *119*, 1264–1270.
38. Huang, R.C.; Burke, V.; Newnham, J.P.; Stanley, F.J.; Kendall, G.E.; Landau, L.I.; Oddy, W.H.; Blake, K.V.; Palmer, L.J.; Beilin, L.J. Perinatal and childhood origins of cardiovascular disease. *Int. J. Obes. (Lond.)* **2007**, *31*, 236–244.
39. Huxley, R.R.; Shiell, A.W.; Law, C.M. The role of size at birth and postnatal catch-up growth in determining systolic blood pressure: A systematic review of the literature. *J. Hypertens.* **2000**, *18*, 815–831.
40. Barker, D.J.; Thornburg, K.L. Placental programming of chronic diseases, cancer and lifespan: A review. *Placenta* **2013**, *34*, 841–845.
41. Taylor, S.J.; Whincup, P.H.; Cook, D.G.; Papacosta, O.; Walker, M. Size at birth and blood pressure: Cross sectional study in 8–11 year old children. *BMJ* **1997**, *314*, 475–480.
42. Yiu, V.; Buka, S.; Zurakowski, D.; McCormick, M.; Brenner, B.; Jabs, K. Relationship between birthweight and blood pressure in childhood. *Am. J. Kidney Dis.* **1999**, *33*, 253–260.
43. Blake, K.V.; Gurrin, L.C.; Evans, S.F.; Beilin, L.J.; Landau, L.I.; Stanley, F.J.; Newnham, J.P. Maternal cigarette smoking during pregnancy, low birth weight and subsequent blood pressure in early childhood. *Early Hum. Dev.* **2000**, *57*, 137–147.
44. Adair, L.; Dahly, D. Developmental determinants of blood pressure in adults. *Annu. Rev. Nutr.* **2005**, *25*, 407–434.
45. Law, C.M.; de Swiet, M.; Osmond, C.; Fayers, P.M.; Barker, D.J.; Cruddas, A.M.; Fall, C.H. Initiation of hypertension in utero and its amplification throughout life. *BMJ* **1993**, *306*, 24–27.
46. Leon, D.A.; Koupilova, I.; Lithell, H.O.; Berglund, L.; Mohsen, R.; Vagero, D.; Lithell, U.B.; McKeigue, P.M. Failure to realise growth potential in utero and adult obesity in relation to blood pressure in 50 year old swedish men. *BMJ* **1996**, *312*, 401–406.
47. Koupilova, I.; Leon, D.A.; Lithell, H.O.; Berglund, L. Size at birth and hypertension in longitudinally followed 50–70-year-old men. *Blood Press.* **1997**, *6*, 223–228.
48. Curhan, G.C.; Willett, W.C.; Rimm, E.B.; Spiegelman, D.; Ascherio, A.L.; Stampfer, M.J. Birth weight and adult hypertension, diabetes mellitus, and obesity in us men. *Circulation* **1996**, *94*, 3246–3250.

49. Uiterwaal, C.S.; Anthony, S.; Launer, L.J.; Witteman, J.C.; Trouwborst, A.M.; Hofman, A.; Grobbee, D.E. Birth weight, growth, and blood pressure: An annual follow-up study of children aged 5 through 21 years. *Hypertension* **1997**, *30*, 267–271.
50. Leon, D.A.; Johansson, M.; Rasmussen, F. Gestational age and growth rate of fetal mass are inversely associated with systolic blood pressure in young adults: An epidemiologic study of 165,136 swedish men aged 18 years. *Am. J. Epidemiol.* **2000**, *152*, 597–604.
51. Hales, C.N.; Ozanne, S.E. The dangerous road of catch-up growth. *J. Physiol.* **2003**, *547*, 5–10.
52. Singhal, A.; Cole, T.J.; Fewtrell, M.; Deanfield, J.; Lucas, A. Is slower early growth beneficial for long-term cardiovascular health? *Circulation* **2004**, *109*, 1108–1113.
53. Lucas, A. Programming by early nutrition: An experimental approach. *J. Nutr.* **1998**, *128*, 401–406.
54. Singhal, A.; Lucas, A. Early origins of cardiovascular disease: Is there a unifying hypothesis? *Lancet* **2004**, *363*, 1642–1645.
55. Lucas, A.; Fewtrell, M.S.; Cole, T.J. Fetal origins of adult disease-the hypothesis revisited. *BMJ* **1999**, *319*, 245–249.
56. Law, C.M.; Shiell, A.W.; Newsome, C.A.; Syddall, H.E.; Shinebourne, E.A.; Fayers, P.M.; Martyn, C.N.; de Swiet, M. Fetal, infant, and childhood growth and adult blood pressure: A longitudinal study from birth to 22 years of age. *Circulation* **2002**, *105*, 1088–1092.
57. Jarvelin, M.R.; Sovio, U.; King, V.; Lauren, L.; Xu, B.; McCarthy, M.I.; Hartikainen, A.L.; Laitinen, J.; Zitting, P.; Rantakallio, P.; *et al.* Early life factors and blood pressure at age 31 years in the 1966 northern finland birth cohort. *Hypertension* **2004**, *44*, 838–846.
58. Estourgie-van Burk, G.F.; Bartels, M.; Hoekstra, R.A.; Polderman, T.J.; Delemarre-van de Waal, H.A.; Boomsma, D.I. A twin study of cognitive costs of low birth weight and catch-up growth. *J. Pediatr.* **2009**, *154*, 29–32.
59. Crispi, F.; Hernandez-Andrade, E.; Pelsers, M.M.; Plasencia, W.; Benavides-Serralde, J.A.; Eixarch, E.; Le Noble, F.; Ahmed, A.; Glatz, J.F.; Nicolaides, K.H.; *et al.* Cardiac dysfunction and cell damage across clinical stages of severity in growth-restricted fetuses. *Am. J. Obstet. Gynecol.* **2008**, *199*, 251–258.
60. Kaijser, M.; Bonamy, A.K.; Akre, O.; Cnattingius, S.; Granath, F.; Norman, M.; Ekbom, A. Perinatal risk factors for ischemic heart disease: Disentangling the roles of birth weight and preterm birth. *Circulation* **2008**, *117*, 405–410.
61. Crispi, F.; Bijnens, B.; Figueras, F.; Bartrons, J.; Eixarch, E.; Le Noble, F.; Ahmed, A.; Gratacos, E. Fetal growth restriction results in remodeled and less efficient hearts in children. *Circulation* **2010**, *121*, 2427–2436.
62. Soto, N.; Bazaes, R.A.; Pena, V.; Salazar, T.; Avila, A.; Iniguez, G.; Ong, K.K.; Dunger, D.B.; Mericq, M.V. Insulin sensitivity and secretion are related to catch-up growth in small-for-gestational-age infants at age 1 year: Results from a prospective cohort. *J. Clin. Endocrinol. Metab.* **2003**, *88*, 3645–3650.
63. Forsen, T.; Eriksson, J.; Tuomilehto, J.; Reunanen, A.; Osmond, C.; Barker, D. The fetal and childhood growth of persons who develop type 2 diabetes. *Ann. Intern. Med.* **2000**, *133*, 176–182.

64. Ong, K.K.; Ahmed, M.L.; Emmett, P.M.; Preece, M.A.; Dunger, D.B. Association between postnatal catch-up growth and obesity in childhood: Prospective cohort study. *BMJ* **2000**, *320*, 967–971.
65. Eriksson, J.; Forsen, T.; Tuomilehto, J.; Osmond, C.; Barker, D. Fetal and childhood growth and hypertension in adult life. *Hypertension* **2000**, *36*, 790–794.
66. Fagerberg, B.; Bondjers, L.; Nilsson, P. Low birth weight in combination with catch-up growth predicts the occurrence of the metabolic syndrome in men at late middle age: The atherosclerosis and insulin resistance study. *J. Intern. Med.* **2004**, *256*, 254–259.
67. Valman, H.B. Infants of low birth weight. *Br. Med. J.* **1979**, *2*, 1431–1432.
68. Luke, B.; Petrie, R.H. Intrauterine growth: Correlation of infant birth weight and maternal postpartum weight. *Am. J. Clin. Nutr.* **1980**, *33*, 2311–2317.
69. Kiely, J.L.; Susser, M. Preterm birth, intrauterine growth retardation, and perinatal mortality. *Am. J. Public Health* **1992**, *82*, 343–345.
70. Resnik, R. Intrauterine growth restriction. *Obstet. Gynecol.* **2002**, *99*, 490–496.
71. Wollmann, H.A. Intrauterine growth restriction: Definition and etiology. *Horm. Res.* **1998**, *49*, 1–6.
72. Lockwood, C.J.; Weiner, S. Assessment of fetal growth. *Clin. Perinatol.* **1986**, *13*, 3–35.
73. Malamitsi-Puchner, A.; Nikolaou, K.E.; Puchner, K.P. Intrauterine growth restriction, brain-sparing effect, and neurotrophins. *Ann. N. Y. Acad. Sci.* **2006**, *1092*, 293–296.
74. Beeby, A.R.; Dunlop, W.; Hunter, S. Evidence of redistribution of cardiac output in asymmetrical growth retardation. *Br. J. Obstet. Gynaecol.* **1989**, *96*, 1453–1454.
75. Patterson, R.M.; Pouliot, M.R. Neonatal morphometrics and perinatal outcome: Who is growth retarded? *Am. J. Obstet. Gynecol.* **1987**, *157*, 691–693.
76. Peleg, D.; Kennedy, C.M.; Hunter, S.K. Intrauterine growth restriction: Identification and management. *Am. Fam. Physician* **1998**, *58*, 453–470.
77. Zadik, Z. Maternal nutrition, fetal weight, body composition and disease in later life. *J. Endocrinol. Investig.* **2003**, *26*, 941–945.
78. Widdowson, E.M. Trace elements in foetal and early postnatal development. *Proc. Nutr. Soc.* **1974**, *33*, 275–284.
79. Bergmann, R.L.; Bergmann, K.E.; Dudenhausen, J.W. Undernutrition and growth restriction in pregnancy. *Nestle Nutr. Workshop Ser. Pediatr. Program* **2008**, *61*, 103–121.
80. Barker, D.J. Outcome of low birthweight. *Horm. Res.* **1994**, *42*, 223–230.
81. Barker, D.J.; Bergmann, R.L.; Ogra, P.L. Concluding remarks. The window of opportunity: Pre-pregnancy to 24 months of age. *Nestle Nutr. Workshop Ser. Pediatr. Program* **2008**, *61*, 255–260.
82. Desai, M.; Crowther, N.J.; Lucas, A.; Hales, C.N. Organ-selective growth in the offspring of protein-restricted mothers. *Br. J. Nutr.* **1996**, *76*, 591–603.
83. Crews, F.; He, J.; Hodge, C. Adolescent cortical development: A critical period of vulnerability for addiction. *Pharmacol. Biochem. Behav.* **2007**, *86*, 189–199.
84. Gluckman, P.D.; Hanson, M.A.; Low, F.M. The role of developmental plasticity and epigenetics in human health. *Birth Defects Res. C Embryo Today* **2011**, *93*, 12–18.

85. Godfrey, K.M.; Barker, D.J. Fetal nutrition and adult disease. *Am. J. Clin. Nutr.* **2000**, *71*, 1344–1352.
86. Symonds, M.E.; Sebert, S.P.; Hyatt, M.A.; Budge, H. Nutritional programming of the metabolic syndrome. *Nat. Rev. Endocrinol.* **2009**, *5*, 604–610.
87. Lucas, A. Programming by early nutrition in man. *Ciba Found. Symp.* **1991**, *156*, 38–50.
88. Godfrey, K.M.; Barker, D.J. Maternal nutrition in relation to fetal and placental growth. *Eur. J. Obstet. Gynecol. Reprod. Biol.* **1995**, *61*, 15–22.
89. Langley-Evans, S.C. Developmental programming of health and disease. *Proc. Nutr. Soc.* **2006**, *65*, 97–105.
90. Gluckman, P.D.; Cutfield, W.; Hofman, P.; Hanson, M.A. The fetal, neonatal, and infant environments-the long-term consequences for disease risk. *Early Hum. Dev.* **2005**, *81*, 51–59.
91. Edwards, L.J.; McFarlane, J.R.; Kauter, K.G.; McMillen, I.C. Impact of periconceptional nutrition on maternal and fetal leptin and fetal adiposity in singleton and twin pregnancies. *Am. J. Physiol. Regul. Integr. Comp. Physiol.* **2005**, *288*, 39–45.
92. Edwards, L.J.; McMillen, I.C. Periconceptional nutrition programs development of the cardiovascular system in the fetal sheep. *Am. J. Physiol. Regul. Integr. Comp. Physiol.* **2002**, *283*, 669–679.
93. Woods, L.L.; Weeks, D.A.; Rasch, R. Programming of adult blood pressure by maternal protein restriction: Role of nephrogenesis. *Kidney Int.* **2004**, *65*, 1339–1348.
94. Zimanyi, M.A.; Denton, K.M.; Forbes, J.M.; Thallas-Bonke, V.; Thomas, M.C.; Poon, F.; Black, M.J. A developmental nephron deficit in rats is associated with increased susceptibility to a secondary renal injury due to advanced glycation end-products. *Diabetologia* **2006**, *49*, 801–810.
95. Hoppe, C.C.; Evans, R.G.; Bertram, J.F.; Moritz, K.M. Effects of dietary protein restriction on nephron number in the mouse. *Am. J. Physiol. Regul. Integr. Comp. Physiol.* **2007**, *292*, 1768–1774.
96. Briscoe, T.A.; Rehn, A.E.; Dieni, S.; Duncan, J.R.; Wlodek, M.E.; Owens, J.A.; Rees, S.M. Cardiovascular and renal disease in the adolescent guinea pig after chronic placental insufficiency. *Am. J. Obstet. Gynecol.* **2004**, *191*, 847–855.
97. Bassan, H.; Trejo, L.L.; Kariv, N.; Bassan, M.; Berger, E.; Fattal, A.; Gozes, I.; Harel, S. Experimental intrauterine growth retardation alters renal development. *Pediatr. Nephrol.* **2000**, *15*, 192–195.
98. Zohdi, V.; Moritz, K.M.; Bubb, K.J.; Cock, M.L.; Wreford, N.; Harding, R.; Black, M.J. Nephrogenesis and the renal renin-angiotensin system in fetal sheep: Effects of intrauterine growth restriction during late gestation. *Am. J. Physiol. Regul. Integr. Comp. Physiol.* **2007**, *293*, 1267–1273.
99. Corstius, H.B.; Zimanyi, M.A.; Maka, N.; Herath, T.; Thomas, W.; van der Laarse, A.; Wreford, N.G.; Black, M.J. Effect of intrauterine growth restriction on the number of cardiomyocytes in rat hearts. *Pediatr. Res.* **2005**, *57*, 796–800.
100. Stacy, V.; de Matteo, R.; Brew, N.; Sozo, F.; Probyn, M.E.; Harding, R.; Black, M.J. The influence of naturally occurring differences in birthweight on ventricular cardiomyocyte number in sheep. *Anat. Rec. (Hoboken)* **2009**, *292*, 29–37.

101. Bedi, K.S.; Birzgalis, A.R.; Mahon, M.; Smart, J.L.; Wareham, A.C. Early life undernutrition in rats. 1. Quantitative histology of skeletal muscles from underfed young and refed adult animals. *Br. J. Nutr.* **1982**, *47*, 417–431.
102. Tilley, R.E.; McNeil, C.J.; Ashworth, C.J.; Page, K.R.; McArdle, H.J. Altered muscle development and expression of the insulin-like growth factor system in growth retarded fetal pigs. *Domest. Anim. Endocrinol.* **2007**, *32*, 167–177.
103. Fahey, A.J.; Brameld, J.M.; Parr, T.; Buttery, P.J. The effect of maternal undernutrition before muscle differentiation on the muscle fiber development of the newborn lamb. *J. Anim. Sci.* **2005**, *83*, 2564–2571.
104. Snoeck, A.; Remacle, C.; Reusens, B.; Hoet, J.J. Effect of a low protein diet during pregnancy on the fetal rat endocrine pancreas. *Biol. Neonate* **1990**, *57*, 107–118.
105. Vonnahme, K.A.; Zhu, M.J.; Borowicz, P.P.; Geary, T.W.; Hess, B.W.; Reynolds, L.P.; Caton, J.S.; Means, W.J.; Ford, S.P. Effect of early gestational undernutrition on angiogenic factor expression and vascularity in the bovine placentome. *J. Anim. Sci.* **2007**, *85*, 2464–2472.
106. Langley-Evans, S.C.; Gardner, D.S.; Jackson, A.A. Maternal protein restriction influences the programming of the rat hypothalamic-pituitary-adrenal axis. *J. Nutr.* **1996**, *126*, 1578–1585.
107. Leonhardt, M.; Lesage, J.; Dufourny, L.; Dickes-Coopman, A.; Montel, V.; Dupouy, J.P. Perinatal maternal food restriction induces alterations in hypothalamo-pituitary-adrenal axis activity and in plasma corticosterone-binding globulin capacity of weaning rat pups. *Neuroendocrinology* **2002**, *75*, 45–54.
108. Brans, Y.W.; Kuehl, T.J.; Hayashi, R.H.; Andrew, D.S.; Reyes, P. Amniotic fluid in baboon pregnancies with normal *versus* growth-retarded fetuses. *Am. J. Obstet. Gynecol.* **1986**, *155*, 216–219.
109. Oyama, K.; Padbury, J.; Chappell, B.; Martinez, A.; Stein, H.; Humme, J. Single umbilical artery ligation-induced fetal growth retardation: Effect on postnatal adaptation. *Am. J. Physiol.* **1992**, *263*, 575–583.
110. Cock, M.L.; Harding, R. Renal and amniotic fluid responses to umbilicoplacental embolization for 20 days in fetal sheep. *Am. J. Physiol.* **1997**, *273*, 1094–1102.
111. Louey, S.; Cock, M.L.; Stevenson, K.M.; Harding, R. Placental insufficiency and fetal growth restriction lead to postnatal hypotension and altered postnatal growth in sheep. *Pediatr. Res.* **2000**, *48*, 808–814.
112. Cock, M.L.; Joyce, B.J.; Hooper, S.B.; Wallace, M.J.; Gagnon, R.; Brace, R.A.; Louey, S.; Harding, R. Pulmonary elastin synthesis and deposition in developing and mature sheep: Effects of intrauterine growth restriction. *Exp. Lung Res.* **2004**, *30*, 405–418.
113. Mitchell, E.K.; Louey, S.; Cock, M.L.; Harding, R.; Black, M.J. Nephron endowment and filtration surface area in the kidney after growth restriction of fetal sheep. *Pediatr. Res.* **2004**, *55*, 769–773.
114. Bubb, K.J.; Cock, M.L.; Black, M.J.; Dodic, M.; Boon, W.M.; Parkington, H.C.; Harding, R.; Tare, M. Intrauterine growth restriction delays cardiomyocyte maturation and alters coronary artery function in the fetal sheep. *J. Physiol.* **2007**, *578*, 871–881.
115. Merlet-Benichou, C.; Gilbert, T.; Muffat-Joly, M.; Lelievre-Pegorier, M.; Leroy, B. Intrauterine growth retardation leads to a permanent nephron deficit in the rat. *Pediatr. Nephrol.* **1994**, *8*, 175–180.

116. Langley-Evans, S.C.; Welham, S.J.; Jackson, A.A. Fetal exposure to a maternal low protein diet impairs nephrogenesis and promotes hypertension in the rat. *Life Sci.* **1999**, *64*, 965–974.
117. Zimanyi, M.A.; Bertram, J.F.; Black, M.J. Does a nephron deficit in rats predispose to salt-sensitive hypertension? *Kidney Blood Press. Res.* **2004**, *27*, 239–247.
118. Cheema, K.K.; Dent, M.R.; Saini, H.K.; Aroutiounova, N.; Tappia, P.S. Prenatal exposure to maternal undernutrition induces adult cardiac dysfunction. *Br. J. Nutr.* **2005**, *93*, 471–477.
119. Langley-Evans, S.C. Nutrition in early life and the programming of adult disease: A review. *J. Hum. Nutr. Diet.* **2014**, *28*, 1–14.
120. Turner, M.R. Perinatal mortality, growth and survival to weaning in offspring of rats reared on diets moderately deficient in protein. *Br. J. Nutr.* **1973**, *29*, 139–147.
121. Ozanne, S.E.; Wang, C.L.; Coleman, N.; Smith, G.D. Altered muscle insulin sensitivity in the male offspring of protein-malnourished rats. *Am. J. Physiol.* **1996**, *271*, 1128–1134.
122. Woods, L.L.; Ingelfinger, J.R.; Nyengaard, J.R.; Rasch, R. Maternal protein restriction suppresses the newborn renin-angiotensin system and programs adult hypertension in rats. *Pediatr. Res.* **2001**, *49*, 460–467.
123. Bellinger, L.; Sculley, D.V.; Langley-Evans, S.C. Exposure to undernutrition in fetal life determines fat distribution, locomotor activity and food intake in ageing rats. *Int. J. Obes. (Lond.)* **2006**, *30*, 729–738.
124. Plank, C.; Ostreicher, I.; Hartner, A.; Marek, I.; Struwe, F.G.; Amann, K.; Hilgers, K.F.; Rascher, W.; Dotsch, J. Intrauterine growth retardation aggravates the course of acute mesangioproliferative glomerulonephritis in the rat. *Kidney Int.* **2006**, *70*, 1974–1982.
125. Alwasel, S.H.; Ashton, N. Prenatal programming of renal sodium handling in the rat. *Clin. Sci. (Lond.)* **2009**, *117*, 75–84.
126. Boubred, F.; Daniel, L.; Buffat, C.; Feuerstein, J.M.; Tsimaratos, M.; Oliver, C.; Dignat-George, F.; Lelievre-Pegorier, M.; Simeoni, U. Early postnatal overfeeding induces early chronic renal dysfunction in adult male rats. *Am. J. Physiol. Renal Physiol.* **2009**, *297*, 943–951.
127. Sherman, R.C.; Langley-Evans, S.C. Antihypertensive treatment in early postnatal life modulates prenatal dietary influences upon blood pressure in the rat. *Clin. Sci. (Lond.)* **2000**, *98*, 269–275.
128. Swali, A.; McMullen, S.; Langley-Evans, S.C. Prenatal protein restriction leads to a disparity between aortic and peripheral blood pressure in wistar male offspring. *J. Physiol.* **2010**, *588*, 3809–3818.
129. Kwong, W.Y.; Wild, A.E.; Roberts, P.; Willis, A.C.; Fleming, T.P. Maternal undernutrition during the preimplantation period of rat development causes blastocyst abnormalities and programming of postnatal hypertension. *Development* **2000**, *127*, 4195–4202.
130. Manning, J.; Beutler, K.; Knepper, M.A.; Vehaskari, V.M. Upregulation of renal bsc1 and tsc in prenatally programmed hypertension. *Am. J. Physiol. Renal Physiol.* **2002**, *283*, 202–206.
131. Sathishkumar, K.; Elkins, R.; Yallampalli, U.; Yallampalli, C. Protein restriction during pregnancy induces hypertension and impairs endothelium-dependent vascular function in adult female offspring. *J. Vasc. Res.* **2009**, *46*, 229–239.
132. Dagan, A.; Habib, S.; Gattineni, J.; Dwarakanath, V.; Baum, M. Prenatal programming of rat thick ascending limb chloride transport by low-protein diet and dexamethasone. *Am. J. Physiol. Regul. Integr. Comp. Physiol.* **2009**, *297*, 93–99.

133. Habib, S.; Gattineni, J.; Twombley, K.; Baum, M. Evidence that prenatal programming of hypertension by dietary protein deprivation is mediated by fetal glucocorticoid exposure. *Am. J. Hypertens.* **2011**, *24*, 96–101.
134. Langley, S.C.; Jackson, A.A. Increased systolic blood pressure in adult rats induced by fetal exposure to maternal low protein diets. *Clin. Sci. (Lond.)* **1994**, *86*, 217–222.
135. Manning, J.; Vehaskari, V.M. Low birth weight-associated adult hypertension in the rat. *Pediatr. Nephrol.* **2001**, *16*, 417–422.
136. Tonkiss, J.; Trzcinska, M.; Galler, J.R.; Ruiz-Opazo, N.; Herrera, V.L. Prenatal malnutrition-induced changes in blood pressure: Dissociation of stress and nonstress responses using radiotelemetry. *Hypertension* **1998**, *32*, 108–114.
137. Vehaskari, V.M.; Aviles, D.H.; Manning, J. Prenatal programming of adult hypertension in the rat. *Kidney Int.* **2001**, *59*, 238–245.
138. Coupe, B.; Grit, I.; Darmaun, D.; Parnet, P. The timing of "catch-up growth" affects metabolism and appetite regulation in male rats born with intrauterine growth restriction. *Am. J. Physiol. Regul. Integr. Comp. Physiol.* **2009**, *297*, 813–824.
139. Plank, C.; Grillhosl, C.; Ostreicher, I.; Meissner, U.; Struwe, F.G.; Rauh, M.; Hartner, A.; Rascher, W.; Dotsch, J. Transient growth hormone therapy to rats with low protein-inflicted intrauterine growth restriction does not prevent elevated blood pressure in later life. *Growth Factors* **2008**, *26*, 355–364.
140. Zeng, Y.; Gu, P.; Liu, K.; Huang, P. Maternal protein restriction in rats leads to reduced pgc-1alpha expression via altered DNA methylation in skeletal muscle. *Mol. Med. Rep.* **2013**, *7*, 306–312.
141. Menendez-Castro, C.; Fahlbusch, F.; Cordasic, N.; Amann, K.; Munzel, K.; Plank, C.; Wachtveitl, R.; Rascher, W.; Hilgers, K.F.; Hartner, A. Early and late postnatal myocardial and vascular changes in a protein restriction rat model of intrauterine growth restriction. *PLoS One* **2011**, *6*, doi:10.1371/journal.pone.0020369.
142. Woods, L.L.; Ingelfinger, J.R.; Rasch, R. Modest maternal protein restriction fails to program adult hypertension in female rats. *Am. J. Physiol. Regul. Integr. Comp. Physiol.* **2005**, *289*, 1131–1136.
143. Lim, K.; Zimanyi, M.A.; Black, M.J. Effect of maternal protein restriction in rats on cardiac fibrosis and capillarization in adulthood. *Pediatr. Res.* **2006**, *60*, 83–87.
144. Lim, K.; Zimanyi, M.A.; Black, M.J. Effect of maternal protein restriction during pregnancy and lactation on the number of cardiomyocytes in the postproliferative weanling rat heart. *Anat. Rec. (Hoboken)* **2010**, *293*, 431–437.
145. Lim, K.; Armitage, J.A.; Stefanidis, A.; Oldfield, B.J.; Black, M.J. IUGR in the absence of postnatal "catch-up" growth leads to improved whole body insulin sensitivity in rat offspring. *Pediatr. Res.* **2011**, *70*, 339–344.
146. Lim, K.; Lombardo, P.; Schneider-Kolsky, M.; Hilliard, L.; Denton, K.M.; Black, M.J. Induction of hyperglycemia in adult intrauterine growth-restricted rats: Effects on renal function. *Am. J. Physiol. Renal. Physiol.* **2011**, *301*, 288–294.
147. Lim, K.; Lombardo, P.; Schneider-Kolsky, M.; Black, M.J. Intrauterine growth restriction coupled with hyperglycemia: Effects on cardiac structure in adult rats. *Pediatr. Res.* **2012**, *72*, 344–351.

148. Zohdi, V.; Jane Black, M.; Pearson, J.T. Elevated vascular resistance and afterload reduce the cardiac output response to dobutamine in early growth-restricted rats in adulthood. *Br. J. Nutr.* **2011**, *106*, 1374–1382.
149. Zohdi, V.; Wood, B.R.; Pearson, J.T.; Bambery, K.R.; Black, M.J. Evidence of altered biochemical composition in the hearts of adult intrauterine growth-restricted rats. *Eur. J. Nutr.* **2013**, *52*, 749–758.
150. Zohdi, V.; Pearson, J.T.; Kett, M.M.; Lombardo, P.; Schneider, M.; Black, M.J. When early life growth restriction in rats is followed by attenuated postnatal growth: Effects on cardiac function in adulthood. *Eur. J. Nutr.* **2014**, *13*, doi:10.1007/s00394-014-0752-6.
151. Brawley, L.; Itoh, S.; Torrens, C.; Barker, A.; Bertram, C.; Poston, L.; Hanson, M. Dietary protein restriction in pregnancy induces hypertension and vascular defects in rat male offspring. *Pediatr. Res.* **2003**, *54*, 83–90.
152. Elmes, M.J.; Gardner, D.S.; Langley-Evans, S.C. Fetal exposure to a maternal low-protein diet is associated with altered left ventricular pressure response to ischaemia-reperfusion injury. *Br. J. Nutr.* **2007**, *98*, 93–100.
153. Gardner, D.S.; Jackson, A.A.; Langley-Evans, S.C. Maintenance of maternal diet-induced hypertension in the rat is dependent on glucocorticoids. *Hypertension* **1997**, *30*, 1525–1530.
154. Harrison, M.; Langley-Evans, S.C. Intergenerational programming of impaired nephrogenesis and hypertension in rats following maternal protein restriction during pregnancy. *Br. J. Nutr.* **2009**, *101*, 1020–1030.
155. Langley-Evans, S.C.; Phillips, G.J.; Jackson, A.A. In utero exposure to maternal low protein diets induces hypertension in weanling rats, independently of maternal blood pressure changes. *Clin. Nutr.* **1994**, *13*, 319–324.
156. Langley-Evans, S.C.; Phillips, G.J.; Benediktsson, R.; Gardner, D.S.; Edwards, C.R.; Jackson, A.A.; Seckl, J.R. Protein intake in pregnancy, placental glucocorticoid metabolism and the programming of hypertension in the rat. *Placenta* **1996**, *17*, 169–172.
157. McMullen, S.; Langley-Evans, S.C. Maternal low-protein diet in rat pregnancy programs blood pressure through sex-specific mechanisms. *Am. J. Physiol. Regul. Integr. Comp. Physiol.* **2005**, *288*, 85–90.
158. McMullen, S.; Gardner, D.S.; Langley-Evans, S.C. Prenatal programming of angiotensin ii type 2 receptor expression in the rat. *Br. J. Nutr.* **2004**, *91*, 133–140.
159. Mehta, G.; Roach, H.I.; Langley-Evans, S.; Taylor, P.; Reading, I.; Oreffo, R.O.; Aihie-Sayer, A.; Clarke, N.M.; Cooper, C. Intrauterine exposure to a maternal low protein diet reduces adult bone mass and alters growth plate morphology in rats. *Calcif. Tissue Int.* **2002**, *71*, 493–498.
160. Nwagwu, M.O.; Cook, A.; Langley-Evans, S.C. Evidence of progressive deterioration of renal function in rats exposed to a maternal low-protein diet in utero. *Br. J. Nutr.* **2000**, *83*, 79–85.
161. Pladys, P.; Sennlaub, F.; Brault, S.; Checchin, D.; Lahaie, I.; Le, N.L.; Bibeau, K.; Cambonie, G.; Abran, D.; Brochu, M.; *et al.* Microvascular rarefaction and decreased angiogenesis in rats with fetal programming of hypertension associated with exposure to a low-protein diet in utero. *Am. J. Physiol. Regul. Integr. Comp. Physiol.* **2005**, *289*, 1580–1588.

162. Tappia, P.S.; Nijjar, M.S.; Mahay, A.; Aroutiounova, N.; Dhalla, N.S. Phospholipid profile of developing heart of rats exposed to low-protein diet in pregnancy. *Am. J. Physiol. Regul. Integr. Comp. Physiol.* **2005**, *289*, 1400–1406.
163. Tappia, P.S.; Thliveris, J.; Xu, Y.J.; Aroutiounova, N.; Dhalla, N.S. Effects of amino acid supplementation on myocardial cell damage and cardiac function in diabetes. *Exp. Clin. Cardiol.* **2011**, *16*, 17–22.
164. Torrens, C.; Brawley, L.; Anthony, F.W.; Dance, C.S.; Dunn, R.; Jackson, A.A.; Poston, L.; Hanson, M.A. Folate supplementation during pregnancy improves offspring cardiovascular dysfunction induced by protein restriction. *Hypertension* **2006**, *47*, 982–987.
165. Ohishi, T.; Wang, L.; Akane, H.; Shiraki, A.; Sato, A.; Uematsu, M.; Suzuki, K.; Mitsumori, K.; Shibutani, M. Adolescent hyperactivity of offspring after maternal protein restriction during the second half of gestation and lactation periods in rats. *J. Toxicol. Sci.* **2012**, *37*, 345–352.
166. Reyes-Castro, L.A.; Rodriguez, J.S.; Rodriguez-Gonzalez, G.L.; Wimmer, R.D.; McDonald, T.J.; Larrea, F.; Nathanielsz, P.W.; Zambrano, E. Pre- and/or postnatal protein restriction in rats impairs learning and motivation in male offspring. *Int. J. Dev. Neurosci.* **2011**, *29*, 177–182.
167. Zambrano, E.; Bautista, C.J.; Deas, M.; Martinez-Samayoa, P.M.; Gonzalez-Zamorano, M.; Ledesma, H.; Morales, J.; Larrea, F.; Nathanielsz, P.W. A low maternal protein diet during pregnancy and lactation has sex- and window of exposure-specific effects on offspring growth and food intake, glucose metabolism and serum leptin in the rat. *J. Physiol.* **2006**, *571*, 221–230.
168. Li, F.; Wang, X.; Capasso, J.M.; Gerdes, A.M. Rapid transition of cardiac myocytes from hyperplasia to hypertrophy during postnatal development. *J. Mol. Cell. Cardiol.* **1996**, *28*, 1737–1746.
169. Oliver, M.H.; Hawkins, P.; Harding, J.E. Periconceptional undernutrition alters growth trajectory and metabolic and endocrine responses to fasting in late-gestation fetal sheep. *Pediatr. Res.* **2005**, *57*, 591–598.
170. Oliver, M.H.; Jaquiery, A.L.; Bloomfield, F.H.; Harding, J.E. The effects of maternal nutrition around the time of conception on the health of the offspring. *Soc. Reprod. Fertil. Suppl.* **2007**, *64*, 397–410.
171. Chavatte-Palmer, P.; Al Gubory, K.; Picone, O.; Heyman, Y. Maternal nutrition: Effects on offspring fertility and importance of the periconceptional period on long-term development. *Gynecol. Obstet. Fertil.* **2008**, *36*, 920–929.
172. Zhang, S.; Rattanatray, L.; McMillen, I.C.; Suter, C.M.; Morrison, J.L. Periconceptional nutrition and the early programming of a life of obesity or adversity. *Prog. Biophys. Mol. Biol.* **2011**, *106*, 307–314.
173. McMillen, I.C.; MacLaughlin, S.M.; Muhlhausler, B.S.; Gentili, S.; Duffield, J.L.; Morrison, J.L. Developmental origins of adult health and disease: The role of periconceptional and foetal nutrition. *Basic Clin. Pharmacol. Toxicol.* **2008**, *102*, 82–89.
174. Rumball, C.W.; Bloomfield, F.H.; Oliver, M.H.; Harding, J.E. Different periods of periconceptional undernutrition have different effects on growth, metabolic and endocrine status in fetal sheep. *Pediatr. Res.* **2009**, *66*, 605–613.

175. Gamborg, M.; Byberg, L.; Rasmussen, F.; Andersen, P.K.; Baker, J.L.; Bengtsson, C.; Canoy, D.; Droyvold, W.; Eriksson, J.G.; Forsen, T.; *et al.* Birth weight and systolic blood pressure in adolescence and adulthood: Meta-regression analysis of sex- and age-specific results from 20 nordic studies. *Am. J. Epidemiol.* **2007**, *166*, 634–645.
176. Chen, W.; Srinivasan, S.R.; Berenson, G.S. Amplification of the association between birthweight and blood pressure with age: The bogalusa heart study. *J. Hypertens.* **2010**, *28*, 2046–2052.
177. Chen, W.; Srinivasan, S.R.; Ruan, L.; Mei, H.; Berenson, G.S. Adult hypertension is associated with blood pressure variability in childhood in blacks and whites: The bogalusa heart study. *Am. J. Hypertens.* **2011**, *24*, 77–82.
178. O'Regan, D.; Kenyon, C.J.; Seckl, J.R.; Holmes, M.C. Prenatal dexamethasone "programmes" hypotension, but stress-induced hypertension in adult offspring. *J. Endocrinol.* **2008**, *196*, 343–352.
179. Gluckman, P.D.; Hanson, M.A. The developmental origins of the metabolic syndrome. *Trends Endocrinol. Metab.* **2004**, *15*, 183–187.
180. Armitage, J.A.; Khan, I.Y.; Taylor, P.D.; Nathanielsz, P.W.; Poston, L. Developmental programming of the metabolic syndrome by maternal nutritional imbalance: How strong is the evidence from experimental models in mammals? *J. Physiol.* **2004**, *561*, 355–377.
181. McMillen, I.C.; Robinson, J.S. Developmental origins of the metabolic syndrome: Prediction, plasticity, and programming. *Physiol. Rev.* **2005**, *85*, 571–633.
182. Stocker, C.J.; Arch, J.R.; Cawthorne, M.A. Fetal origins of insulin resistance and obesity. *Proc. Nutr. Soc.* **2005**, *64*, 143–151.
183. Gluckman, P.D.; Hanson, M.A.; Cooper, C.; Thornburg, K.L. Effect of in utero and early-life conditions on adult health and disease. *N. Engl. J. Med.* **2008**, *359*, 61–73.
184. Augustyniak, R.A.; Singh, K.; Zeldes, D.; Singh, M.; Rossi, N.F. Maternal protein restriction leads to hyperresponsiveness to stress and salt-sensitive hypertension in male offspring. *Am. J. Physiol. Regul. Integr. Comp. Physiol.* **2010**, *298*, 1375–1382.
185. Van Abeelen, A.F.; Veenendaal, M.V.; Painter, R.C.; de Rooij, S.R.; Thangaratinam, S.; van Der Post, J.A.; Bossuyt, P.M.; Elias, S.G.; Uiterwaal, C.S.; Grobbee, D.E.; *et al.* The fetal origins of hypertension: A systematic review and meta-analysis of the evidence from animal experiments of maternal undernutrition. *J. Hypertens.* **2012**, *30*, 2255–2267.
186. Grassi, G.; Facchetti, R.; Seravalle, G.; Cuspidi, C.; Mancia, G. Home and ambulatory blood pressure in resistant hypertension. *EuroIntervention* **2013**, *9*, 35–41.
187. Mancia, G.; Bombelli, M.; Brambilla, G.; Facchetti, R.; Sega, R.; Toso, E.; Grassi, G. Long-term prognostic value of white coat hypertension: An insight from diagnostic use of both ambulatory and home blood pressure measurements. *Hypertension* **2013**, *62*, 168–174.
188. Martin, U.; Holder, R.; Hodgkinson, J.; McManus, R. Inter-arm blood pressure differences compared with ambulatory monitoring: A manifestation of the "white-coat" effect? *Br. J. Gen. Pract.* **2013**, *63*, 97–103.

189. R Rios, M.T.; Dominguez-Sardina, M.; Ayala, D.E.; Gomara, S.; Sineiro, E.; Pousa, L.; Callejas, P.A.; Fontao, M.J.; Fernandez, J.R.; Hermida, R.C. Prevalence and clinical characteristics of isolated-office and true resistant hypertension determined by ambulatory blood pressure monitoring. *Chronobiol. Int.* **2013**, *30*, 207–220.
190. Sung, S.H.; Cheng, H.M.; Wang, K.L.; Yu, W.C.; Chuang, S.Y.; Ting, C.T.; Lakatta, E.G.; Yin, F.C.; Chou, P.; Chen, C.H. White coat hypertension is more risky than prehypertension: Important role of arterial wave reflections. *Hypertension* **2013**, *61*, 1346–1353.
191. Wight, T.N. Cell biology of arterial proteoglycans. *Arteriosclerosis* **1989**, *9*, 1–20.
192. Halper, J. Proteoglycans and diseases of soft tissues. *Adv. Exp. Med. Biol.* **2014**, *802*, 49–58.
193. Ozanne, S.E.; Hales, C.N. Early programming of glucose-insulin metabolism. *Trends Endocrinol. Metab.* **2002**, *13*, 368–373.
194. Fagundes, A.T.; Moura, E.G.; Passos, M.C.; Santos-Silva, A.P.; de Oliveira, E.; Trevenzoli, I.H.; Casimiro-Lopes, G.; Nogueira-Neto, J.F.; Lisboa, P.C. Temporal evaluation of body composition, glucose homeostasis and lipid profile of male rats programmed by maternal protein restriction during lactation. *Horm. Metab. Res.* **2009**, *41*, 866–873.
195. Devereux, R.B.; Roman, M.J. Left ventricular hypertrophy in hypertension: Stimuli, patterns, and consequences. *Hypertens. Res.* **1999**, *22*, 1–9.
196. Palmieri, V.; Bella, J.N.; DeQuattro, V.; Roman, M.J.; Hahn, R.T.; Dahlof, B.; Sharpe, N.; Lau, C.P.; Chen, W.C.; Paran, E.; *et al.* Relations of diastolic left ventricular filling to systolic chamber and myocardial contractility in hypertensive patients with left ventricular hypertrophy (the preserve study). *Am. J. Cardiol.* **1999**, *84*, 558–562.
197. Elnakish, M.T.; Hassanain, H.H.; Janssen, P.M. Vascular remodeling-associated hypertension leads to left ventricular hypertrophy and contractile dysfunction in profilin-1 transgenic mice. *J. Cardiovasc. Pharmacol.* **2012**, *60*, 544–552.
198. Sanchez-Soria, P.; Broka, D.; Monks, S.L.; Camenisch, T.D. Chronic low-level arsenite exposure through drinking water increases blood pressure and promotes concentric left ventricular hypertrophy in female mice. *Toxicol. Pathol.* **2012**, *40*, 504–512.
199. Nadruz, W. Myocardial remodeling in hypertension. *J. Hum. Hypertens.* **2014**, *29*, 1–6.
200. Sampson, A.K.; Moritz, K.M.; Jones, E.S.; Flower, R.L.; Widdop, R.E.; Denton, K.M. Enhanced angiotensin ii type 2 receptor mechanisms mediate decreases in arterial pressure attributable to chronic low-dose angiotensin ii in female rats. *Hypertension* **2008**, *52*, 666–671.
201. Payne, J.A.; Alexander, B.T.; Khalil, R.A. Decreased endothelium-dependent no-cgmp vascular relaxation and hypertension in growth-restricted rats on a high-salt diet. *Hypertension* **2004**, *43*, 420–427.
202. Sanders, M.W.; Fazzi, G.E.; Janssen, G.M.; Blanco, C.E.; de Mey, J.G. High sodium intake increases blood pressure and alters renal function in intrauterine growth-retarded rats. *Hypertension* **2005**, *46*, 71–75.
203. Myrie, S.B.; McKnight, L.L.; King, J.C.; McGuire, J.J.; van Vliet, B.N.; Bertolo, R.F. Effects of a diet high in salt, fat, and sugar on telemetric blood pressure measurements in conscious, unrestrained adult yucatan miniature swine (sus scrofa). *Comp. Med.* **2012**, *62*, 282–290.

204. Langley-Evans, S.C.; Jackson, A.A. Rats with hypertension induced by in utero exposure to maternal low-protein diets fail to increase blood pressure in response to a high salt intake. *Ann. Nutr. Metab.* **1996**, *40*, 1–9.
205. Yu, H.C.; Burrell, L.M.; Black, M.J.; Wu, L.L.; Dilley, R.J.; Cooper, M.E.; Johnston, C.I. Salt induces myocardial and renal fibrosis in normotensive and hypertensive rats. *Circulation* **1998**, *98*, 2621–2628.
206. Whaley-Connell, A.T.; Habibi, J.; Aroor, A.; Ma, L.; Hayden, M.R.; Ferrario, C.M.; Demarco, V.G.; Sowers, J.R. Salt loading exacerbates diastolic dysfunction and cardiac remodeling in young female ren2 rats. *Metabolism* **2013**, *62*, 1761–1771.

9

Understanding the Role of Maternal Diet on Kidney Development: An Opportunity to Improve Cardiovascular and Renal Health for Future Generations

Ryan James Wood-Bradley [1], Sanna Barrand [1], Anais Giot [2] and James Andrew Armitage [1,3,*]

[1] School of Medicine, Deakin University, Waurn Ponds, Victoria 3216, Australia;
E-Mails: r.woodbradley@deakin.edu.au (R.J.W.-B.); s.barrand@deakin.edu.au (S.B.)

[2] Insitut Politechnique LaSalle Beauvais, 60026 Beauvais Cedex, Picardie, France;
E-Mail: g.anais@deakin.edu.au

[3] Department of Anatomy and Developmental Biology, Monash University, Clayton, Victoria 3800, Australia

* Author to whom correspondence should be addressed; E-Mail: James.armitage@deakin.edu.au

---

Abstract: The leading causes of mortality and morbidity worldwide are cardiovascular disease (high blood pressure, high cholesterol and renal disease), cancer and diabetes. It is increasingly obvious that the development of these diseases encompasses complex interactions between adult lifestyle and genetic predisposition. Maternal malnutrition can influence the fetal and early life environment and pose a risk factor for the future development of adult diseases, most likely due to impaired organogenesis in the developing offspring. This then predisposes these offspring to cardiovascular disease and renal dysfunction in adulthood. Studies in experimental animals have further illustrated the significant impact maternal diet has on offspring health. Many studies report changes in kidney structure (a reduction in the number of nephrons in the kidney) in offspring of protein-deprived dams. Although the early studies suggested that increased blood pressure was also present in offspring of protein-restricted dams, this is not a universal finding and requires clarification. Importantly, to date, the literature offers little to no understanding of *when* in development these changes in kidney development occur, nor are the cellular and molecular mechanisms that drive these changes well characterised. Moreover, the mechanisms linking maternal nutrition and a suboptimal renal phenotype in offspring are yet to be discerned—one potential mechanism involves epigenetics. This review will focus on recent information on potential mechanisms by which maternal nutrition (focusing on malnutrition due to protein restriction, micronutrient restriction and excessive fat intake) influences kidney development and thereby function in later life.

Keywords: developmental programming; kidney development; maternal diet

---

1. Maternal Nutrition and the Kidney

A plethora of evidence exists for to support the crucial role that the environment plays during development in determining the future health of the offspring. *Developmental programming* refers to the mechanism underlying this phenomenon and is defined as "a permanent change in the structure or function of an organism due to alterations in development that occur in response to an environmental stimulus during critical periods of organ development" [1]. Particularly implicated is maternal nutrition, which has been shown to have an effect on offspring health, with both over- and under-nutrition having negative consequences on offspring health [2–5]. A number of studies have provided evidence to support the hypothesis that maternal nutritional status plays a critical role on the health and wellbeing of the fetus [6–8]. Changes to maternal nutritional status may change the ability of the mother to supply the growing fetus with the required nutrients for optimal growth. Initial studies during early and mid 20th Century documented the nutritional requirements during pregnancy in humans [9,10] as well as animals [11–14], indicating the importance of a diet containing sufficient amounts of essential nutrients (proteins, fats, carbohydrates) and micronutrients (iron and calcium) and a sufficient caloric value. These studies reported that protein or micronutrient restriction in the mother lead to poor offspring growth *in utero* and in early postnatal life. It was much later that we began to appreciate the biological consequences of these fetal trade-offs in response to a sub-optimal maternal diet.

Perturbations to the maternal diet during pregnancy and/or lactation are associated with increased risk of renal, cardiovascular and metabolic disease in the offspring [15,16]. The developing kidney is particularly susceptible to the effects of a suboptimal maternal diet; changes in expression of genes and proteins important for kidney development, are likely to underlie the developmental programming of kidney structure and physiology. This paper will review the literature to describe the role of maternal macro- and micro-nutrient imbalance in influencing fetal and neonatal kidney development, final nephron complement and the effect of these structural abnormalities on adult function. The mechanisms underlying these observations will also be discussed.

In order to understand developmental programming of renal structure and function in humans, animal models using dietary interventions have been established. This is primarily due to the difficulty in quantifying structure of the human kidney by non-invasive methods. For example, the effects of maternal dietary zinc, vitamin A and protein restriction or maternal dietary fat excess all have been shown to have a negative impact on kidney development and later renal disease in the offspring [16–19]. Furthermore, a decrease in nephron number is hypothesized to lead to disrupted fluid and electrolyte balance, which in turn, may lead to volume expansion and finally glomerular hyperfiltration and systemic hypertension [20]. Importantly, restricted maternal protein intake in pregnancy has been linked to reduced birth weight, impaired nephron endowment, elevated blood pressure and reduced glomerular filtration rate (GFR) [21–29].

1.1. Maternal Protein Restriction Programs Reduced Nephron Number but the Physiological Consequences are Unclear

Interestingly, despite there being a consistent observation from several research groups that protein restriction during development results in a reduction in nephron number, the follow-on effects on renal function (characterized by a measurement of glomerular filtration rate; GFR) and blood pressure are far from clear due to inconsistent techniques used. For example, early studies by Woods *et al.* [26] clearly showed that male offspring from protein restricted dams had a 25% nephron deficit, an 11% GFR reduction and a 10 mmHg increase in mean arterial blood pressure compared with control rats. The calculated single nephron glomerular filtration rate in these protein deprived offspring was 20% greater in protein-restricted than in protein-replete controls [26]. Increases in individual nephron GFR can be an indication of renal hyperfiltration, which can ultimately lead to further nephron loss, perpetuating this cycle [20].

Later studies demonstrated that the phenotype induced by maternal protein-deprivation is not invariant. Woods *et al.* [27] reported that maternal diet affected offspring in a sex-specific manner; female offspring of protein restricted *Sprague-Dawley* rats did not demonstrate hypertension or a nephron deficit. This suggests that sex-dependent variations in developmental programming of the kidney exist, are subtle and highly reliant on the concentration of dietary protein or, potentially, timing of the intervention. Furthermore, reductions in nephron endowment associated with intrauterine protein restriction, are not always accompanied by hypertension. For example, Zimanyi *et al.* (2006) reported a nephron deficit in *Wistar-Kyoto* (WKY) rats fed an 8.7% (low) protein diet (control rats were fed a 20% protein diet) with no alteration in blood pressure or evidence of renal hyperfiltration in the protein-restricted group [30]. Maternal low-protein or caloric restricted diets induce low birth weight in the offspring [31,32] and this reduction in body size may correlate with changes in cardiovascular function and growth [33,34]. Catch-up growth may exacerbate the adverse consequences, such as hypertension, of developmental programming [15,35,36]. Together, these data suggest that maternal protein restriction during pregnancy most likely results in altered kidney and morphology but the follow-on effects on physiology and function are currently not well understood. The variability in phenotype may be resultant from exposure to dietary insult at different points of kidney development. Knowledge of the molecular processes involved in controlling kidney development and ultimately adult morphology are essential for understanding the impact of maternal protein restriction and will be discussed in further detail later in the review.

1.2. Maternal Overnutrition Has Subtle Impacts upon Kidney Development and Function in the Offspring

Although early programming studies focused on the role of maternal undernutrition as models for the Dutch Hunger Winter studies [37–39], it is apparent that overnutrition is now a major risk to human health and wellbeing. The concept of maternal malnutrition must therefore be expanded to include excess caloric or fatty acid intake [40–44]. Over nutrition and obesity during pregnancy is risk factor for poor outcomes for offspring health, including the susceptibility to chronic diseases [45,46] as well as mortality from these diseases [42,47]. Investigating neonatal outcomes in obese mothers, Catalano *et al.* [48] report that maternal obesity leads to fetuses with greater fat mass, and insulin resistance. Likewise,

Boney *et al.* [49] reported that children born large-for-gestational-age to obese mothers were at a greater risk of developing metabolic syndrome. In a rabbit model of maternal high-fat feeding (containing 13% fat), Prior *et al.* [50] report greater mean arterial pressure (6 mmHg), heart rate (13 bpm) and renal sympathetic nerve activity (1.3 nU) compared with controls. These animals were slightly heavier throughout postnatal life and at 4 months of age had significantly heavier white adipose tissue (64%) compared with controls. Similarly, Jackson and colleagues report glomerular sclerosis and reduced kidney function (increased urine albumin excretion) in offspring exposed to a maternal diet high in fructose and fat compared to controls [51]. In a rat model of maternal high fat feeding, Armitage *et al.* (2005) report no change in nephron endowment in offspring of fat fed dams compared with controls, but these same high fat offspring had abnormal renal renin activity which the authors hypothesized to underlie the increased mean arterial pressure [52].

The mechanism by which maternal over nutrition leads to poor health outcomes is not fully understood. Obesity is linked to a chronic inflammatory state in both the mother and fetus [53] and it is possible that this is mediating the changes in gene expression and the development of the offspring.

1.3. Maternal Micronutrient Status and Its Impact on Offspring Kidney Health

In utero development is characterized by rapid cell synthesis and therefore the developing fetus has a particularly high demand for nutritional substrate. Micronutrients are critical co-factors in enzymatic pathways of cell synthesis in the fetus and therefore there is a high dietary demand for these compounds during pregnancy. Maternal deficiencies in micronutrients can have lasting detrimental effects on the fetus and again there is evidence that the kidney is preferentially affected. Lelievre-Pegorier *et al.* [54] report a 20% reduction in nephron number in adult rats born to mothers that were fed a vitamin A deficient diet during 3 weeks prior to pregnancy, throughout pregnancy up until day 21 of gestation. The mechanism underlying this abnormal kidney phenotype is most likely the fact the vitamin A is a key ligand for the cRET receptor, which controls the earliest processes of kidney development (see Section 2 for full details).

Although the role of vitamin A is well established, other maternal micronutrient deficiencies are associated with abnormal kidney structure or function in her offspring; but with less clear mechanisms Lisle *et al.* [55] reported that diet-induced maternal iron deficiency is associated with greater systolic blood pressure and reduced glomerular number in adult offspring, when compared with controls. Similarly in a model of maternal zinc restriction, Tomat and colleagues [17,56,57] reported reduced nephron number and kidney function (determined by nitric oxide synthase activity) as well as greater blood pressure (tail cuff plethysmography) when compared with controls. The pathway by which different micronutrient deficiency leads to similar morphological phenotypes remains unknown; zinc deficiency has negative effects on branching morphogenesis; a process key to kidney development, but can also impact upon the development of the placenta, thereby affecting the growth potential of the entire embryo or fetus [58].

Given the great disparity in the forms of maternal dietary challenge it is intriguing that a similar phenotype is observed in the offspring in response to challenges as diverse as zinc or protein deficiency. This prompts the hypothesis that fundamental processes in kidney development may be sensitive to an array of abnormal signals from the environment, eliciting a common adaptive response and resulting in a characteristic phenotype. In order to discuss these mechanisms, we will first consider the factors that underpin the development of the kidney.

2. Kidney Development

2.1. Early Signaling: Specification of the Ureteric Bud and Metanephric Mesenchyme

The kidneys play a vital role in health and disease. In mammals, the kidney develops through three successive stages (Figure 1):

The Pronephros, a rudimentary structure that develops from the lateral plate and intermediate mesoderm and continues to develop into the mesonephros [59].

The Mesonephros, a transient organ, although the mesonephric (nephric) duct is important for the development of the metanephros, the permanent mammalian kidney [59].

The Metanephros which begins to develop at day 35 in human gestation, embryonic day 11.5 (E11.5) in the mouse [60] and embryonic day E12–E13 in rats [61,62].

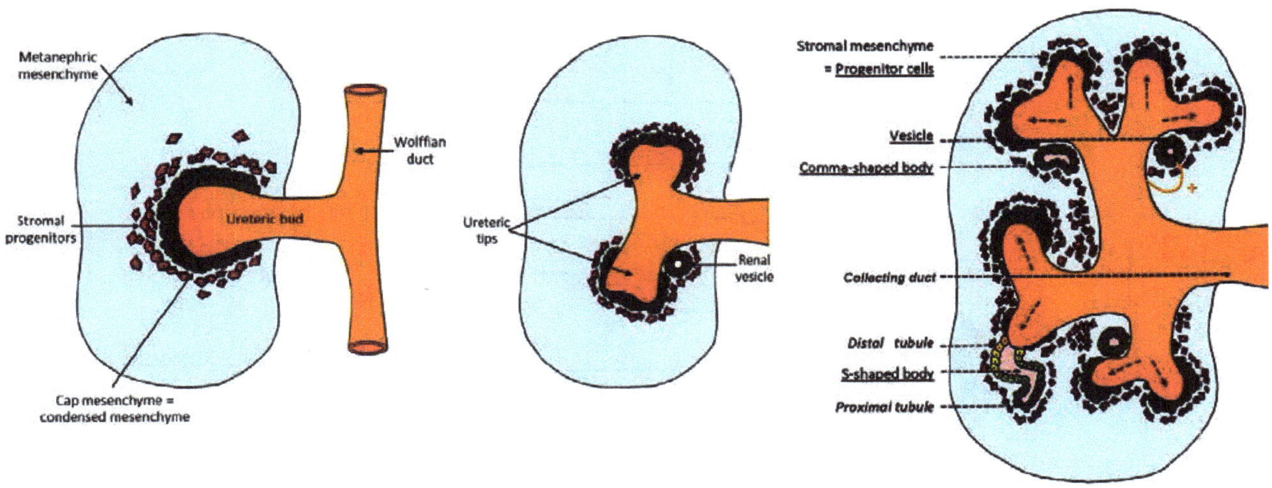

Figure 1. Kidney development. The mammalian kidney develops through three stages (pronephros, mesonephros and metanephros). The pronephros develops from the nephric duct, following which, mesonephric development occurs in conjunction with the degeneration of the pronephros and the formation of the mesonephric tubules. The metanephros develops from the induction of the metanepheric mesenchyme by the ureteric bud from the nephric (Wolffian) duct. As the ureteric bud branches into the metanephric mesenchyme, the mesenchyme around the tips of this branching structure are induced to form renal vesicles. Renal vesicles will progress through the comma-shaped body and S-shaped body stages before connecting to the collecting system of the developing kidney to form a developed nephron.

Nephrogenesis is complete by 36 weeks gestation in humans, by about PN3 (postnatal) in mice [59,63] and PN7 in rats [64]. The metanephros begins to develop when cells from the caudal end grow out from the Wolffian duct (or mesonephric duct) forming the ureteric bud in response to growth factors (discussed in the following sections) secreted by the metanephric mesenchyme [59,64–66]. Under the influence of these growth factors, the ureteric bud invades the metanephric mesenchyme and branches forming the collecting duct system.

2.2. Genetic Control of Kidney Development

2.2.1. Control of Branching: Molecules Involved in Branching and Inhibiting Lateral Branching

Branching morphogenesis is the dichotomous arborisation of ureteric epithelium and is responsible for the development of the collecting duct system of the kidney. The process of branching morphogenesis is tightly regulated by inhibitors (BMP4, bone morphogenic protein 4), promoters (GDNF, glial derived neurotrophic factor and c-RET, c-ret tyrosine kinase receptor) and growth factors (TGF, transforming growth factor β superfamily). These genes are essential regulators of ureteric bud branching and patterning [67] (Figure 2).

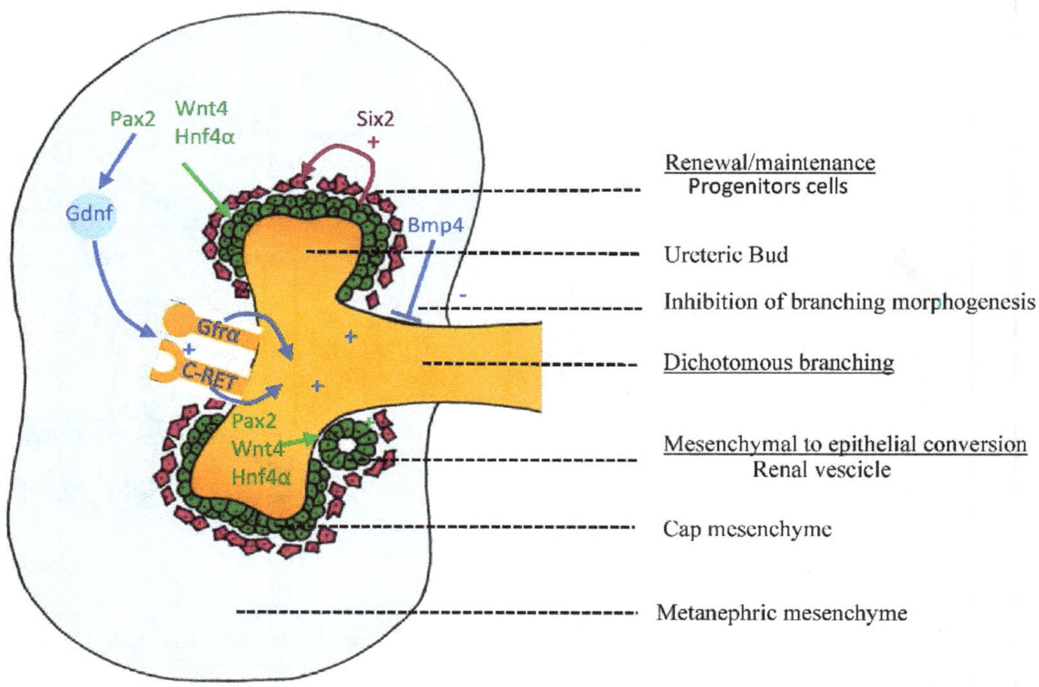

Figure 2. Molecular control of early kidney development. Early development of the metanephros, the permanent mammalian kidney, is under tight molecular control. Outgrowth and branching morphogenesis of the ureteric bud is controlled by the expression of receptors *Gfra1* and *C-ret* to which *Gdnf* binds. Production of *Gdnf* is under the influence of *Pax2*, Together these factors stimulate branching morphogenesis of the kidney. *Bmp4* inhibits lateral branching of the ureteric, which ensures tight control of branching morphogenesis. Induction of the metanephric mesenchyme to undergo epithelial to mesenchymal transition is influenced by *Wnt4* and *Hnf4α*. The formation of renal vesicles (from the cap mesenchyme) is controlled by the number of *Six2* positive cells (denoting renal stem cells). Once committed to forming a nephron, these cells begin to express *Pax2*, *Wnt4* and *Hnf4α*.

Branching morphogenesis begins with the interaction between the metanephric mesenchyme and the ureteric bud, whereby inductive signals from both embryonic derivatives (GDNF is released from the metanephric mesenchyme and binds to its receptors c-RET and GFRα1 at the tips of the ureteric bud) initiate the branching process [68–72]. Tight regulation of branching morphogenesis is essential to both kidney development and function.

2.2.2. Control of Nephrogenesis: Epithelial-Mesenchymal Transition (EMT)

Nephrogenesis is intricately involved with branching morphogenesis. The induction of nephron development occurs only at the tips of the developing ureteric tree. Metanephric mesenchymal cells adjacent to the ureteric branch tips are induced, leading to condensation, epithelialization and proliferation of the cap mesenchyme. This induced mesenchyme expresses genes involved in extracellular matrix formation and remodeling, cell-adhesion molecules, cell survival and proliferation [73–75]. Under influence of the genes *Pax2*, *Wnt4* and *Hnf4α* [76–79] the induced mesenchyme undergoes epithelialisation and differentiates successively into renal vesicles, comma-shaped bodies, S-shaped bodies before the glomerular vascular tuft develops and attaches to the proximal tubule to finally form mature nephrons, the functional units of the kidney.

3. Specification of Nephron Structures

The induced mesenchyme continues to develop through various morphological steps including a comma-shaped body which is characterised by expression of the primitive podocyte marker MNFB and genes involved with *Bmp* signalling including *Bmp2*, *4*, *7* [80–84]. Then, the comma-shaped body develops into an S-shaped body through FGF8 and PAX2 signalling [77,85,86], linking up with the ureteric epithelium. The S-shaped body contains the primitive cells of the glomerulus with the invasion of angiogenic cells. With capillarisation and connecting to the tubule (influenced by FGF2 and LIF expression) [87] the basic structure of the nephron is complete. However, the nephron continues to undergo maturation in the form of tubular elongation.

The metanephric mesenchyme is preserved through the maintenance of a population of progenitor cells. This leads to sufficient support of the progression and development of nephrogenesis. Extensive study, aimed at identifying the genes involved in the maintenance of this cell population, has indicated the importance of Six2, Fgf2 and Bmp7 [88,89]. Self *et al.* [90] reported that knockout of Six2 lead to premature development of renal vesicles. This suggests that Six2 is required to maintain a population of cells required for the development of progenitor cells that form renal vesicles. The generation of Six2 positive cells is related to cortical stromal cells expressing Foxd1, which suggests that there are complex interrelationships between cell subsets that give rise to cells that can control the development of structures within the kidney [91].

4. Arcade Formation

In humans nephrogenesis is complete by approximately 36 weeks of gestation, while in rodents, nephrogenesis continues for a short time after birth [64,92]. Until approximately 14–15 weeks of pregnancy in humans, and the end of gestation in rodents, each tip of the ureteric tip connects to a single nephron produced by the surrounding mesenchyme. When arborisation of the ureteric tree is finished and branching ceases, nephrogenesis continues by a process of nephron arcade formation whereby multiple nephrons attached to the same tip.

A second nephron is induced by the same tip, attaches to this tip and the connecting tubule of the older nephron shifts to the new nephron. Other nephrons are then induced until four to seven nephrons form an arcade arrangement by being attached to the stalk rather than just to the tips forming a common connecting segment. Arcade formation enables deep and mid-cortical nephrons to connect to collecting ducts located in the renal cortex [93]. After 20–22 weeks of gestation in humans, and by the very end of kidney development in rodent, nephrons are attached individually and directly along the entire length of the collecting duct and are not incorporated in the arcade [63,65]. Arcade formation is thought to be underpinned by the activity of a number of genes within the Notch pathway as they are involved in the formation of intercellular connections (such as N-cadherin and integrins), however further elucidation of the mechanism is required [94]. Arcade formation is a period of rapid nephron formation and therefore disruption of kidney development durign this critical window can have a profound impact.

5. Final Nephron Endowment

The processes controlling the time at which nephrogenesis ends are less well described than those controlling active nephrogenesis. One hypothesis is that the population of cells in the metanephric mesenchyme limits the magnitude of cells that can aggregate and differentiate into nephrons. Indeed this has been proposed as a factor underlying the large variability in nephron number in mammals [95–97]. In human, the peak period of nephrogenesis occurs during the last third of pregnancy after the cessation of branching morphogenesis. The progenitor cells of the metanephric mesenchyme provide the basis from which all the cells of the nephron will differentiate. For this reason, as the population of metanephric mesenchyme diminishes there is a natural cessation of nephrogenesis.

Nephron endowment is also dependent upon the branching capacity of the ureteric bud, as nephrons only form adjacent to ureteric tips [54,64,98]. Retarded branching of the ureteric epithelium can therefore manifest in a permanent reduction of nephrons and impaired kidney growth.

In addition, factors involved in the ureteric branching and the epithelisation of the metanephric mesenchyme including growth factors and their receptors, degrading enzyme, proto-oncogenes, transcription factors, suppressor genes extracellular matrix, teratogens and fetal/maternal environment are all involved in the regulation of kidney development and can impinge on nephron endowment [61,99]. It is perhaps not surprising therefore that the number of nephrons in human kidneys varies widely, from 300,000 to nearly 2 million [95,100–106].

Early Investigations Supporting Changes during Kidney Development (Genes and Pathways, Cells and Timing)

Kidney development occurs across a number of periods of plasticity and is therefore subject to a number of "critical periods" when external insults may produce life-long structural and potentially functional changes in kidney. Importantly, once kidney development is complete (at around gestational week 38 in humans and postnatal day 8 in rat), no further nephrons are formed. Therefore, a reduction in nephron number caused by interventions during kidney development persists throughout life and may contribute to the burden of disease in later life. Singh *et al.*, 2007 showed in rats that glucocorticoid exposure during the early stages of kidney development (embryonic day E14 to E15), permanently decreased nephron number at PN30 [98]. This is in agreement with an earlier study by Woods *et al.* (2004), which showed that maternal protein restriction during the second half of the pregnancy, when nephrogenesis is active, is associated with a reduction in nephron endowment [28].

Interestingly, the dietary insult need not occur during the period of active nephrogenesis to promote a reduction in nephron number. Welham *et al.* 2005 demonstrate that exposure low protein maternal diet from start of the pregnancy until day E13 in rats (prior to the onset of nephrogenesis) is sufficient to cause reduction in glomerular numbers by approximately 20% [99]. Additionally, uteroplacental insufficiency and reduction in litter number has similar effect during the late stage kidney development [107,108]. Conversely, removing dietary insult during postnatal life may improve glomerular numbers [107,109] owing to the fact that nephrogenesis in rats proceeds until approximately PN7-8. These studies together suggest that dietary insults during critical developmental window may cause changes, especially, in kidney morphology, which may translate to physiological deficits.

The underlying nephron deficit observed in studies of maternal dietary manipulation must be underpinned by changes in the expression of genes and proteins. However, only few studies have analyzed the early gene expression profiles of the kidney exposed to a suboptimal intrauterine environment and how these changes lead to nephron deficit still remains unclear. Abdel-Hakkem and colleagues (2008) induced global caloric restriction in *Sprague-Dawley* rats, and analyzed 10 critical genes involved in branching morphogenesis and nephrogenesis at E20 [110]. Genes involved in mesenchymal to epithelial transformation (*Wnt4*, *Wt1*, *Fgf2* and *Bmp7*) were found to be up-regulated, while genes involved in branching morphogenesis (*Pax2*, *Gdnf*, *Fgf7*, *Bmp4*, and *Wnt11*) were down-regulated [110]. Additionally, proteins of GDNF and MAPK-ERK pathway (e.g., Gfraα1, phosphorylated ERK1/2 and mitogen-activated protein kinase 1/2) are altered already at E20 by maternal food restriction, indicating the importance of these pathways for normal nephrogenesis [111]. In addition a recent study in rats, adult offspring (16 weeks) of low-protein dams showed up-regulation of TGF-β1 and ZEB2 mRNA in kidneys displaying nephron deficit [112]. The authors further suggested that TGF-β1 may induce ZEB2 expression further leading to down-regulation of specific miRNAs within the glomeruli, leading to altered function [112]. These studies suggest that aberrant gene expression of various pathways may underlie reduced nephron endowment, however, the exact mechanism remain to be determined.

For some time, there have been suggestions that apoptosis of mesenchymal cells in developing kidneys play a role in the reduction of nephron endowment [113]. Rats exposed to a maternal LP diet demonstrated a 20% reduction in adult nephron number and up-regulation of apoptotic pathways (e.g., Bax and Bcl-2) [99]. Apoptotic gene expression is also altered by maternal undernourishment [114] particularly increased levels of proteins in late embryonic life (E20; Fas-receptor and Caspase-9) and early postnatal life (PN1; Fas-receptor and caspase-3). These molecular changes were accompanied with increased apoptosis in the nephrogenic zone (the area of active nephrogenesis) of the kidney [115]. These findings demonstrated that maternal programming might increase apoptosis in the developing kidney, which in turn may contribute to nephron deficit.

Other mechanisms proposed to contribute to the nephron deficit, include dysregulation of the Renin-angiotensin system (RAS). Angiotensin is essential in forming blood vessels and tubules during nephrogenesis as well as the development of smooth muscle in the ureter [116,117]. Thus, deficits in nephron number may be preceded by suppression of RAS further contributing to disturbed fluid and electrolyte balance (dysfunction of kidney) and adulthood hypertension. Interestingly, a recent report suggests sex-specific alteration of RAS system is induced by *in utero* exposure to a low-protein diet [19]. Cooke *et al.* 2014 showed that expression of Angiotensin converting enzyme (ACE) was up-regulated in male, but not in female offspring, as early as at E19 relative to control [19]. Additionally, expression of the G-protein coupled receptor of RAS, AT1R, was observed in male offspring at PN21 [19]. Thus, maternal low protein diet may alter nephron numbers in the developing kidney through altered expression of the RAS system, especially in the male offspring. Another study has highlighted the potential function of the Na co-transporters and the RAS in the developmental programming of the kidney [109]. Na-K-Cl co-transporter and Na-Cl co-transporters display functional role in Na reabsorption in kidney and altering levels of these co-transporter could ultimately lead to development of adulthood hypertension.

The exact mechanism underpinning the programming of a nephron deficit remains unknown, but most likely involve alterations in multiple pathways such as apoptotic-pathways, RAS and specific EMT related pathways. The mechanism underlying these gene modulations is proposed to be heritable but not related to mutations in the genome.

6. Maternal Diet and the Offspring Epigenome

Changed gene expression; not mutations within the genome, but changes in the way that the genome is expressed, is controlled by epigenetic "marks" such as gene methylation, histone modifications and the binding of DNA proteins. These marks can act independently or in concert to modify expression of genes. Epigenetics may play a role in developmental programming of adult disease as it provides a mechanism that explains the change in gene expression, and therefore the change in phenotype. These changes can be brought about through multiple epigenetic pathways.

The maternal environment, before, during and after birth can have a significant impact on the epigenome of the offspring [118–122]. Essentially, the epigenetic profile of the organism is malleable during any stage of development—as during this stage the genome is undergoing modifications and specification. Before the genome becomes heritably stable, changes in the epigenetic profile can be incorporated into the phenotypic profile and therefore be inherited over multiple cellular cycles and alter the gene expression of that cell line or organ system. One of the most well studied models of how the maternal environment affects the offspring genome through epigenetic mechanisms, is that of the *agouti* mouse.

The *agouti* viable yellow (*AvY*) mouse strain has been used extensively to demonstrate the effects of a methyl deficient diet and subsequent disease outcome. The agouti gene is under the control of a methylation sensitive promoter and infers a yellow coat colour and an increased preponderance to obesity, diabetes, cancer and a shorter lifespan when expressed [123–125]. Pregnant *AvY* mice exposed to methyl deficient diets give birth to pups displaying variable coat colours but the majority of offspring present with the agouti phenotype. This phenotype occurs in response to hypomethylation of the agouti locus and an increase in expression. The phenotype is not reversible by later methyl donor supplementation. Where methyl donors are freely available in the maternal diet, the agouti locus remains methylated and the gene repressed, thus the majority of offspring have a brown coat and normal physiology, metabolism and life expectancy.

Studies that have investigated the consequences of maternal dietary manipulation on offspring phenotype, commonly report changes in gene expression and major function in the offspring [126].

Epigenetic control of gene expression is maintained and regulated by three major mechanisms: DNA methylation, histone acetylation and non-protein coding RNA [126]. Few studies have investigated the role of epigenetics in kidney development however there is strong evidence that relatively high level (*i.e.*, changes to enzymes that have wide-reaching effects, rather than those that control a particular process of kidney development) epigenetic changes may drive later kidney disease. Pham *et al.* [127] used uteroplacental insufficiency as a model of intrauterine growth restriction and report that CpG methylation of p53 was altered leading to changes in expression of genes involved in apoptosis within the kidney. While methylation is one form of epigenetic modification, there is also the production and implication of microRNAs. The importance of Dicer; the enzyme which cleaves non-coding microRNAs into active microRNAs during mammalian kidney development has been shown by Nagalakshmi *et al.* [128]. These authors used a transgenic mouse model (Six2Cre) where *Dicer* was conditionally ablated from the progenitors of the nephron epithelium. The removal of Dicer lead to elevated apoptosis and premature termination of nephrogenesis. Ablation of *Dicer* from ureteric bud epithelium (using HoxB7Cre transgenic mice) resulted in disrupted branching morphogenesis and the development of renal cysts [128]. Likewise in a mouse model with the conditional knockout of Dicer1 from the developing urogenital tract, Pastorelli *et al.* [129] report renal abnormalities including hydronephrosis and cyst formation. Furthermore, offspring had increased renal apoptosis combined with reduced glomerular number. These results illustrate the importance of miRNA function during kidney development.

Offspring of rats whose mothers were fed protein restricted diets in pregnancy and lactation demonstrate global changes to the methylation status of whole organs, and important gene pathways that play a major role in kidney development and adult function [130–132]. These studies have further investigated these effects to show that important enzymes involved in setting the methylation profile of the genome are altered (specifically DNMT1, which is involved in maintaining the methylation status of the genome during replication), as well as receptors involved in protein metabolism [133,134]. Given that methylation is highly dependent on dietary intake of methyl donors, it has now been demonstrated that when either the maternal or early postnatal diet are supplemented with methyl donors (such as glycine and folic acid), the deleterious cardiovascular effects of maternal protein restriction may be at least partially ameliorated or rescued. Song *et al.* 2010, suggest that a number of genes underlying ureteric bud formation (including elements of the renin angiotensin system) are controlled by histone acetylation; certainly HDAC inhibitors have a negative impact on kidney development. Interestingly, despite the intense interest in determining epigenetic changes in models of maternal or developmental programming, there is still little direct evidence for an epigenetic modification in the development of kidney disease or morphological abnormality [135]. This is likely due to the complex interplay between histone acetylation, gene methylation and miRNA post-translational modifications.

7. The Impact of Nephron Endowment on Adult Cardiovascular and Renal Health

As nephrons are the functional units of the kidney a reduction in number is theoretically detrimental to kidney function. Low nephron number may result in adult kidney dysfunction including hypervolaemia, electrolyte balance and toxaemia [136] and is implicated in hypertension and renal disease [137].

The mechanism underlying this link between nephron number and cardiovascular/renal function was first described and popularized by Brenner *et al.* [20]. Brenner hypothesised that a reduction in renal filtration surface area (due to either lower nephron number or lower filtration surface area per glomerulus) would lead to limited sodium excretion, secondary hypervolaemia which promotes an increase in glomerular capillary pressure. Over time this excessive pressure results in glomerular sclerosis [20], further reductions filtration surface area a further increase in systemic blood pressure.

There is strong evidence to support the hypothesis that there is an associate between nephron number and blood pressure but due to fact that present methods for estimating human nephron endowment can only be conducted post mortem it is not possible to show causation. Keller *et al.* [105] reported an inverse association between nephron endowment and hypertension in humans. However, it was unclear whether the lower numbers of nephrons in subjects with a history of hypertension were responsible for hypertension or a consequence of hypertension. Keller *et al.* [105] analysed kidneys obtained at autopsy from Caucasian subjects (normotensive and hypertensive patients) between the age of 35 and 59 years, and found that 10 normotensive subjects had a median glomerular number of 1,429,200 while 10 hypertensive subjects had a median glomerular number of 702,379. Although it was unclear whether the lower numbers of nephrons in subjects with a history of hypertension were responsible for hypertension or a consequence of hypertension. The hypertensive patients showed very few obsolescent glomeruli which may suggest that the hypertension had not caused the deficit in nephron number. Douglas-Denton *et al.* [100] also reported that hypertensive subjects have significantly fewer nephrons (746,468 ± 133,240) than normotensive subjects (1,402,360 ± 346,357).

Low birth weight (LBW) is often used as an indication of intra-uterine growth restriction and has been correlated with the incidence of kidney disease [138,139]. For example, Lackland [138] provided evidence that kidney failure and end-stage renal disease demonstrate a racial and geographic disparity. This concept is supported by findings of Hoy *et al.* [101] that the kidneys of Australian Aboriginals contain 30% fewer nephrons than those of non-indigenous Australians. This phenomenon may explain in part why Australian Aborigines in remote areas have a much greater incidence of renal disease (as well as hypertension and cardiovascular disease) than non-Aboriginal peoples in remote areas [140]. A study by Lackland [141] focused on the incidence of hypertension, demonstrating that adults born with LBW had a much higher systolic blood pressure and were more likely to suffer from hypertensive-related end-stage renal disease than those of normal birth weight. Investigating the developing kidney in the human fetus, Lori *et al.* [142] report that IUGR was associated with reduced renal volume compared to gestational-age adjusted controls. While renal volume can be indicative of nephron number, no technique is available for *in situ* measurement of human fetal nephron number. The investigation by Lori *et al.* does provide information on how the human intrauterine environment impacts directly upon the kidney and the finding is repeatable. A more recent investigation by Wang *et al.* [143] in human fetal kidneys also reports that fetal growth restriction is associated with smaller kidneys which appears to be caused by increased apoptosis and reduced expression of renin and angiotensinogen.

Although the limited human data appear to be supportive of an association between low birth weight and reduced kidney size this association is not always observed in animal studies [144] where tighter control over experimental conditions and potential bias are possible. In support of this hypothesis Langley-Evans *et al.* [145] reported that a deficit of 13% in nephron number was associated with a 13 mmHg elevation in arterial pressure of protein-restricted offspring (*Wistar* rats exposed to a 9% protein diet, while controls had a normal 18% protein diet). On the other hand, no relationship between nephron number and blood pressure was found in female offspring from protein restricted *Sprague-Dawley* dams (on a 8.5% protein diet, while controls were on a 19% protein diet) by Woods *et al.* [27].

Investigations into the relationship between nephron number and cardiovascular health do not support the Brenner Hypothesis unconditionally (see review by Kett and Denton [146]. Nephron deficiency is not always associated with elevated arterial pressure. For example, Zimanyi *et al.* (2006) reported a nephron deficit in offspring of *WKY* rats fed an 8.7% (low) protein diet (while control rats were fed a 20% protein diet) but blood pressure and renal filtration were normal [30]. The absence of change in blood pressure between the dietary groups may also be a product of offspring exposed to maternal protein restriction failing to demonstrate catch-up growth.

Moreover, reduced nephron endowment does not necessarily underlie systemic high blood pressure, in a model of hypertension unrelated to maternal nutrition. Investigating the *Spontaneously Hypertensive Rat* (SHR), Black and colleagues [147] report no change in nephron number but a 29 mmHg increase in blood pressure (measured via tail cuff plethysmography). This is in contrast to the findings of Skov *et al.* [148] who reported reduced nephron number in the *SHR* compared to normotensive *WKY* rats. While it is understood that the hypertension that develops in the *SHR* is multifactorial, the relationship that nephron endowment may play is unclear. The results from these studies indicate that the relationship between nephron number and blood pressure is not direct and may be influenced by other factors including the renin-angiotensin-aldosterone systems and aberrant sympathetic nerve activity. The other potential confounding factor is the blood pressure measurement technique. Tail-cuff plethysmography is known to induce a stress response in animals that may lead to increased blood pressure [149,150]. Further studies are required using less stressful techniques, such as radiotelemetry [149,150], to further elucidate the underlying mechanism of hypertension within the *SHR*.

Tonkiss and colleagues, using radiotelemetry devices, reported that malnourished rat offspring (6% maternal LP diet) demonstrated a 4 mmHg increase in diastolic blood pressure compared with controls, however offspring of protein-restricted rats elicited a greater cardiovascular arousal response (increased systolic pressure) to acute stress compared with controls [151]. This same study did not report nephron number in malnourished offspring, but did find that malnourished offspring weighed the same as controls at the time of blood pressure measurement. In a rat model of maternal caloric restriction, Brennan and colleagues reported a nephron deficit and no change in adult blood pressure (recorded using radiotelemetry) [152]. Lim *et al.* [153] report that in rats exposed to maternal protein restriction that while there was no change in mean arterial pressure (consciously measured with indwelling catheters) there was greater filtration of the kidney. Therefore, the question still remains about the relative contribution of postnatal growth and nephron number to adult blood pressure.

Although multiple studies have reported low nephron number in offspring of dams exposed to a protein-restricted diet, the renal physiological effects of this reduction in nephron number have received less attention and findings have been contradictory. Alwasel and Ashton [154] reported no change in GFR in male or female rat offspring exposed to maternal LP diet (no nephron number reported), while Nwagwu *et al.* [23] reported reduced GFR in rat offspring exposed to maternal LP diet (no nephron number reported). Hoppe *et al.* [22] using a model of life long protein restriction in rats reported no change in GFR with a 31% reduction in nephron number.

Sidduque *et al.* (2014) show no association between hypertension and low nephron number in the offspring of Sprague Dawley rats fed 6% protein from 12 days of gestation [109]. Neonates of these dams were cross-fostered and studied. Offspring exposed to a high protein diet (20% w/w) *in utero* and cross-fostered to a mother fed a low-protein (6% protein) diet showed increased blood pressure and expression of the co-transporters after birth relative to control animals (20% protein throughout life) [109]. Surprisingly, these animal maintained similar nephron number and blood pressure compared with controls [109]. On the other hand, animals that were maintained on a protein restricted diet throughout the pregnancy and suckling recorded increased blood pressure, increased expression of renin and ANGII, had reduced nephron number, but did not show alteration in the Na co-transporter expression relative to controls [109]. This study indicates that dietary impact at different time points indeed could affect kidney development through different pathways. In summary, suboptimal maternal diet may alter gene and protein expression in the developing kidney leading to permanent reduction of nephron number but whether or not this results in hypertension is clearly dependent on other, yet to be identified factors.

There is also evidence that pre- *vs.* post-natal nutritional planes have differing effects on kidney development in altricial species such as rats and mice. Jennings and colleagues used a cross-fostering method in rats to compare the contributions of the fetal and postnatal environments on offspring growth [155]. Pups that were exposed to protein restriction *in utero* then switched to a control dam post birth underwent catch-up growth and had similar weight to control pups by PN21, while pups that were maintained on a low protein diet postnatally did not. In fact, pups that underwent catch-up growth had reduced longevity. Investigations into catch-up growth also report changes in insulin sensitivity [156] and reduced β-cell proliferation and islet size during fetal life [157]. Wlodek *et al.* [107] using an uteroplacental insufficiency model in rats to induce fetal growth restriction report that offspring that were growth restricted in utero and postnatally had higher blood pressure as well as a nephron deficit, compared to controls. Meanwhile, offspring that were restricted in utero and were then cross-fostered to control dams did not have a reduced nephron endowment or increased blood pressure [107]. These studies indicate that postnatal nutrition of offspring is critical to the development of disease. Many studies that have linked maternal low protein diet to reduced nephron endowment and hypertension also observed accelerated growth postnatally [26,158,159].

The difficulty in translating these rodent studies back to the human condition is that rats and mice are born immature and nephrogenesis proceeds for up to a week postnatal. In humans, this process of nephrogenesis occurs *in utero* until 38 weeks gestation, therefore the postnatal period has little impact upon term infants. In the premature infant, however, the situation may be very different because these children are born whilst nephrogenesis is ongoing. Moreover, in many cases, the supply of breast milk is constrained in mothers of premature infants and formula supplementation may be required.

Investigating the impact of preterm birth in humans on kidney development and function, Gubhaju *et al.* 2014 report that renal function was affected by gestational age and may be linked to renal maturity [160]. Assessing the maturity of preterm kidneys, Sutherland *et al.* (2011) report that while there is a renal maturation in infants born preterm (before the cessation of nephrogenesis) this accelerated maturation is associated with morphologically small glomeruli [161]. These data further illustrate that in both animals and humans there is great potential for the kidney to be influenced by the environment, whether that be maternal or postnatal.

8. Conclusions

The dietary intake and nutritional status of pregnant and breastfeeding mothers is a major public health concern given the robust evidence from human and animal studies which indicates that a healthy pregnancy (normal birth weight and absence of congenital defects) predicts a healthy start to life that will continue into the offspring's adult life. Indeed, maternal malnutrition is still a major health concern world-wide, in both developing nations (malnutrition) and developed nations (over-nutrition). The consequence of poor maternal diets can potentially affect future generations, leading to them developing hypertension, diabetes, obesity or the metabolic syndrome. Of particular interest is the susceptibility of the kidney to the *in utero* environment because this organ develops slowly and across most of fetal life. The molecular control of the kidney has been well-reported (www.gudmap.org), however the impact of maternal diet on these molecular targets not been. It remains to be discovered *when* the maternal diet influences kidney development, *what* molecular processes are effected and *if* the phenotype can be rescued or halted. While the current generation's *in utero* experience cannot be altered, there are protective measures that can be encouraged to minimise the potential for the *in utero* environment to be deleterious to future health.

Author Contributions

All authors contributed original text to the first draft of the manuscript. In addition AG prepared figures and RJWB/JAA had editorial input and revised the manuscript.

References

1. Lucas, A. Programming by early nutrition in man. *Ciba Found. Symp.* **1991**, *156*, 38–50.
2. Yajnik, C.S.; Deshpande, S.S.; Jackson, A.A.; Refsum, H.; Rao, S.; Fisher, D.J.; Bhat, D.S.; Naik, S.S.; Coyaji, K.J.; Joglekar, C.V.; *et al.* Vitamin B12 and folate concentrations during pregnancy and insulin resistance in the offspring: The pune maternal nutrition study. *Diabetologia* **2008**, *51*, 29–38.
3. Cleal, J.K.; Poore, K.R.; Boullin, J.P.; Khan, O.; Chau, R.; Hambidge, O.; Torrens, C.; Newman, J.P.; Poston, L.; Noakes, D.E.; *et al.* Mismatched pre- and postnatal nutrition leads to cardiovascular dysfunction and altered renal function in adulthood. *PNAS* **2007**, *104*, 9529–9533.
4. Poston, L. Influences of maternal nutritional status on vascular function in the offspring. *Curr. Drug Targets* **2007**, *8*, 914–922.
5. Pettitt, D.J.; Jovanovic, L. Birth weight as a predictor of type 2 diabetes mellitus: The U-shaped curve. *Curr. Diab. Rep.* **2001**, *1*, 78–81.
6. Van der Spuy, Z.M. Nutrition and reproduction. *Clin. Obstet. Gynaecol.* **1985**, *12*, 579–604.
7. Van der Spuy, Z.M.; Jones, D.L.; Wright, C.S.; Piura, B.; Paintin, D.B.; James, V.H.; Jacobs, H.S. Inhibition of 3-beta-hydroxy steroid dehydrogenase activity in first trimester human pregnancy with trilostane and win 32729. *Clin. Endocrinol. (Oxf.)* **1983**, *19*, 521–531.
8. Imdad, A.; Bhutta, Z.A. Maternal nutrition and birth outcomes: Effect of balanced protein-energy supplementation. *Paediatr. Perinat. Epidemiol.* **2012**, *26* (Suppl. 1), 178–190.

9. Widdowson, E.M. Prenatal nutrition. *Ann. New York Acad. Sci.* **1977**, *300*, 188–196.
10. McCance, R.A.; Widdowson, E.M.; Verdon-Roe, C.M. A study of english diets by the individual method: III. Pregnant women at different economic levels. *J. Hyg. (Lond.)* **1938**, *38*, 596–622.
11. Widdowson, E.M.; McCance, R.A. The effect of finite periods of undernutrition at different ages on the composition and subsequent development of the rat. *Proc. R. Soc. Lond. Ser. B Containing Papers Biol. Character. R. Soc.* **1963**, *158*, 329–342.
12. Baird, A.; Widdowson, E.M.; Cowley, J.J. Effects of calorie and protein deficiencies early in life on the subsequent learning ability of rats. *Br. J. Nutr.* **1971**, *25*, 391–403.
13. Dickerson, J.W.; Merat, A.; Widdowson, E.M. Intra-uterine growth retardation in the pig. 3. The chemical structure of the brain. *Biol. Neonate* **1971**, *19*, 354–362.
14. Widdowson, E.M. Changes in pigs due to undernutrition before birth, and for one, two, and three years afterwards, and the effects of rehabilitation. *Adv. Exp. Med. Biol.* **1974**, *49*, 165–181.
15. Armitage, J.A.; Khan, I.Y.; Taylor, P.D.; Nathanielsz, P.W.; Poston, L. Developmental programming of the metabolic syndrome by maternal nutritional imbalance: How strong is the evidence from experimental models in mammals? *J. Physiol.* **2004**, *561*, 355–377.
16. Armitage, J.A.; Lakasing, L.; Taylor, P.D.; Balachandran, A.A.; Jensen, R.I.; Dekou, V.; Ashton, N.; Nyengaard, J.R.; Poston, L. Developmental programming of aortic and renal structure in offspring of rats fed fat-rich diets in pregnancy. *J. Physiol.* **2005**, *565*, 171–184.
17. Tomat, A.L.; Costa Mde, L.; Arranz, C.T. Zinc restriction during different periods of life: Influence in renal and cardiovascular diseases. *Nutrition* **2011**, *27*, 392–398.
18. El-Khashab, E.K.; Hamdy, A.M.; Maher, K.M.; Fouad, M.A.; Abbas, G.Z. Effect of maternal vitamin A deficiency during pregnancy on neonatal kidney size. *J. Perinat. Med.* **2013**, *41*, 199–203.
19. Cooke, C.L.; Zhao, L.; Gysler, S.; Arany, E.; Regnault, T.R. Sex-specific effects of low protein diet on *in utero* programming of renal g-protein coupled receptors. *J. Dev. Orig. Health Dis.* **2014**, *5*, 36–44.
20. Brenner, B.M.; Garcia, D.L.; Anderson, S. Glomeruli and blood pressure: Less of one, more the other? *Am. J. Hypertens.* **1988**, *1*, 335–347.
21. Hoppe, C.C.; Evans, R.G.; Bertram, J.F.; Moritz, K.M. Effects of dietary protein restriction on nephron number in the mouse. *Ame. J. Physiol. Regul. Integr. Comp. Physiol.* **2007**, *292*, R1768–R1774.
22. Hoppe, C.C.; Evans, R.G.; Moritz, K.M.; Cullen-McEwen, L.A.; Fitzgerald, S.M.; Dowling, J.; Bertram, J.F. Combined prenatal and postnatal protein restriction influences adult kidney structure, function, and arterial pressure. *Am. J. Physiol. Regul. Integr. Comp. Physiol.* **2007**, *292*, R462–R469.
23. Nwagwu, M.O.; Cook, A.; Langley-Evans, S.C. Evidence of progressive deterioration of renal function in rats exposed to a maternal low-protein diet *in utero*. *Br. J. Nutr.* **2000**, *83*, 79–85.
24. Vehaskari, V.M.; Aviles, D.H.; Manning, J. Prenatal programming of adult hypertension in the rat. *Kidney Int.* **2001**, *59*, 238–245.
25. Vehaskari, V.M.; Woods, L.L. Prenatal programming of hypertension: Lessons from experimental models. *J. Am. Soc. Nephrol.* **2005**, *16*, 2545–2556.

26. Woods, L.L.; Ingelfinger, J.R.; Nyengaard, J.R.; Rasch, R. Maternal protein restriction suppresses the newborn renin-angiotensin system and programs adult hypertension in rats. *Pediatr. Res.* **2001**, *49*, 460–467.
27. Woods, L.L.; Ingelfinger, J.R.; Rasch, R. Modest maternal protein restriction fails to program adult hypertension in female rats. *Am. J. Physiol. Regul. Integr. Comp. Physiol.* **2005**, *289*, R1131–R1136.
28. Woods, L.L.; Weeks, D.A.; Rasch, R. Programming of adult blood pressure by maternal protein restriction: Role of nephrogenesis. *Kidney Int.* **2004**, *65*, 1339–1348.
29. Chong, E.; Yosypiv, I.V. Developmental programming of hypertension and kidney disease. *Int. J. Nephrol.* **2012**, *2012*, 760580.
30. Zimanyi, M.A.; Denton, K.M.; Forbes, J.M.; Thallas-Bonke, V.; Thomas, M.C.; Poon, F.; Black, M.J. A developmental nephron deficit in rats is associated with increased susceptibility to a secondary renal injury due to advanced glycation end-products. *Diabetologia* **2006**, *49*, 801–810.
31. Do Carmo Franco, M.; Ponzio, B.F.; Gomes, G.N.; Gil, F.Z.; Tostes, R.; Carvalho, M.H.; Fortes, Z.B. Micronutrient prenatal supplementation prevents the development of hypertension and vascular endothelial damage induced by intrauterine malnutrition. *Life Sci.* **2009**, *85*, 327–333.
32. Reyes-Castro, L.A.; Rodriguez, J.S.; Charco, R.; Bautista, C.J.; Larrea, F.; Nathanielsz, P.W.; Zambrano, E. Maternal protein restriction in the rat during pregnancy and/or lactation alters cognitive and anxiety behaviors of female offspring. *Int. J. Dev. Neurosci.* **2011**, *30*, 39–45.
33. Bertram, C.; Trowern, A.R.; Copin, N.; Jackson, A.A.; Whorwood, C.B. The maternal diet during pregnancy programs altered expression of the glucocorticoid receptor and type 2 11beta-hydroxysteroid dehydrogenase: Potential molecular mechanisms underlying the programming of hypertension *in utero*. *Endocrinology* **2001**, *142*, 2841–2853.
34. Dagan, A.; Habib, S.; Gattineni, J.; Dwarakanath, V.; Baum, M. Prenatal programming of rat thick ascending limb chloride transport by low-protein diet and dexamethasone. *Am. J. Physiol. Regul. Integr. Comp. Physiol.* **2009**, *297*, R93–R99.
35. Ozanne, S.E.; Hales, C.N. Lifespan: Catch-up growth and obesity in male mice. *Nature* **2004**, *427*, 411–412.
36. Ozanne, S.E.; Hales, C.N. Poor fetal growth followed by rapid postnatal catch-up growth leads to premature death. *Mech. Ageing Dev.* **2005**, *126*, 852–854.
37. Roseboom, T.J.; van der Meulen, J.H.; Osmond, C.; Barker, D.J.; Ravelli, A.C.; Schroeder-Tanka, J.M.; van Montfrans, G.A.; Michels, R.P.; Bleker, O.P. Coronary heart disease after prenatal exposure to the Dutch famine, 1944–1945. *Heart* **2000**, *84*, 595–598.
38. Roseboom, T.J.; van der Meulen, J.H.; Ravelli, A.C.; Osmond, C.; Barker, D.J.; Bleker, O.P. Effects of prenatal exposure to the Dutch famine on adult disease in later life: An overview. *Twin Res.* **2001**, *4*, 293–298.
39. Roseboom, T.J.; van der Meulen, J.H.; Ravelli, A.C.; van Montfrans, G.A.; Osmond, C.; Barker, D.J.; Bleker, O.P. Blood pressure in adults after prenatal exposure to famine. *J. Hypertens.* **1999**, *17*, 325–330.
40. Jarvie, E.; Hauguel-de-Mouzon, S.; Nelson, S.M.; Sattar, N.; Catalano, P.M.; Freeman, D.J. Lipotoxicity in obese pregnancy and its potential role in adverse pregnancy outcome and obesity in the offspring. *Clin. Sci. (Lond.)* **2010**, *119*, 123–129.

41. Zhang, S.; Rattanatray, L.; McMillen, I.C.; Suter, C.M.; Morrison, J.L. Periconceptional nutrition and the early programming of a life of obesity or adversity. *Prog. Biophys. Mol. Biol.* **2011**, *106*, 307–314.
42. Taylor, P.D.; Samuelsson, A.M.; Poston, L. Maternal obesity and the developmental programming of hypertension: A role for leptin. *Acta Physiol. (Oxf.)* **2014**, *210*, 508–523.
43. Henry, S.L.; Barzel, B.; Wood-Bradley, R.J.; Burke, S.L.; Head, G.A.; Armitage, J.A. Developmental origins of obesity-related hypertension. *Clin. Exp. Pharmacol. Physiol.* **2012**, *39*, 799–806.
44. Henry, S.L.; Bensley, J.G.; Wood-Bradley, R.J.; Cullen-McEwen, L.A.; Bertram, J.F.; Armitage, J.A. White adipocytes: More than just fat depots. *Int. J. Biochem. Cell Biol.* **2012**, *44*, 435–440.
45. Tarantal, A.F.; Berglund, L. Obesity and lifespan health—Importance of the fetal environment. *Nutrients* **2014**, *6*, 1725–1736.
46. Shasa, D.R.; Odhiambo, J.F.; Long, N.M.; Tuersunjiang, N.; Nathanielsz, P.W.; Ford, S.P. Multigenerational impact of maternal overnutrition/obesity in the sheep on the neonatal leptin surge in granddaughters. *Int. J. Obes. (Lond.)* **2014**, doi:10.1038/ijo.2014.190.
47. Reynolds, R.M.; Allan, K.M.; Raja, E.A.; Bhattacharya, S.; McNeill, G.; Hannaford, P.C.; Sarwar, N.; Lee, A.J.; Bhattacharya, S.; Norman, J.E. Maternal obesity during pregnancy and premature mortality from cardiovascular event in adult offspring: Follow-up of 1,323,275 person years. *BMJ* **2013**, *347*, f4539.
48. Catalano, P.M.; Presley, L.; Minium, J.; Hauguel-de Mouzon, S. Fetuses of obese mothers develop insulin resistance *in utero*. *Diabetes Care* **2009**, *32*, 1076–1080.
49. Boney, C.M.; Verma, A.; Tucker, R.; Vohr, B.R. Metabolic syndrome in childhood: Association with birth weight, maternal obesity, and gestational diabetes mellitus. *Pediatrics* **2005**, *115*, e290–e296.
50. Prior, L.J.; Davern, P.J.; Burke, S.L.; Lim, K.; Armitage, J.A.; Head, G.A. Exposure to a high-fat diet during development alters leptin and ghrelin sensitivity and elevates renal sympathetic nerve activity and arterial pressure in rabbits. *Hypertension* **2013**, *63*, 338–345.
51. Jackson, C.M.; Alexander, B.T.; Roach, L.; Haggerty, D.; Marbury, D.C.; Hutchens, Z.M.; Flynn, E.R.; Maric-Bilkan, C. Exposure to maternal overnutrition and a high-fat diet during early postnatal development increases susceptibility to renal and metabolic injury later in life. *Am. J. Physiol. Renal Physiol.* **2012**, *302*, F774–F783.
52. Armitage, J.A.; Pearce, A.D.; Sinclair, A.J.; Vingrys, A.J.; Weisinger, R.S.; Weisinger, H.S. Increased blood pressure later in life may be associated with perinatal *n*-3 fatty acid deficiency. *Lipids* **2003**, *38*, 459–464.
53. Schmatz, M.; Madan, J.; Marino, T.; Davis, J. Maternal obesity: The interplay between inflammation, mother and fetus. *J. Perinatol.* **2010**, *30*, 441–446.
54. Lelievre-Pegorier, M.; Vilar, J.; Ferrier, M.-L.; Moreau, E.; Freund, N.; Gilbert, T.; Merlet-Benichou, C. Mild vitamin A deficiency leads to inborn nephron deficit in the rat. *Kidney Int.* **1998**, *54*, 1455–1462.
55. Lisle, S.J.M.; Lewis, R.M.; Petry, C.J.; Ozanne, S.E.; Hales, C.N.; Forhead, A.J. Effect of maternal iron restriction during pregnancy on renal morphology in the adult rat offspring. *Br. J. Nutr.* **2003**, *90*, 33–39.

56. Tomat, A.L.; Costa, M.A.; Girgulsky, L.C.; Veiras, L.; Weisstaub, A.R.; Inserra, F.; Balaszczuk, A.M.; Arranz, C.T. Zinc deficiency during growth: Influence on renal function and morphology. *Life Sci.* **2007**, *80*, 1292–1302.
57. Tomat, A.L.; Veiras, L.C.; Aguirre, S.; Fasoli, H.; Elesgaray, R.; Caniffi, C.; Costa, M.A.; Arranz, C.T. Mild zinc deficiency in male and female rats: Early postnatal alterations in renal nitric oxide system and morphology. *Nutrition* **2013**, *29*, 568–573.
58. Tian, X.; Anthony, K.; Neuberger, T.; Diaz, F.J. Preconception zinc deficiency disrupts postimplantation fetal and placental development in mice. *Biol. Reprod.* **2014**, *90*, 83.
59. Dressler, G.R. The cellular basis of kidney development. *Annu. Rev. Cell Dev. Biol.* **2006**, *22*, 509–529.
60. Caruana, G.; Young, R.J.; Bertram, J.F. Imaging the embryonic kidney. *Nephron. Exp. Nephrol.* **2006**, *103*, e62–e68.
61. Moritz, K.M.; Wintour, E.M. Functional development of the meso- and metanephros. *Pediatr. Nephrol.* **1999**, *13*, 171–178.
62. Ortiz, L.A.; Quan, A.; Weinberg, A.; Baum, M. Effect of prenatal dexamethasone on rat renal development. *Kidney Int.* **2001**, *59*, 1663–1669.
63. Hartman, H.A.; Lai, H.L.; Patterson, L.T. Cessation of renal morphogenesis in mice. *Dev. Biol.* **2007**, *310*, 379–387.
64. Cullen-McEwen, L.A.; Armitage, J.A.; Nyengaard, J.R.; Moritz, K.M.; Bertram, J.F. A design-based method for estimating glomerular number in the developing kidney. *Am. J. Physiol. Renal Physiol.* **2011**, *300*, F1448–F1453.
65. Moritz, K.M.; Wintour, E.M.; Black, M.J.; Bertram, J.F.; Caruana, G. Factors influencing mammalian kidney development: Implications for health in adult life. *Adv. Anat. Embryol. Cell Biol.* **2008**, *196*, 1–78.
66. Zohdi, V.; Sutherland, M.R.; Lim, K.; Gubhaju, L.; Zimanyi, M.A.; Black, M.J. Low birth weight due to intrauterine growth restriction and/or preterm birth: Effects on nephron number and long-term renal health. *Int. J. Nephrol.* **2012**, *2012*, 136942.
67. Davies, J.A.; Fisher, C.E. Genes and proteins in renal development. *Exp. Nephrol.* **2002**, *10*, 102–113.
68. Jain, S. The many faces of ret dysfunction in kidney. *Organogenesis* **2009**, *5*, 177–190.
69. Little, M.; Georgas, K.; Pennisi, D.; Wilkinson, L. Kidney development: Two tales of tubulogenesis. *Curr. Top. Dev. Biol.* **2010**, *90*, 193–229.
70. Michos, O. Kidney development: From ureteric bud formation to branching morphogenesis. *Curr. Opin. Genet. Dev.* **2009**, *19*, 484–490.
71. Popsueva, A.; Poteryaev, D.; Arighi, E.; Meng, X.; Angers-Loustau, A.; Kaplan, D.; Saarma, M.; Sariola, H. GDNF promotes tubulogenesis of GFRalpha1-expressing MDCK cells by Src-mediated phosphorylation of Met receptor tyrosine kinase. *J. Cell Biol.* **2003**, *161*, 119–129.
72. Schedl, A. Renal abnormalities and their developmental origin. *Nat. Rev. Genet.* **2007**, *8*, 791–802.
73. Schwab, K.; Patterson, L.T.; Aronow, B.J.; Luckas, R.; Liang, H.C.; Potter, S.S. A catalogue of gene expression in the developing kidney. *Kidney Int.* **2003**, *64*, 1588–1604.
74. Stuart, R.O.; Bush, K.T.; Nigam, S.K. Changes in global gene expression patterns during development and maturation of the rat kidney. *Proc. Natl. Acad. Sci. USA* **2001**, *98*, 5649–5654.

75. Stuart, R.O.; Bush, K.T.; Nigam, S.K. Changes in gene expression patterns in the ureteric bud and metanephric mesenchyme in models of kidney development. *Kidney Int.* **2003**, *64*, 1997–2008.
76. Sariola, H. Nephron induction revisited: From caps to condensates. *Curr. Opin. Nephrol. Hypertens.* **2002**, *11*, 17–21.
77. Torban, E.; Dziarmaga, A.; Iglesias, D.; Chu, L.L.; Vassilieva, T.; Little, M.; Eccles, M.; Discenza, M.; Pelletier, J.; Goodyer, P. Pax2 activates wnt4 expression during mammalian kidney development. *J. Biol. Chem.* **2006**, *281*, 12705–12712.
78. Kanazawa, T.; Ichii, O.; Otsuka, S.; Namiki, Y.; Hashimoto, Y.; Kon, Y. Hepatocyte nuclear factor 4 alpha is associated with mesenchymal-epithelial transition in developing kidneys of c57bl/6 mice. *J. Vet. Medical Sci./Jpn. Soc. Vet. Sci.* **2011**, *73*, 601–607.
79. Kanazawa, T.; Konno, A.; Hashimoto, Y.; Kon, Y. Hepatocyte nuclear factor 4 alpha is related to survival of the condensed mesenchyme in the developing mouse kidney. *Dev. Dyn.* **2010**, *239*, 1145–1154.
80. Brunskill, E.W.; Aronow, B.J.; Georgas, K.; Rumballe, B.; Valerius, M.T.; Aronow, J.; Kaimal, V.; Jegga, A.G.; Yu, J.; Grimmond, S.; *et al.* Atlas of gene expression in the developing kidney at microanatomic resolution. *Dev. Cell* **2008**, *15*, 781–791.
81. Goncalves, A.; Zeller, R. Genetic analysis reveals an unexpected role of bmp7 in initiation of ureteric bud outgrowth in mouse embryos. *PLoS One* **2011**, *6*, e19370.
82. Martinez, G.; Bertram, J.F. Organisation of bone morphogenetic proteins in renal development. *Nephron. Exp. Nephrol.* **2003**, *93*, e18–e22.
83. Martinez, G.; Loveland, K.L.; Clark, A.T.; Dziadek, M.; Bertram, J.F. Expression of bone morphogenetic protein receptors in the developing mouse metanephros. *Exp. Nephrol.* **2001**, *9*, 372–379.
84. Hartwig, S.; Hu, M.C.; Cella, C.; Piscione, T.; Filmus, J.; Rosenblum, N.D. Glypican-3 modulates inhibitory Bmp2-Smad signaling to control renal development *in vivo*. *Mech. Dev.* **2005**, *122*, 928–938.
85. Grieshammer, U.; Cebrian, C.; Ilagan, R.; Meyers, E.; Herzlinger, D.; Martin, G.R. Fgf8 is required for cell survival at distinct stages of nephrogenesis and for regulation of gene expression in nascent nephrons. *Development* **2005**, *132*, 3847–3857.
86. Perantoni, A.O.; Timofeeva, O.; Naillat, F.; Richman, C.; Pajni-Underwood, S.; Wilson, C.; Vainio, S.; Dove, L.F.; Lewandoski, M. Inactivation of fgf8 in early mesoderm reveals an essential role in kidney development. *Development* **2005**, *132*, 3859–3871.
87. Plisov, S.Y.; Yoshino, K.; Dove, L.F.; Higinbotham, K.G.; Rubin, J.S.; Perantoni, A.O. TGF beta 2, LIF and FGF2 cooperate to induce nephrogenesis. *Development* **2001**, *128*, 1045–1057.
88. Dudley, A.T.; Godin, R.E.; Robertson, E.J. Interaction between fgf and bmp signaling pathways regulates development of metanephric mesenchyme. *Genes Dev.* **1999**, *13*, 1601–1613.
89. Kobayashi, A.; Valerius, M.T.; Mugford, J.W.; Carroll, T.J.; Self, M.; Oliver, G.; McMahon, A.P. Six2 defines and regulates a multipotent self-renewing nephron progenitor population throughout mammalian kidney development. *Cell Stem Cell* **2008**, *3*, 169–181.
90. Self, M.; Lagutin, O.V.; Bowling, B.; Hendrix, J.; Cai, Y.; Dressler, G.R.; Oliver, G. Six2 is required for suppression of nephrogenesis and progenitor renewal in the developing kidney. *EMBO J.* **2006**, *25*, 5214–5228.

91. Kobayashi, A.; Mugford, J.W.; Krautzberger, A.M.; Naiman, N.; Liao, J.; McMahon, A.P. Identification of a multipotent self-renewing stromal progenitor population during mammalian kidney organogenesis. *Stem Cell Rep.* **2014**, *3*, 650–662.
92. Charlton, J.R.; Norwood, V.F.; Kiley, S.C.; Gurka, M.J.; Chevalier, R.L. Evolution of the urinary proteome during human renal development and maturation: Variations with gestational and postnatal age. *Pediatr Res* **2012**, *72*, 179–185.
93. Kishore, B.K.; Mandon, B.; Oza, N.B.; DiGiovanni, S.R.; Coleman, R.A.; Ostrowski, N.L.; Wade, J.B.; Knepper, M.A. Rat renal arcade segment expresses vasopressin-regulated water channel and vasopressin v2 receptor. *J. Clin. Investig.* **1996**, *97*, 2763–2771.
94. Zent, R.; Pozzi, A. Connecting the segments. *J. Am. Soc. Nephrol.* **2012**, *23*, 1603–1605.
95. Hughson, M.D.; Douglas-Denton, R.; Bertram, J.F.; Hoy, W.E. Hypertension, glomerular number, and birth weight in african americans and white subjects in the southeastern united states. *Kidney Int.* **2006**, *69*, 671–678.
96. Merlet-Benichou, C. Influence of fetal environment on kidney development. *Int. J. Dev. Biol.* **1999**, *43*, 453–456.
97. Rumballe, B.A.; Georgas, K.M.; Combes, A.N.; Ju, A.L.; Gilbert, T.; Little, M.H. Nephron formation adopts a novel spatial topology at cessation of nephrogenesis. *Dev. Biol.* **2011**, *360*, 110–122.
98. Singh, R.R.; Moritz, K.M.; Bertram, J.F.; Cullen-McEwen, L.A. Effects of dexamethasone exposure on rat metanephric development: *In vitro* and *in vivo* studies. *Am. J. Physiol. Renal Physiol.* **2007**, *293*, F548–F554.
99. Welham, S.J.; Riley, P.R.; Wade, A.; Hubank, M.; Woolf, A.S. Maternal diet programs embryonic kidney gene expression. *Physiol. Genomics* **2005**, *22*, 48–56.
100. Douglas-Denton, R.N.; McNamara, B.J.; Hoy, W.E.; Hughson, M.D.; Bertram, J.F. Does nephron number matter in the development of kidney disease? *Ethn. Dis.* **2006**, *16*, 40–45.
101. Hoy, W.E.; Hughson, M.D.; Singh, G.R.; Douglas-Denton, R.; Bertram, J.F. Reduced nephron number and glomerulomegaly in australian aborigines: A group at high risk for renal disease and hypertension. *Kidney Int.* **2006**, *70*, 104–110.
102. Hoy, W.E.; Hughson, M.D.; Bertram, J.F.; Douglas-Denton, R.; Amann, K. Nephron number, hypertension, renal disease, and renal failure. *J. Am. Soc. Nephrol.* **2005**, *16*, 2557–2564.
103. Hoy, W.E.; Samuel, T.; Hughson, M.D.; Nicol, J.L.; Bertram, J.F. How many glomerular profiles must be measured to obtain reliable estimates of mean glomerular areas in human renal biopsies? *J. Am. Soc. Nephrol.* **2006**, *17*, 556–563.
104. Hughson, M.D.; Gobe, G.C.; Hoy, W.E.; Manning, R.D., Jr.; Douglas-Denton, R.; Bertram, J.F. Associations of glomerular number and birth weight with clinicopathological features of African Americans and whites. *Am. J. Kidney Dis.* **2008**, *52*, 18–28.
105. Keller, G.; Zimmer, G.; Mall, G.; Ritz, E.; Amann, K. Nephron number in patients with primary hypertension. *N. Engl. J. Med.* **2003**, *348*, 101–108.
106. Nyengaard, J.R.; Bendsten, T.F. Glomerular number and size in relation to age, kidney weight, and body surface in normal man. *Anat. Rec.* **1992**, *232*, 194–201.

107. Wlodek, M.E.; Mibus, A.; Tan, A.; Siebel, A.L.; Owens, J.A.; Moritz, K.M. Normal lactational environment restores nephron endowment and prevents hypertension after placental restriction in the rat. *J. Am. Soc. Nephrol.* **2007**, *18*, 1688–1696.
108. Wlodek, M.E.; Westcott, K.; Siebel, A.L.; Owens, J.A.; Moritz, K.M. Growth restriction before or after birth reduces nephron number and increases blood pressure in male rats. *Kidney Int.* **2008**, *74*, 187–195.
109. Siddique, K.; Guzman, G.L.; Gattineni, J.; Baum, M. Effect of postnatal maternal protein intake on prenatal programming of hypertension. *Reprod. Sci.* **2014**, *21*, 1499–1507.
110. Abdel-Hakeem, A.K.; Henry, T.Q.; Magee, T.R.; Desai, M.; Ross, M.G.; Mansano, R.Z.; Torday, J.S.; Nast, C.C. Mechanisms of impaired nephrogenesis with fetal growth restriction: Altered renal transcription and growth factor expression. *Am. J. Obstet. Gynecol.* **2008**, *199*, 252.e1–252.e7.
111. Henry, T.Q.; Mansano, R.Z.; Nast, C.C.; Lakshmanan, J.; Abdallah, M.; Abdel-Hakeem, A.K.; Desai, M.; Ross, M.G.; Magee, T.R. Gdnf and MAPK-ERK pathway signaling is reduced during nephrogenesis following maternal under-nutrition. *J. Dev. Orig. Health Dis.* **2010**, *1*, 67–74.
112. Sene, L.D.B.; Mesquita, F.F.; de Moraes, L.N.; Santos, D.C.; Carvalho, R.; Gontijo, J.A.; Boer, P.A. Involvement of renal corpuscle microrna expression on epithelial-to-mesenchymal transition in maternal low protein diet in adult programmed rats. *PLoS One* **2013**, *8*, e71310.
113. Welham, S.J.; Wade, A.; Woolf, A.S. Protein restriction in pregnancy is associated with increased apoptosis of mesenchymal cells at the start of rat metanephrogenesis. *Kidney Int.* **2002**, *61*, 1231–1242.
114. Magee, T.R.; Tafti, S.A.; Desai, M.; Liu, Q.; Ross, M.G.; Nast, C.C. Maternal undernourished fetal kidneys exhibit differential regulation of nephrogenic genes including downregulation of the notch signaling pathway. *Reprod. Sci.* **2011**, *18*, 563–576.
115. Tafti, S.A.; Nast, C.C.; Desai, M.; Amaya, K.E.; Ross, M.G.; Magee, T.R. Maternal undernutrition upregulates apoptosis in offspring nephrogenesis. *J. Dev. Orig. Health Dis.* **2011**, *2*, 226–235.
116. Barker, D.J.P.; Bagpy, S.P.; Hanson, M.A. Mechanisms of disease; *in utero* programming in the pathogenesis of hypertension. *Nat. Clin. Pract. Nephrol.* **2006**, *2*, 700–707.
117. Burrow, C.R. Regulatory molecules in kidney development. *Pediatr. Nephrol.* **2000**, *14*, 240–253.
118. Dolinoy, D.C.; Jirtle, R.L. Environmental epigenomics in human health and disease. *Environ. Mol. Mutagen.* **2008**, *49*, 4–8.
119. Hales, B.F.; Grenier, L.; Lalancette, C.; Robaire, B. Epigenetic programming: From gametes to blastocyst. *Birth Defects Res. Part A Clin. Mol. Teratol.* **2011**, *91*, 652–665.
120. Hochberg, Z.; Feil, R.; Constancia, M.; Fraga, M.; Junien, C.; Carel, J.C.; Boileau, P.; le Bouc, Y.; Deal, C.L.; Lillycrop, K.; *et al.* Child health, developmental plasticity, and epigenetic programming. *Endocr. Rev.* **2011**, *32*, 159–224.
121. Ikeda, S.; Koyama, H.; Sugimoto, M.; Kume, S. Roles of one-carbon metabolism in preimplantation period—Effects on short-term development and long-term programming. *J. Reprod. Dev.* **2012**, *58*, 38–43.
122. Romagnolo, D.F.; Dashwood, R.; Stover, P.J.; Waterland, R.A.; Ziegler, T.R. Nutritional regulation of epigenetic changes. *Adv. Nutr.* **2012**, *3*, 749–750.
123. Burdge, G.C.; Hanson, M.A.; Slater-Jefferies, J.L.; Lillycrop, K.A. Epigenetic regulation of transcription: A mechanism for inducing variations in phenotype (fetal programming) by differences in nutrition during early life? *Br. J. Nutr.* **2007**, *97*, 1036–1046.

124. Cooney, C.A.; Dave, A.A.; Wolff, G.L. Maternal methyl supplements in mice affect epigenetic variation and DNA methylation of offspring. *J. Nutr.* **2002**, *132*, 2393S–2400S.

125. Wolff, G.L.; Kodell, R.L.; Moore, S.R.; Cooney, C.A. Maternal epigenetics and methyl supplements affect agouti gene expression in Avy/a mice. *Faseb J.* **1998**, *12*, 949–957.

126. Waterland, R.A.; Michels, K.B. Epigenetic epidemiology of the developmental origins hypothesis. *Annu. Rev. Nutr.* **2007**, *27*, 363–388.

127. Pham, T.D.; MacLennan, N.K.; Chiu, C.T.; Laksana, G.S.; Hsu, J.L.; Lane, R.H. Uteroplacental insufficiency increases apoptosis and alters p53 gene methylation in the full-term iugr rat kidney. *Am. J. Physiol. Regul. Integr. Comp. Physiol.* **2003**, *285*, R962–R970.

128. Nagalakshmi, V.K.; Ren, Q.; Pugh, M.M.; Valerius, M.T.; McMahon, A.P.; Yu, J. Dicer regulates the development of nephrogenic and ureteric compartments in the mammalian kidney. *Kidney Int.* **2011**, *79*, 317–330.

129. Pastorelli, L.M.; Wells, S.; Fray, M.; Smith, A.; Hough, T.; Harfe, B.D.; McManus, M.T.; Smith, L.; Woolf, A.S.; Cheeseman, M.; *et al.* Genetic analyses reveal a requirement for Dicer1 in the mouse urogenital tract. *Mamm. Genome* **2009**, *20*, 140–151.

130. Lillycrop, K.A.; Phillips, E.S.; Jackson, A.A.; Hanson, M.A.; Burdge, G.C. Dietary protein restriction of pregnant rats induces and folic acid supplementation prevents epigenetic modification of hepatic gene expression in the offspring. *J. Nutr.* **2005**, *135*, 1382–1386.

131. Rees, W.D.; Hay, S.M.; Brown, D.S.; Antipatis, C.; Palmer, R.M. Maternal protein deficiency causes hypermethylation of DNA in the livers of rat fetuses. *J. Nutr.* **2000**, *130*, 1821–1826.

132. Bogdarina, I.; Welham, S.; King, P.J.; Burns, S.P.; Clark, A.J. Epigenetic modification of the renin-angiotensin system in the fetal programming of hypertension. *Circ. Res.* **2007**, *100*, 520–526.

133. Lillycrop, K.A.; Phillips, E.S.; Torrens, C.; Hanson, M.A.; Jackson, A.A.; Burdge, G.C. Feeding pregnant rats a protein-restriction diet persistently alters the methylation of specific cytosines in the hepatic PPAR[alpha] promoter of the offspring. *Br. J. Nutr.* **2008**. *100*, 278–282.

134. Lillycrop, K.A.; Slater-Jefferies, J.L.; Hanson, M.A.; Godfrey, K.M.; Jackson, A.A.; Burdge, G.C. Induction of altered epigenetic regulation of the hepatic glucocorticoid receptor in the offspring of rats fed a protein restricted diet during pregnancy suggests that reduced DNA methyltransferase-1 expression is involved in impaired DNA methylation and changes in histone modifications. *Br. J. Nutr.* **2007**, *97*, 1064–1073.

135. Song, R.; van Buren, T.; Yosypiv, I.V. Histone deacetylases are critical regulators of the renin-angiotensin system during ureteric bud branching morphogenesis. *Pediatr. Res.* **2010**, *67*, 573–578.

136. Koleganova, N.; Piecha, G.; Ritz, E.; Becker, L.E.; Muller, A.; Weckbach, M.; Nyengaard, J.R.; Schirmacher, P.; Gross-Weissmann, M.L. Both high and low maternal salt intake in pregnancy alter kidney development in the offspring. *Am. J. Physiol. Renal Physiol.* **2011**, *301*, F344–F354.

137. Cebrian, C.; Asai, N.; D'Agati, V.; Costantini, F. The number of fetal nephron progenitor cells limits ureteric branching and adult nephron endowment. *Cell Rep.* **2014**, *7*, 127–137.

138. Lackland, D.T. Mechanisms and fetal origins of kidney disease. *J. Am. Soc. Nephrol.* **2005**, *16*, 2531–2532.

139. Lackland, D.T.; Bendall, H.E.; Osmond, C.; Egan, B.M.; Barker, D.J. Low birth weights contribute to the high rates of early-onset chronic renal failure in the southeastern United States. *Arch. Intern. Med.* **2000**, *160*, 1472–1476.

140. Hoy, W.E.; Kincaid-Smith, P.; Hughson, M.D.; Fogo, A.B.; Sinniah, R.; Dowling, J.; Samuel, T.; Mott, S.A.; Douglas-Denton, R.N.; Bertram, J.F. Ckd in aboriginal australians. *Am. J. Kidney Dis.* **2010**, *56*, 983–993.

141. Lackland, D.T. Fetal and early life determinants of hypertension in adults: Implications for study. *Hypertension* **2004**, *44*, 811–812.

142. Silver, L.E.; Decamps, P.J.; Korst, L.M.; Platt, L.D.; Castro, L. Intrauterine growth restriction is accompanied by decreased renal volume in the human fetus. *Am. J. Obstet. Gynecol.* **2003**, *188*, 1320–1325.

143. Wang, Y.P.; Chen, X.; Zhang, Z.K.; Cui, H.Y.; Wang, P.; Wang, Y. Effects of a restricted fetal growth environment on human kidney morphology, cell apoptosis and gene expression. *J. Renin Angiotensin Aldosterone Syst.* **2014**, doi:10.1177/1470320314543808.

144. Moritz, K.M.; Singh, R.R.; Probyn, M.E.; Denton, K.M. Developmental programming of a reduced nephron endowment: More than just a baby's birth weight. *Am. J. Physiol. Renal Physiol.* **2009**, *296*, F1–F9.

145. Langley-Evans, S.C.; Welham, S.J.M.; Jackson, A.A. Fetal exposure to a maternal low protein diet impairs nephrogenesis and promotes hypertension in the rat. *Life Sci.* **1999**, *64*, 965–974.

146. Kett, M.M.; Denton, K.M. Renal programming: Cause for concern? *Am. J. Physiol. Regul. Integr. Comp. Physiol.* **2011**, *300*, R791–R803.

147. Black, M.J.; Briscoe, T.A.; Constantinou, M.; Kett, M.M.; Bertram, J.F. Is there an association between level of adult blood pressure and nephron number or renal filtration surface area? *Kidney Int.* **2004**, *65*, 582–588.

148. Skov, K.; Nyengaard, J.R.; Korsgaard, N.; Mulvany, M.J. Number and size of renal glomeruli in spontaneously hypertensive rats. *J. Hypertens.* **1994**, *12*, 1373–1376.

149. Kramer, K.; Kinter, L.; Brockway, B.P.; Voss, H.P.; Remie, R.; van Zutphen, B.L. The use of radiotelemetry in small laboratory animals: Recent advances. *Contemp. Top. Lab. Anim. Sci.* **2001**, *40*, 8–16.

150. Kramer, K.; Remie, R. Measuring blood pressure in small laboratory animals. *Methods Mol. Med.* **2005**, *108*, 51–62.

151. Tonkiss, J.; Trzcinska, M.; Galler, J.R.; Ruiz-Opazo, N.; Herrera, V.L. Prenatal malnutrition-induced changes in blood pressure: Dissociation of stress and nonstress responses using radiotelemetry. *Hypertension* **1998**, *32*, 108–114.

152. Brennan, K.A.; Kaufman, S.; Reynolds, S.W.; McCook, B.T.; Kan, G.; Christiaens, I.; Symonds, M.E.; Olson, D.M. Differential effects of maternal nutrient restriction through pregnancy on kidney development and later blood pressure control in the resulting offspring. *Am. J. Physiol. Regul. Integr. Comp. Physiol.* **2008**, *295*, R197–R205.

153. Lim, K.; Lombardo, P.; Schneider-Kolsky, M.; Hilliard, L.; Denton, K.M.; Black, M.J. Induction of hyperglycemia in adult intrauterine growth-restricted rats: Effects on renal function. *Am. J. Physiol. Renal Physiol.* **2011**, *301*, F288–F294.
154. Alwasel, S.H.; Ashton, N. Prenatal programming of renal sodium handling in the rat. *Clin. Sci.* **2009**, *117*, 75–84.
155. Jennings, B.J.; Ozanne, S.E.; Dorling, M.W.; Hales, C.N. Early growth determines longevity in male rats and may be related to telomere shortening in the kidney. *FEBS Lett.* **1999**, *448*, 4–8.
156. Petry, C.J.; Desai, M.; Ozanne, S.E.; Hales, C.N. Early and late nutritional windows for diabetes susceptibility. *Proc. Nutr. Soc.* **1997**, *56*, 233–242.
157. Snoeck, A.; Remacle, C.; Reusens, B.; Hoet, J.J. Effect of a low protein diet during pregnancy on the fetal rat endocrine pancreas. *Biol. Neonate* **1990**, *57*, 107–118.
158. Langley-Evans, S.C.; Phillips, G.J.; Jackson, A.A. *In utero* exposure to maternal low protein diets induces hypertension in weanling rats, independently of maternal blood pressure changes. *Clin. Nutr.* **1994**, *13*, 319–324.
159. Langley-Evans, S.C.; Welham, S.J.; Sherman, R.C.; Jackson, A.A. Weanling rats exposed to maternal low-protein diets during discrete periods of gestation exhibit differing severity of hypertension. *Clin. Sci. (Lond.)* **1996**, *91*, 607–615.
160. Gubhaju, L.; Sutherland, M.R.; Horne, R.S.; Medhurst, A.; Kent, A.L.; Ramsden, A.; Moore, L.; Singh, G.; Hoy, W.E.; Black, M.J. Assessment of renal functional maturation and injury in preterm neonates during the first month of life. *Am. J. Physiol. Renal. Physiol.* **2014**, *307*, F149–F158.
161. Sutherland, M.R.; Gubhaju, L.; Moore, L.; Kent, A.L.; Dahlstrom, J.E.; Horne, R.S.; Hoy, W.E.; Bertram, J.F.; Black, M.J. Accelerated maturation and abnormal morphology in the preterm neonatal kidney. *J. Am. Soc. Nephrol.* **2011**, *22*, 1365–1374.

10

Association between Dietary Patterns during Pregnancy and Birth Size Measures in a Diverse Population in Southern US

Uriyoán Colón-Ramos [1,*], Susan B. Racette [2], Jody Ganiban [3], Thuy G. Nguyen [4], Mehmet Kocak [5], Kecia N. Carroll [6], Eszter Völgyi [7] and Frances A. Tylavsky [4]

[1] Department of Global Health, Milken Institute School of Public Health, George Washington University, 950 New Hampshire Avenue, Washington, DC 20037, USA

[2] Program in Physical Therapy, Department of Medicine, and Institute for Public Health, Washington University School of Medicine, 4444 Forest Park Avenue, Campus Box 8502, St. Louis, MO 63108, USA; E-Mail: racettes@wustl.edu

[3] Clinical and Developmental Psychology, Department of Psychology, Columbian College of Arts and Sciences, George Washington University, Room 304 Building GG 2125 St. NW, Washington, DC 20052, USA; E-Mail: ganiban@gwu.edu

[4] Department of Preventive Medicine, University of Tennessee Health Science Center, 600 Jefferson St. Room 337 Memphis, TN 38105, USA; E-Mails: tnguye41@uthsc.edu (T.G.N.); ftylavsky@uthsc.edu (F.A.T.)

[5] Division of Biostatistics and Epidemiology, Department of Preventive Medicine, College of Medicine, University of Tennessee Health Science Center, 66 N. Pauline Street, Suite-633, Office 619, Memphis, TN 38105, USA; E-Mail: mkocak1@uthsc.edu

[6] Division of General Pediatrics, Department of Pediatrics, Vanderbilt University School of Medicine, 313 Oxford House, Nashville, TN 37232-4313, USA; E-Mail: kecia.carroll@vanderbilt.edu

[7] Department of Pediatrics (primary), Department of Preventive Medicine, University of Tennessee Health Science Center, Le Bonheur Children's Hospital, Research Building, 50 North Dunlap Street, Room 477R, Memphis, TN 38103, USA; E-Mail: evoelgyi@uthsc.edu

* Author to whom correspondence should be addressed; E-Mail: uriyoan@gwu.edu

---

Abstract: Despite increased interest in promoting nutrition during pregnancy, the association between maternal dietary patterns and birth outcomes has been equivocal. We examined maternal dietary patterns during pregnancy as a determinant of offspring's birth weight-for-length (WLZ), weight-for-age (WAZ), length-for-age (LAZ), and head circumference (HCZ) Z-scores in Southern United States (n = 1151). Maternal diet during pregnancy was assessed by seven dietary patterns. Multivariable linear regression models described the association of WLZ, WAZ, LAZ, and HCZ with diet patterns controlling for other maternal and child characteristics. In bivariate analyses, WAZ and HCZ were significantly lower for processed and processed-Southern compared to healthy dietary patterns, whereas LAZ was significantly higher for these patterns. In the multivariate models, mothers who consumed a healthy-processed dietary pattern had children with significantly higher HCZ compared to the ones who consumed a healthy dietary pattern (HCZ β: 0.36; $p = 0.019$). No other dietary pattern was significantly associated with any of the birth outcomes. Instead, the major outcome determinants were: African American race, pre-pregnancy BMI, and gestational weight gain. These findings justify further investigation about socio-environmental and genetic factors related to race and birth outcomes in this population.

Keywords: nutrition; pregnancy; birth weight; birth length; birth head circumference; African American; diet patterns

---

1. Introduction

Pregnancy is a critical period for the offspring's metabolic development [1]. Inadequate maternal nutrient or energy intake during pregnancy is thought to lead to low birth size [2–4], a risk factor for infant and child mortality and morbidity, and potential risk factor for predisposition to cardiometabolic diseases later in life [5–8]. In the context of an increasingly energy-dense, nutrient-poor food environment in the US [9–11], there is increased interest in the promotion of nutrient-rich diets during pregnancy, with emphasis on iron-rich foods, folic acid, calcium-rich foods, and plenty of fruits and vegetables [12,13]. Dietary patterns are a way to capture the quality of the entire diet consumed by study populations.

Dietary patterns integrate dietary behaviors of a population through food and nutrient-group analyses. They are therefore more intuitive to public health nutrition recommendations than analyses that focus on single nutrients. Dietary patterns consider beneficial or harmful interactions among nutrients in different foods consumed together, as well as different food sources of the same nutrient [14]. The two most common approaches to study dietary patterns are *a priori* and *a posteriori* approaches [15]. The first one establishes *a priori* scores of foods and nutrients based on a hypothesis (e.g., adherence to the Mediterranean Diet Score [16], the Healthy Eating Index [17,18] or a score for junk food intake [19]). The second approach is exploratory, usually employing principal component analysis or factor analysis to generate patterns that maximally explain the variance in food intake in a population, where the results are data-driven and context-specific. Both approaches have been shown to be biologically meaningful [20,21]. For example, patterns characterized by a high intake of nutrient-poor, highly refined foods containing added sugar or unhealthy fats have been associated with biomarkers of inflammation and increased risk factors for cardiovascular disease, type 2 diabetes, and obesity compared to patterns characterized by high intake of lean proteins, vegetables, fruits and whole-grain cereals [15,22–29].

Few studies have examined the association between pregnancy or preconception dietary patterns and birth outcomes; most used principal component analysis or factor analysis [21,30–35] and approaches such as *a priori* scores [16–19,36–38]. In general, these studies suggest that energy-dense, nutrient-poor dietary patterns characterized by foods high in saturated and trans fats, refined sugar, or sodium are negatively associated with birth size outcomes [30,31,34,35,39], and that patterns characterized with nutrient-rich foods such as fruits, vegetables, and whole grains, were positively associated with birth size outcomes [30,31,33–35,39]. However, there are some inconsistencies in findings, probably due to the variation in birth size outcome measures, context of the population and resulting dietary patterns [31,32,39]. The majority of these studies have been conducted among white European or European American populations and, to date, no study has examined the association between maternal dietary patterns and birth size outcomes in a population with a high burden of low birth weight.

Due to the important differences in eating patterns by geography, culture and other context-specific characteristics of the population, we sought to determine the influence of specific dietary patterns on birth size outcomes in a diverse, largely black African-American and low-income population residing in the South of the US. The objective of this study was to examine the extent to which maternal dietary patterns are associated with offspring size at birth (birth weight, length, and head circumference). Dietary patterns were used to describe patterns that emerge from the data and display the unique features of that population which may not be captured by any predefined score. We hypothesized that dietary patterns characterized by energy-dense, nutrient-poor processed foods that are high in saturated and trans fats, sodium, and refined sugars would be associated with lower birth weight, length, and head circumference compared to healthy dietary patterns during pregnancy.

2. Materials and Methods

This analysis was conducted in a pregnancy cohort of 1151 women who were followed from the second trimester of pregnancy until delivery.

2.1. Setting

The Conditions Affecting Neurocognitive Development and Learning in Early Childhood (CANDLE) study is a longitudinal cohort study set in Shelby County, the southwestern corner of the state of Tennessee. Shelby County is largely African-American with mid-level education, and low income status (<200% poverty level). The CANDLE study aims to investigate the effects of different exposures such as mother's prenatal habits and characteristics, home environment and childhood experiences, genetics, and exposure to potentially harmful substances on the neurocognitive development of children from birth to age three years. The study was conducted in accordance with the Helsinki Declaration and was approved and reviewed by the Institutional Review Board of the University of Tennessee Health Science Center on 17 June 2014 (approval code: 06-08495-FB).

2.2. Participants

Women were eligible to enroll in the CANDLE study if they were between 16–28 weeks pregnant, were a resident of Shelby County, had a low medical risk pregnancy, were between the ages of 16–40 years, spoke and understood English, had a single pregnancy and were willing to give consent. The CANDLE study recruited a total of 1503 pregnant women; 1474 mother-child dyads were available for follow up after excluding post-consent ineligibilities, pre-delivery withdrawals, and fetal demises. Of the 1474 participants, 1151 had diet data at the visit between 16–26 weeks, when their diet was assessed.

2.3. Variables

Outcomes were Z-scores for weight-for-length (WLZ), weight-for-age (WAZ), length-for-age (LAZ), and head circumference (HCZ). Exposure of interest was the maternal dietary patterns that have been previously assessed via factor analysis [40]. Independent variables were socio-demographic, behavioral, and medical history characteristics that would be considered as confounding variables in the association between pregnancy outcomes and diet.

2.4. Data Sources

Data used for this study were collected during the second trimester and at birth. During the second trimester, participants completed questionnaires asking about demographics, health status, diet, and medical history. At birth, research assistants conducted medical chart abstractions for birth outcomes (weight, length, head circumference).

Diet Instrument: Diet was assessed at enrollment (16–26 weeks of pregnancy) using the Block 2005 food frequency questionnaire (FFQ) that asks consumption of 111 food and drink items during the previous three months [41–43]. The Block FFQ has been shown to be a valid and reliable instrument to rank individuals according to dietary and nutrient intake [44]. Interviewers were trained by registered dietitians and re-certified by a registered dietitian based on a taped interview every six months to estimate the frequency and quantity of intake. Nutrient values were obtained from NutritionQuest (Berkeley, CA, USA). Over and under-reporters of total caloric intake (>5000 kcal per day or <1000 kcal per day) were excluded ($n = 152$).

Dietary patterns: Seven dietary patterns were identified previously using exploratory factor analysis with principal component extraction and varimax rotation method to determine the frequency of 111 food and beverage groups that made up distinct dietary patterns. Volgyi *et al.* [40] describe these patterns as: healthy (characterized by high factor loadings of vegetables, fruits, non-fried fish and chicken, and water); processed (*i.e.*, processed meat, fast food items, snacks, sweets, and soft drinks); Southern (*i.e.*, cooked cereals, peaches, corn, fried fish, beans, greens, pig's feet, neck bones oxtails, tongue, pork); healthy-processed; healthy-Southern; Southern-processed, and mixed. The "mixed" pattern reflects foods from all of the other patterns together. In brief, to create the patterns, Volgyi and colleagues [40] estimated a factor score for each participant as a sum of daily frequency of intake of each food group, multiplied by the loading score for the food group. A large segment of the population belonged to mixed patterns rather than to single pure patterns (such as healthy, processed or Southern), so they then created combined food patterns based on the individual's rank order in each single factor. Dietary patterns were assigned based on the individuals' scoring in the quintiles for each food factor. These dietary patterns are distinct from each other in their content of energy-adjusted nutrients and explain more than 80% of the variance in macronutrient intake for this study population [40].

The demographic survey: Administered during enrollment asked respondents about formal education, medical insurance, annual household income, age, race and ethnicity.

Maternal baseline data form: At the time of enrollment, researchers collected the participant's self-reported pre-pregnancy length and weight, tobacco use, alcohol use, and total number of pregnancies (including abortions, miscarriages, stillbirths and current pregnancy). Pre-pregnancy body mass index (BMI) was calculated using the self-reported heights and weights.

Labor and delivery forms and neonatal summary forms: At the time of labor and delivery, the following information was abstracted from the medical charts: maternal weight and newborn birth weight, length, and head circumference.

2.5. Data Analyses

For full term infants (≥37 weeks), WHO Child Growth Standards were used to calculate Z-scores for each outcome WLZ, WAZ, LAZ and HCZ [45]. Normal distribution of scores was assessed via Q-Q plots of residuals for each birth outcome. Descriptive statistics (*i.e.*, mean, standard deviation, frequencies and percent frequencies) were reported for all socio-demographic, behavior, and health characteristics. These variables were cross-tabulated by race, dietary patterns, and birth outcomes, and significant differences were assessed. Pearson correlations were conducted to assess linear relationship between birth outcomes and dietary patterns. Bivariate associations (least square means comparisons) were conducted between outcomes of interest (WLZ, WAZ, LAZ, HCZ) and maternal socio-demographic (age, length, race, education, health insurance) and health characteristics (BMI, tobacco use, gestational age, gravidity, total pregnancy weight gain, alcohol use, dietary patterns, use of multivitamin) and sex of the newborn.

Multivariable models for each outcome variable were constructed to describe their association with the exposure of interest (e.g., dietary patterns). These models were adjusted for any maternal socio-demographic or health characteristic that was independently and significantly associated with the outcomes of interest and with the exposure of interest in bivariate models. An alpha level of 0.05 was used for all statistical tests and p-values reported were not adjusted for multiplicity; therefore, the results must be considered in a hypothesis generating context. All analyses were performed using SAS version 9.3.

3. Results

3.1. Dietary Patterns and Nutrient Content

Table 1 describes each dietary pattern by its nutrient content and MyPyramid equivalents [46]. All of the dietary patterns were distinct in their macro and micronutrient contents. Below is a description of the most notable differences between patterns. The processed-Southern dietary pattern had the highest content in energy, total fat (% energy and total grams, including saturated, omega 3 fatty acids, monounsaturated, and polyunsaturated fats), total sugar, iron, zinc, sodium, and meats, and had the lowest content in whole grains. The processed dietary pattern was the highest *in trans* fats, total grains and potato servings. In contrast, the healthy-Southern dietary pattern had the highest content of fiber, folate, egg-meat equivalents, oils, vegetables (including dark green and orange vegetables, and tomatoes, excluding legumes and potatoes) and fruits (including fruit juice). The healthy-processed was characterized by high intake of nuts, seeds, whole grains, and dairy, as well as highly refined foods that are higher in simple sugars and fat. The healthy dietary pattern had the lowest energy, fat, total sugar, sodium, egg-meat equivalents and meats, and highest content of protein, carbohydrate, and soy legumes.

3.2. CANDLE Study Population Characteristics

Table 2 shows the socioeconomic characteristics of the CANDLE population sample for this study by race. There were significant differences in socio-demographic and behavioral characteristics of the racial groups. The African American mothers tended to be younger, have a higher body mass index (mean 28.8 kg/m^2), be less likely to smoke, less likely to have completed higher education, and more likely to have Medicaid/Medicare insurance compared to the European Americans. Dietary patterns were significantly different by racial group, with European Americans and other race more likely to report a healthy dietary pattern. Mean birth weight for age, length for age, and head circumferences were significantly lower for African American offspring. European Americans were less likely to have more than one pregnancy.

3.3. Modeling

In bivariate analyses, eating processed and processed-Southern dietary patterns compared to healthy dietary pattern were negatively associated ($p < 0.05$) with weight-for-age Z-Score (WAZ), and head circumference Z-Score (HCZ), and positively associated with length-for-age Z-score (LAZ).

Variables that were associated with the various outcomes of interest in the bivariate analyses and also with the exposure of interest were included in the final multivariable model using race as a control variable. We also constructed each model for each race sub-group independently, controlling for potential confounders identified in the bivariate analyses. Since results by race groups were similar, we show the multivariable model that includes race as a control variable (Table 3), which is more powerful than the race-based analysis. For the outcome of HCZ, the healthy-processed dietary pattern was a positive significant predictor (HCZ β: 0.36; p = 0.019 compared to the healthy dietary pattern). None of the other dietary patterns were significant predictors of any birth size outcome after adjusting for confounders.

Table 1. Nutrient and MyPyramid values (per day) for dietary patterns in the Conditions Affecting Neurocognitive Development and Learning in Early Childhood (CANDLE) cohort. Values are means (SE).

Nutrient Values	Healthy (n = 135)	Healthy-Southern (n = 98)	Southern (n = 116)	Mixed (n = 440)	Healthy-Processed (n = 130)	Processed Southern (n = 136)	Processed (n = 99)	p-value
Energy (kcal)	1807 (38.6)	2319 (84.7)	1899 (62.1)	2337 (46.8)	2653.93 (72.31)	3051.51 (76.17)	2945.14 (85.79)	<0.0001
Fat (% energy)	34.3 (0.44)	35.8 (0.53)	36.3 (0.56)	36.3 (0.24)	36.36 (0.37)	37.97 (0.39)	37.66 (0.48)	<0.0001
Protein (% energy)	16.6 (0.20)	15.9 (0.26)	14.7 (0.21)	14.9 (0.12)	14.85 (0.17)	14.27 (0.19)	13.31 (0.24)	<0.0001
Carbohydrate (% energy)	52.02 (0.53)	50.71 (00.72)	50.95 (0.74)	50.64 (0.30)	50.73 (0.45)	49.01 (0.54)	50.46 (0.68)	0.0259
Total fat (g)	69.01 (1.78)	92.44 (3.7)	77.22 (2.91)	94.94 (2.06)	107.58 (3.18)	129.10 (3.60)	123.37 (3.95)	<0.0001
Omega 3 fatty acids (g)	1.67 (0.05)	2.36 (0.11)	1.66 (0.07)	2.05 (0.05)	2.28 (0.07)	2.39 (0.08)	2.19 (0.10)	<0.0001
Saturated fat (g)	21.78 (0.64)	28.63 (1.28)	25.61 (1.04)	31.15 (0.69)	35.21 (1.11)	42.86 (1.30)	41.32 (1.42)	<0.0001
Monounsaturated fat (g)	26.89 (0.72)	35.07 (1.4)	29.25 (1.13)	36.21 (0.80)	41.36 (1.24)	49.90 (1.39)	47.32 (1.51)	<0.0001
Polyunsaturated fat (g)	15.35 (0.44)	21.17 (0.87)	15.96 (0.60)	20.12 (0.46)	22.94 (0.70)	25.74 (0.73)	25.08 (0.85)	<0.0001
Trans fats (g)	2.22 (0.07)	2.82 (0.15)	2.84 (0.14)	3.67 (0.10)	4.41 (0.19)	5.15 (0.18)	5.36 (0.22)	<0.0001
Total sugar (g)	109.19 (2.97)	141.99 (6.74)	123.77 (5.49)	145.90 (3.26)	158.5 (5.60)	193.36 (6.75)	191.75 (8.46)	<0.0001
Fiber (g)	22.81 (0.73)	25.66 (0.99)	16.79 (0.64)	19.96 (0.42)	24.19 (0.83)	20.20 (0.62)	19.40 (0.65)	<0.0001
Fe (mg)	15.01 (0.44)	18.92 (0.77)	14.07 (0.47)	17.31 (0.38)	19.59 (0.60)	20.71 (0.56)	19.26 (0.66)	<0.0001
Zn (mg)	11.34 (0.33)	13.04 (0.48)	10.22(0.34)	12.91 (0.27)	14.38 (0.38)	15.88 (0.45)	14.77 (0.50)	<0.0001
Folate (ug)	352.91 (10.57)	439.75 (19.48)	250.90 (10.38)	306.41 (7.46)	359.08 (14.06)	279.95 (8.95)	251.20 (9.13)	<0.0001
Sodium (mg)	3058.62 (73.51)	4050.77 (157.30)	3190.14 (109.85)	3891.66 (85.42)	4393.10 (122.54)	5113.76 (136.66)	4636.01 (143.01)	<0.0001

Table 1. *Cont.*

MyPyramid Values	Healthy ($n = 135$)	Healthy-Southern ($n = 98$)	Southern ($n = 116$)	Mixed ($n = 440$)	Healthy-Processed ($n = 130$)	Processed Southern ($n = 136$)	Processed ($n = 99$)	*p*-value
Dairy-milk, cheese (1 cup equivalent)	1.90 (0.09)	1.79 (0.11)	1.35 (0.08)	1.84 (0.05)	2.06 (0.09)	1.73 (0.08)	1.68 (0.09)	<0.0001
Eggs-meat equivalent (1 egg = 1 oz)	0.35 (0.03)	0.92 (0.08)	0.71 (0.06)	0.61 (0.03)	0.47 (0.05)	0.89 (0.07)	0.61 (0.06)	<0.0001
Grain-total (1-oz equivalents)	5.52 (0.15)	6.67 (0.33)	5.41 (0.23)	7.00 (0.17)	8.45 (0.26)	8.49 (0.25)	8.6 (0.29)	<0.0001
Grain-whole (1-oz equivalent)	1.66 (0.07)	1.88 (0.12)	1.30 (0.09)	1.58 (0.05)	2.03 (0.09)	1.53 (0.08)	1.57 (0.10)	<0.0001
Legumes, soy (cup equivalent)	0.22 (0.03)	0.16 (0.03)	0.05 (0.01)	0.10 (0.01)	0.18 (0.04)	0.07 (0.01)	0.06 (0.01)	<0.0001
Meat-fish, chicken, meat (1 oz)	3.23 (0.13)	4.53 (0.27)	3.79 (0.17)	4.61 (0.13)	4.84 (0.19)	6.98 (0.27)	5.75 (0.28)	<0.0001
Nuts, seeds-(1-oz meat equivalent)	0.69 (0.06)	0.64 (0.07)	0.26 (0.04)	0.48 (0.03)	0.79 (0.05)	0.30 (0.03)	0.40 (0.05)	<0.0001
Beneficial Oils-dressings, fish, nuts, avocado (1 tsp)	2.66 (0.14)	3.06 (0.20)	1.71 (0.11)	2.48 (0.08)	3.00 (0.13)	2.37 (0.13)	2.42 (0.17)	<0.0001
Vegetables-dark green (cups)	0.62 (0.03)	0.81 (0.05)	0.37 (0.03)	0.45 (0.02)	0.50 (0.04)	0.29 (0.02)	0.23 (0.02)	<0.0001
Vegetables-not legumes/potatoes (cups)	1.92 (0.08)	2.39 (0.12)	1.24 (0.07)	1.50 (0.04)	1.75 (0.09)	1.25 (0.06)	1.10 (0.06)	<0.0001
Vegetables-orange (cups)	0.16 (0.01)	0.22 (0.02)	0.11 (0.01)	0.10 (0.004)	0.10 (0.01)	0.08 (0.01)	0.06 (0.01)	<0.0001
Vegetables-other, including tomatoes (cups)	1.14 (0.05)	1.36 (0.07)	0.74 (0.04)	0.94 (0.03)	1.13 (0.05)	0.84 (0.04)	0.76 (0.04)	<0.0001
Vegetables-potato (cups)	0.22 (0.01)	0.28 (0.03)	0.25 (0.02)	0.37 (0.01)	0.45 (0.03)	0.57 (0.03)	0.60 (0.03)	<0.0001
Fruit-total, including juice (cups)	1.68 (0.07)	2.55 (0.13)	1.82 (0.11)	1.68 (0.05)	1.65 (0.10)	1.78 (0.09)	1.43 (0.10)	<0.0001

Table 2. Population characteristics of mothers and newborns of the CANDLE study (n = 1151). Values are number (%) or means (standard deviation).

Characteristics	African American (n = 718)	European American (n = 401)	Other Race (n = 32)	p-value
Maternal characteristics				
Length, m	1.64 (0.07)	1.65 (0.07)	1.64 (0.06)	0.002
Age, years	25.13 (5.32)	28.65 (4.78)	30.00 (4.59)	<0.0001
Total weight gain, kg	14.78 (7.67)	14.83 (6.48)	13.41 (5.34)	0.80
Multivitamin, (% yes)	656 (91.4)	391 (97.5)	31 (96.9)	0.015
Body Mass Index, kg/m^2	28.75 (8.07)	25.69 (6.02)	25.75 (5.58)	<0.0001
Tobacco, (% yes)	49 (6.8)	49 (12.2)	5 (15.6)	0.004
>1 pregnancy, (% yes)	512 (71.3)	254 (63.3)	23 (71.9)	0.021
Education, n (%)				<0.0001
≤High school	489 (69.4)	123(30.7)	12 (37.5)	
>High school	219 (30.5)	278 (69.3)	20 (62.5)	
Insurance, *n* (%)				<0.0001
No insurance	15 (2.1)	4 (1.0)	2 (6.3)	
Medicaid/Medicare	511 (71.2)	86 (21.4)	9 (28.1)	
Private	192 (26.7)	311 (77.6)	21 (65.6)	
Alcohol use (% yes)	43 (6.0)	59 (14.7)	3 (9.4)	<0.0001
Premature delivery (% yes) *	68 (9.5)	26 (6.5)	2 (6.3)	0.18
Diet Pattern, n (%)				<0.0001
Healthy	7 (1.0)	121 (30.2)	7 (21.9)	
Healthy-Southern	74 (10.3)	13 (3.2)	11 (34.4)	
Southern	109 (15.2)	5 (1.2)	2 (6.3)	
Mixed	286 (39.8)	143 (35.7)	9 (28.1)	
Healthy-processed	30 (4.2)	98 (24.4)	2(6.3)	
Processed-Southern	131 (18.2)	3 (0.7)	1 (3.1)	
Processed	81 (11.3)	18 (4.5)	0 (0)	
Newborn characteristics, mean (SD)				
Weight-for-Length Z-score	−0.60 (1.23)	−0.57 (1.19)	−0.63 (0.98)	0.92
Weight-for-Age Z-score	−0.12 (0.91)	0.35 (0.92)	0.32 (0.91)	<0.0001
Length-for-Age Z-score	0.35 (1.18)	0.91 (1.23)	0.87 (1.27)	<0.0001
Head Circumference Z-score	−0.27 (1.22)	0.33 (1.23)	0.36 (1.22)	<0.0001

Significant differences across groups were tested using Chi-square or Kruskal Wallis. * Premature delivery defined as gestational age <37 weeks.

Table 3. Crude least square means (standard errors) and adjusted βeta estimates (standard errors) from generalized linear models of dietary patterns of mothers and newborn birth outcomes in Z-scores.

Dietary Patterns	Weight-for-Length Z-score (WLZ) (*n* = 923)	Weight-for-Age Z-score (WAZ) (*n* = 1011)	Length-for-Age Z-score (LAZ) (*n* = 1008)	Head Circumference Z-score (HCZ) (*n* = 999)
Healthy	Crude: −0.66 (0.10)	0.33 (0.08)	0.93 (0.12)	0.19 (0.11)
	Adjusted: Ref	Ref	Ref	Ref
Healthy Processed	Crude: −0.49 (0.11)	0.36 (0.08)	0.89 (0.10)	0.45 (0.10)
	Adjusted: 0.16 (0.16)	0.12 (0.11)	0.07 (0.15)	0.36 (0.15) *
Healthy Southern	Crude: −0.76 (0.13)	−0.00 (0.09) *	0.60 (0.12)	−0.08 (0.13)
	Adjusted: 0.17 (0.19)	−0.09 (0.14)	0.05 (0.18)	0.04 (0.18)
Mixed	Crude: −0.45 (0.06)	0.06 (0.05) *	0.47 (0.06) *	−0.02 (0.06)
	Adjusted: 0.15 (0.14)	−0.01 (0.10)	−0.09 (0.14)	0.09 (0.14)
Processed	Crude: −0.5 (0.15)	−0.05 (0.09) *	0.32 (0.13) *	−0.33 (0.14) *
	Adjusted: 0.23 (0.19)	−0.03 (0.14)	−0.17 (0.19)	−0.18 (0.19)
Processed Southern	Crude: −0.74 (0.12)	−0.26 (0.08) *	0.30 (0.11) *	−0.39 (0.11) *
	Adjusted: −0.07 (0.19)	−0.15 (0.14)	−0.12 (0.18)	−0.06 (0.19)
Southern	Crude: −0.89 (0.12)	−0.10 (0.09) *	0.59 (0.11)	−0.25 (0.12) *
	Adjusted: −0.28 (0.19)	−0.07 (0.14)	0.17 (0.18)	0.05 (0.18)

This model was adjusted for age, race, pre-pregnancy BMI, education, alcohol and total weight gain. * $p \leq 0.05$.

4. Discussion

This study examined the potential association between maternal dietary patterns during pregnancy and birth outcomes in a diverse population with historical high burden of low birth weight and other adverse birth outcomes [47–49]. The dietary patterns examined emerged from the foods that this population eats, and captured cultural food items related to traditional Southern cuisine, including fried fish, pig's feet, tongue, pork, and dark green vegetables [40]. However, after controlling for confounders, our results do not offer strong evidence for the association between dietary patterns and birth outcomes in this population. Our findings indicate that only one dietary pattern (healthy-processed) characterized by intake of nuts, seeds, whole grains, and dairy, as well as highly refined foods that are higher in simple sugars and fat, is uniquely associated with higher HCZ compared to a healthy dietary patterns characterized by water, fruits and vegetables.

Our findings are somewhat comparable to those from previous publications in which dietary patterns characterized with nutrient-rich foods such as fruits and vegetables, whole grains, and water were associated with larger birth size outcomes[30,31,33–35,39]. The healthy-processed pattern was rich in whole grains, although one of the lowest in terms of dark green or orange vegetables. Our findings do not offer any evidence that either the "healthy" dietary pattern or the "processed" dietary pattern in this population was uniquely associated with birth weight or any other outcome, which is in contrast to what has been observed in other populations [30,31,34,35,39].

A potential explanation for this discrepancy is the antagonistic interaction among nutrients and food sources in the combined dietary patterns consumed by this population. For example, the healthy dietary pattern in the current study includes vegetables, fruits, non-fried fish and chicken, and water, similar to other studies, with the caveat that other studies have also included oils in their healthy pattern [16,17,33,34,50], contrary to the current study. In addition, the "healthy-Southern" pattern, but not the healthy pattern, is characterized by the highest intake of fruits, dark green and orange vegetables, fiber and folate. This division between healthy and "healthy-Southern" perhaps diluted the potential beneficial effects that a healthy diet may have had on birth outcomes. Similarly, the "healthy-processed" pattern, was characterized by high intake of nuts, seeds, dairy, whole grains, but also included processed and red meats, relatively high levels of saturated and trans fats, and refined sugars, which may have diluted some of the beneficial effects of the healthy foods on the other birth outcomes. Nuts, seeds and whole grains have high concentrations of unsaturated fats, protein, fiber, a variety of micronutrients and phytonutrients [51], and have been identified as part of a healthy diet pattern that was associated with favorable birth outcomes in other population studies [30,33,52]. The healthy-processed pattern was also characterized by dairy; dairy intake from milk and cheese can potentially provide optimum amounts of calcium and vitamin D. A few studies suggest that low calcium intake could have effects on the skeletal growth of the fetus, affecting birth, length and weight [53]. Optimum intake of calcium and vitamin D and low levels of parathyroid hormone are associated with decreased risk of SGA birth and a significantly higher birth weight, birth length, and head circumference [54]. These potentially antagonistic relationships could be assessed in a future study by nutrient-based patterns.

Although each dietary pattern has a variety of foods containing nutrients that have been shown to be antagonistic in their health effects, these dietary patterns were distinct in their nutrient profile and explained a large variance in food intake. Other potential explanations for our findings may have to do with socioeconomic or racial characteristics of the study population. Volgyi and colleagues [40] showed that women who were older and had higher level of education were more likely to eat a healthy dietary pattern than processed, Southern or mixed. Only seven African-American mothers consumed a healthy dietary pattern, whereas most European Americans consumed healthy or mixed patterns. Twenty-four percent of European American compared to only 4% of African American mothers consumed a healthy processed diet. Although our analyses statistically controlled for race, there may be contextual factors that affect birth weight and that are covariant with race, but are not completely captured by race.

The results of this study are limited by their reliance on self-reported dietary intake, the inherent limitations of quantifying dietary intake with a food frequency questionnaire, and the inevitable overlap between different dietary patterns. However, we took measures to overcome some of these limitations by excluding from the analyses all potential over and under-reporters of total caloric intake. In addition, the dietary patterns did show distinct factor loadings, suggesting that this population does eat diet patterns that combine "healthy" and "unhealthy" food items in an overlapping manner (*i.e.*, the mixed diet patterns).

5. Conclusions

In sum, our findings do not provide sufficient evidence that either the healthy or the processed dietary pattern in this population is uniquely associated with positive or negative birth outcomes. The mixed dietary patterns consumed by this study population may provide antagonistic relationships between foods and nutrients that result in null associations with birth outcomes. To further investigate this hypothesis, it would be necessary to discriminate the population by nutrient or micronutrient status, perhaps using biomarkers to potentially disentangle any antagonistic effects in foods or preparations. Our results also imply that there are other socio-environmental and maybe genetic aspects related to race in the Southern US that require careful further investigation in their association with birth outcomes.

Author Contributions

Uriyoán Colón-Ramos conceptualized and designed the study, and led the drafting and revisions of the manuscript. Susan B. Racette and Jody Ganiban contributed to the design of the study, interpretation and presentation of results. Thuy G. Nguyen led the acquisition of data, completed the analyses, and drafted the methods section. Mehmet Kocak contributed importantly to the interpretation and revisions of analysis and tables, as well as redrafting of methods section. Frances A. Tylavsky, Kecia N. Carroll, and Eszter Völgyi provided substantial guidance on analysis and interpretation of the data. All authors were involved in revising the manuscript for important intellectual content, and have given final approval of the version to the published.

References

1. Barker, D.J.; Bergmann, R.L.; Ogra, P.L. Concluding remarks. The Window of Opportunity: Pre-pregnancy to 24 months of age. *Nestle Nutr. Workshop Ser. Pediatr. Program* **2008**, *61*, 255–260.
2. Godfrey, K.; Robinson, S.; Barker, D.J.; Osmond, C.; Cox, V. Maternal nutrition in early and late pregnancy in relation to placental and fetal growth. *BMJ* **1996**, *312*, 410–414.
3. Godfrey, K.M.; Barker, D.J. Maternal nutrition in relation to fetal and placental growth. *Eur. J. Obstet. Gynecol. Reprod. Biol.* **1995**, *61*, 15–22.
4. Godfrey, K.; Robinson, S. Maternal nutrition, placental growth and fetal programming. *Proc. Nutr. Soc.* **1998**, *57*, 105–111.
5. Hales, C.N.; Barker, D.J. Type 2 (non-insulin-dependent) diabetes mellitus: The thrifty phenotype hypothesis. *Diabetologia* **1992**, *35*, 595–601.
6. Whincup, P.H.; Kaye, S.J.; Owen, C.G.; Huxley, R.; Cook, D.G.; Anazawa, S.; Barrett-Connor, E.; Bhargava, S.K.; Birgisdottir, B.E.; Carlsson, S.; *et al*. Birth weight and risk of type 2 diabetes: A systematic review. *JAMA* **2008**, *300*, 2886–2897.
7. White, S.L.; Perkovic, V.; Cass, A.; Chang, C.L.; Poulter, N.R.; Spector, T.; Haysom, L.; Craig, J.C.; Salmi, I.A.; Chadban, S.J.; *et al*. Is low birth weight an antecedent of CKD in later life? A systematic review of observational studies. *Am. J. Kidney Dis.* **2009**, *54*, 248–261.
8. Huxley, R.R.; Shiell, A.W.; Law, C.M. The role of size at birth and postnatal catch-up growth in determining systolic blood pressure: A systematic review of the literature. *J. Hypertens.* **2000**, *18*, 815–831.
9. Ervin, R.B.; Ogden, C.L. *Consumption of Added Sugars among U.S. Adults, 2005–2010*; NCHS Data Brief No. 122; National Center for Health Statistics: Hyattsville, MD, USA, 2013.
10. Briefel, R.R.; Johnson, C.L. Secular trends in dietary intake in the United States. *Annu. Rev. Nutr.* **2004**, *24*, 401–431.

11. Wang, H.; Steffen, L.M.; Zhou, X.; Harnack, L.; Luepker, R.V. Consistency between increasing trends in added-sugar intake and body mass index among adults: The Minnesota Heart Survey, 1980–1982 to 2007–2009. *Am. J. Public Health* **2013**, *103*, 501–507.

12. Kramer, M.S. Maternal nutrition, pregnancy outcome and public health policy. *CMAJ* **1998**, *159*, 663–665.

13. Fowles, E.R. What's a pregnant woman to eat? A review of current USDA dietary guidelines and MyPyramid. *J. Perinat. Educ.* **2006**, *15*, 28–33.

14. Hu, F.B. Dietary pattern analysis: A new direction in nutritional epidemiology. *Curr. Opin. Lipidol.* **2002**, *13*, 3–9.

15. Barbaresko, J.; Koch, M.; Schulze, M.B.; Nothlings, U. Dietary pattern analysis and biomarkers of low-grade inflammation: A systematic literature review. *Nutr. Rev.* **2013**, *71*, 511–527.

16. Timmermans, S.; Steegers-Theunissen, R.P.; Vujkovic, M.; den Breeijen, H.; Russcher, H.; Lindemans, J.; Mackenbach, J.; Hofman, A.; Lesaffre, E.E.; Jaddoe, V.V.; *et al*. The Mediterranean diet and fetal size parameters: The Generation R Study. *Br. J. Nutr.* **2012**, *108*, 1399–1409.

17. Rodriguez-Bernal, C.L.; Rebagliato, M.; Iniguez, C.; Vioque, J.; Navarrete-Munoz, E.M.; Murcia, M.; Bolumar, F.; Marco, A.; Ballester, F. Diet quality in early pregnancy and its effects on fetal growth outcomes: The Infancia y Medio Ambiente (Childhood and Environment) Mother and Child Cohort Study in Spain. *Am. J. Clin. Nutr.* **2010**, *91*, 1659–1666.

18. Rifas-Shiman, S.L.; Rich-Edwards, J.W.; Kleinman, K.P.; Oken, E.; Gillman, M.W. Dietary quality during pregnancy varies by maternal characteristics in Project Viva: A US cohort. *J. Am. Diet. Assoc.* **2009**, *109*, 1004–1011.

19. Wen, L.M.; Simpson, J.M.; Rissel, C.; Baur, L.A. Maternal "junk food" diet during pregnancy as a predictor of high birthweight: Findings from the healthy beginnings trial. *Birth* **2013**, *40*, 46–51.

20. Hu, F.B.; Rimm, E.; Smith-Warner, S.A.; Feskanich, D.; Stampfer, M.J.; Ascherio, A.; Sampson, L.; Willett, W.C. Reproducibility and validity of dietary patterns assessed with a food-frequency questionnaire. *Am. J. Clin. Nutr.* **1999**, *69*, 243–249.

21. Northstone, K.; Ness, A.R.; Emmett, P.M.; Rogers, I.S. Adjusting for energy intake in dietary pattern investigations using principal components analysis. *Eur. J. Clin. Nutr.* **2008**, *62*, 931–938.

22. Schulze, M.B.; Fung, T.T.; Manson, J.E.; Willett, W.C.; Hu, F.B. Dietary patterns and changes in body weight in women. *Obesity (Silver Spring)* **2006**, *14*, 1444–1453.

23. Martinez-Ortiz, J.A.; Fung, T.T.; Baylin, A.; Hu, F.B.; Campos, H. Dietary patterns and risk of nonfatal acute myocardial infarction in Costa Rican adults. *Eur. J. Clin. Nutr.* **2006**, *60*, 770–777.

24. Fung, T.T.; Schulze, M.; Manson, J.E.; Willett, W.C.; Hu, F.B. Dietary patterns, meat intake, and the risk of type 2 diabetes in women. *Arch. Intern. Med.* **2004**, *164*, 2235–2240.

25. Lopez-Garcia, E.; Schulze, M.B.; Fung, T.T.; Meigs, J.B.; Rifai, N.; Manson, J.E.; Hu, F.B. Major dietary patterns are related to plasma concentrations of markers of inflammation and endothelial dysfunction. *Am. J. Clin. Nutr.* **2004**, *80*, 1029–1035.

26. Fung, T.T.; Stampfer, M.J.; Manson, J.E.; Rexrode, K.M.; Willett, W.C.; Hu, F.B. Prospective study of major dietary patterns and stroke risk in women. *Stroke* **2004**, *35*, 2014–2019.

27. Fung, T.; Hu, F.B.; Fuchs, C.; Giovannucci, E.; Hunter, D.J.; Stampfer, M.J.; Colditz, G.A.; Willett, W.C. Major dietary patterns and the risk of colorectal cancer in women. *Arch. Intern. Med.* **2003**, *163*, 309–314.
28. Fung, T.T.; Willett, W.C.; Stampfer, M.J.; Manson, J.E.; Hu, F.B. Dietary patterns and the risk of coronary heart disease in women. *Arch. Intern. Med.* **2001**, *161*, 1857–1862.
29. Fung, T.T.; Rimm, E.B.; Spiegelman, D.; Rifai, N.; Tofler, G.H.; Willett, W.C.; Hu, F.B. Association between dietary patterns and plasma biomarkers of obesity and cardiovascular disease risk. *Am. J. Clin. Nutr.* **2001**, *73*, 61–67.
30. Grieger, J.A.; Grzeskowiak, L.E.; Clifton, V.L. Preconception dietary patterns in human pregnancies are associated with preterm delivery. *J. Nutr.* **2014**, doi:10.3945/jn.114.190686.
31. Knudsen, V.K.; Orozova-Bekkevold, I.M.; Mikkelsen, T.B.; Wolff, S.; Olsen, S.F. Major dietary patterns in pregnancy and fetal growth. *Eur. J. Clin. Nutr.* **2008**, *62*, 463–470.
32. Thompson, J.M.; Wall, C.; Becroft, D.M.; Robinson, E.; Wild, C.J.; Mitchell, E.A. Maternal dietary patterns in pregnancy and the association with small-for-gestational-age infants. *Br. J. Nutr.* **2010**, *103*, 1665–1673.
33. Englund-Ogge, L.; Brantsaeter, A.L.; Sengpiel, V.; Haugen, M.; Birgisdottir, B.E.; Myhre, R.; Meltzer, H.M.; Jacobsson, B. Maternal dietary patterns and preterm delivery: Results from large prospective cohort study. *BMJ* **2014**, *348*, g1446, doi:10.1136/bmj.g1446.
34. Okubo, H.; Miyake, Y.; Sasaki, S.; Tanaka, K.; Murakami, K.; Hirota, Y.; Osaka Maternal and Child Health Study Group; Kanzaki, H.; Kitada, M.; Horikoshi, Y.; *et al.* Maternal dietary patterns in pregnancy and fetal growth in Japan: The Osaka Maternal and Child Health Study. *Br. J. Nutr.* **2012**, *107*, 1526–1533.
35. Wolff, C.B.; Wolff, H.K. Maternal eating patterns and birth weight of Mexican American infants. *Nutr. Health* **1995**, *10*, 121–134.
36. Ferland, S.; O'Brien, H.T. Maternal dietary intake and pregnancy outcome. *J. Reprod. Med.* **2003**, *48*, 86–94.
37. Rao, S.; Yajnik, C.S.; Kanade, A.; Fall, C.H.D.; Margetts, B.M.; Jackson, A.A.; Shier, R.; Joshi, S.; Rege, S.; Lubree, H.; *et al.* Intake of micronutrient-rich foods in rural Indian mothers is associated with the size of their babies at birth: Pune maternal nutrition study. *J. Nutr.* **2001**, *131*, 1217–1224.
38. Moore, V.M.; Davies, M.J.; Willson, K.J.; Worsley, A.; Robinson, J.S. Dietary composition of pregnant women is related to size of the baby at birth. *J. Nutr.* **2004**, *134*, 1820–1826.
39. Northstone, K.; Emmett, P.M.; Rogers, I. Dietary patterns in pregnancy and associations with nutrient intakes. *Br. J. Nutr.* **2008**, *99*, 406–415.
40. Volgyi, E.; Carroll, K.N.; Hare, M.E.; Ringwald-Smith, K.; Piyathilake, C.; Yoo, W.; Tylavsky, F.A. Dietary patterns in pregnancy and effects on nutrient intake in the Mid-South: The Conditions Affecting Neurocognitive Development and Learning in Early Childhood (CANDLE) study. *Nutrients* **2013**, *5*, 1511–1530.
41. Block, G.; Coyle, L.M.; Hartman, A.M.; Scoppa, S.M. Revision of dietary analysis software for the Health Habits and History Questionnaire. *Am. J. Epidemiol.* **1994**, *139*, 1190–1196.
42. Block, G.; Hartman, A.M.; Dresser, C.M.; Carroll, M.D.; Gannon, J.; Gardner, L. A data-based approach to diet questionnaire design and testing. *Am. J. Epidemiol.* **1986**, *124*, 453–469.

43. Block, G.; Sinha, R.; Gridley, G. Collection of dietary-supplement data and implications for analysis. *Am. J. Clin. Nutr.* **1994**, *59* (Suppl. 1), 232S–239S.
44. Subar, A.F.; Thompson, F.E.; Kipnis, V.; Midthune, D.; Hurwitz, P.; McNutt, S.; McIntosh, A.; Rosenfeld, S. Comparative validation of the Block, Willett, and National Cancer Institute food frequency questionnaires: The Eating at America's Table Study. *Am. J. Epidemiol.* **2001**, *154*, 1089–1099.
45. The WHO Child Growth Standards. Available online: http://www.who.int/childgrowth/standards/en/ (accessed on 15 January 2015).
46. United States Department of Agriculture and Agricultural Research Service. MyPyramid Equivalents. Available online: www.ars.usda.gov/News/docs.htm?docid=8503 (accessed on 15 January 2015).
47. David, R.J.; Collins, J.W., Jr. Differing birth weight among infants of U.S.-born blacks, African-born blacks, and U.S.-born whites. *N. Engl. J. Med.* **1997**, *337*, 1209–1214.
48. Kleinman, J.C.; Kessel, S.S. Racial differences in low birth weight. Trends and risk factors. *N. Engl. J. Med.* **1987**, *317*, 749–753.
49. Kessel, S.S.; Kleinman, J.C.; Koontz, A.M.; Hogue, C.J.; Berendes, H.W. Racial differences in pregnancy outcomes. *Clin. Perinatol.* **1988**, *15*, 745–754.
50. Bouwland-Both, M.I.; Steegers-Theunissen, R.P.; Vujkovic, M.; Lesaffre, E.M.; Mook-Kanamori, D.O.; Hofman, A.; Lindemans, J.; Russcher, H.; Jaddoe, V.W.; Steegers, E.A.; *et al*. A periconceptional energy-rich dietary pattern is associated with early fetal growth: The Generation R study. *BJOG* **2013**, *120*, 435–445.
51. Slavin, J.L.; Martini, M.C.; Jacobs, D.R., Jr.; Marquart, L. Plausible mechanisms for the protectiveness of whole grains. *Am. J. Clin. Nutr.* **1999**, *70*, 459S–463S.
52. Hillesund, E.R.; Bere, E.; Haugen, M.; Overby, N.C. Development of a New Nordic Diet score and its association with gestational weight gain and fetal growth—A study performed in the Norwegian Mother and Child Cohort Study (MoBa). *Public Health Nutr.* **2014**, *17*, 1909–1918.
53. Buppasiri, P.; Lumbiganon, P.; Thinkhamrop, J.; Ngamjarus, C.; Laopaiboon, M. Calcium supplementation (other than for preventing or treating hypertension) for improving pregnancy and infant outcomes. *Cochrane Database Syst. Rev.* **2011**, doi:10.1002/14651858.CD007079.pub2.
54. Scholl, T.O.; Chen, X.; Stein, T.P. Maternal calcium metabolic stress and fetal growth. *Am. J. Clin. Nutr.* **2014**, *99*, 918–925.

11

Reducing Postpartum Weight Retention and Improving Breastfeeding Outcomes in Overweight Women

Julia Martin [1], Lesley MacDonald-Wicks [1], Alexis Hure [2], Roger Smith [3] and Clare E Collins [1,4,*]

1 School of Health Sciences, Faculty of Health and Medicine, University of Newcastle, Callaghan, Newcastle 2308, New South Wales, Australia; E-Mails: Julia.Martin@hnehealth.gov.au (J.M.); Lesley.Wicks@newcastle.edu.au (L.M.-W.)

2 School of Medicine and Public Health, Faculty of Health and Medicine, University of Newcastle, Callaghan, Newcastle 2308, New South Wales, Australia; E-Mail: Alexis.Hure@newcastle.edu.au

3 Mothers and Babies Research Centre, Hunter Medical Research Institute, John Hunter Hospital, Level 3, Endocrinology, Locked Bag 1, Hunter Region Mail Centre, Newcastle 2310, New South Wales, Australia; E-Mail: Roger.Smith@newcastle.edu.au

4 Priority Research Centre in Physical Activity and Nutrition, Faculty of Health and Medicine, University of Newcastle, Callaghan, Newcastle 2308, New South Wales, Australia

* Author to whom correspondence should be addressed; E-Mail: Clare.Collins@newcastle.edu.au

---

Abstract: Overweight and obesity is prevalent among women of reproductive age (42% BMI > 25 kg/m^2) and parity is associated with risk of weight gain. Weight gain greater than that recommended by the Institute of Medicine (IOM)is also associated with lower rates of breastfeeding initiation and duration in women. The aim of this pilot randomised controlled trial is to examine the feasibility of recruiting and maintaining a cohort of pregnant women with the view of reducing postpartum weight retention and improving breastfeeding outcomes. Women (BMI of 25–35 kg/m^2 (n = 36)) were recruited from the John Hunter Hospital antenatal clinic in New South Wales, Australia. Participants were stratified by BMI and randomised to one of three groups with follow-up to six months postpartum. Women received a dietary intervention with or without breastfeeding support from a lactation consultant, or were assigned to a wait-list control group where the dietary intervention was issued at three months postpartum. Feasibility and acceptability was assessed by participation rates and questionnaire. Analysis of variance and covariance was conducted to determine any differences between groups. Sixty-nine per cent of the participants were still enrolled at six months postpartum. This pilot demonstrated some difficulties in recruiting women from antenatal clinics and retaining them in the trial. Although underpowered; the results on weight; biomarkers and breastfeeding outcomes indicated improved metabolic health.

Keywords: maternal; pregnancy; dietary intake; breastfeeding; postpartum weight retention

---

1. Introduction

Overweight and obesity is prevalent among women of reproductive age (25–34 years) with 42% having a BMI > 25 kg/m^2 [1]. Having children is associated with maternal weight gain, particularly in the long-term [2]. Fifty to eighty percent of women retain 1.4–5 kg up to 12 months postpartum, with 20%–50% retaining 5 kg or more [3–7]. Weight gain increases the risk of developing diabetes and heart disease [8,9]. The amount of weight retained after pregnancy can shift women from the healthy weight category into the overweight or obese BMI categories. Starting the next pregnancy at a higher weight increases the risk for poor pregnancy outcomes [9,10], such as gestational diabetes (RR = 2.09 for BMI > 30 kg/m^2) [11], delivery intervention [10], macrosomia (OR = 1.57 for BMI >25–30 kg/m^2 and 2.36 for BMI > 30 kg/m^2) [12,13] and lower rates of breastfeeding initiation and duration [14]. Women with a high BMI have been reported to have a 7% lower breastfeeding initiation rate and breastfeed for six weeks less on average, compared to women with a normal BMI (18.5 to 24.9 kg/m^2) [15]. Concomitantly, evidence from a nationally representative sample of Australian women indicate that women are not eating in a manner compliant with national food group recommendations, and therefore, may not be meeting their nutrient intake targets [16].

Childbearing presents an opportunity to facilitate behaviour change towards a healthy lifestyle [17]. Recently, mothers who had a BMI of >25 kg/m^2 were consulted to determine barriers to postpartum weight loss [18]. The 10 face-to-face interviews reported that the major barriers included a lack of time, maternal low energy levels, the low priority of weight loss, overall low motivation and psychological concerns [18]. Despite this, there is evidence to suggest that women can be motivated to make healthy choices for themselves and their families, and frequently seek advice and support from family, friends and health professionals during pregnancy and after birth [19,20]. Women at this life-stage have frequent contact with clinicians, which provide potential opportunities to implement lifestyle education.

There is growing evidence that overweight and obese women have reduced rates of breastfeeding initiation and breastfeed for a shorter duration, likely due to the physical size of the breast and diminished lactogenesis [21–24]. In a longitudinal cohort (USA, n = 405), overweight and obese women were 1.8 and 2.2 times more likely to have delayed lactogenesis compared to underweight and normal weight women [22]. In a similar study (n > 37,000), overweight and obese Danish women had a shorter breastfeeding duration compared to normal weight women (RR: 1.12, 95% CI: 1.09–1.16 for overweight and RR: 1.39, 95% CI: 1.19–1.63 for obese) [25]. Lactation adds to energy expenditure, and therefore could assist with weight loss in the postpartum period [5]. In combination, this suggests that women with a higher BMI may need to be targeted for additional breastfeeding support.

Two Cochrane systematic reviews assessed a range of antenatal and postnatal educational methods used to enhance breastfeeding initiation [26] and duration [27]. These included formal and informal education, one-on-one and group education, workshops, peer counseling, discussion groups, practical skills and were provided individually and in combination. The antenatal interventions that improved breastfeeding initiation included peer counseling and regular education from an International Board Certified Lactation Consultant (IBCLC) [26,27]. The reviewers concluded that there was a lack of well-conducted Randomised Controlled Trials (RCTs) in this area, and this research was needed to determine the best ways to improve breastfeeding initiation and duration rates, in particular with a focus on those at risk of suboptimal initiation and duration rates such as overweight and obese women.

The aim of this study was to determine the feasibility of delivering an intervention during pregnancy (at week 35), which aimed to reduce weight retention in women up to 12 months postpartum, who were overweight and obese before pregnancy and who were intending to breastfeed. While interventions for postpartum weight loss or to optimise breastfeeding have been trialed as separate interventions, to the best of the authors' knowledge, there has not been a randomised controlled trial combining both. In the current study a dietary intervention for weight loss, with and without lactation support, was compared to a wait-list control group with patterns of breastfeeding also compared between groups. The intent on including a lactation consultant (IBCLC) was to increase the duration of breastfeeding in overweight and obese women to positively impact on energy balance.

2. Experimental Section

A pilot, RCT was undertaken at a public tertiary obstetrics hospital in Newcastle, Australia, from October 2010 to September 2011. The approved study protocol prohibited direct recruitment by research staff, therefore flyers were distributed in clinic which encouraged potential participants to seek further information. Eligible participants were randomised to one of three groups: (i) antenatal dietary intervention for postpartum weight loss; (ii) antenatal dietary intervention and breastfeeding support for postpartum weight loss; or (iii) wait-listed control, where dietary intervention for weight loss was offered at three months postpartum. The baseline study visit was conducted at approximately 26 weeks gestation followed by a study visit at 35 weeks gestation (study visit 2) and then three months postpartum (study visit 3) as outlined in Figure 1.The fourth and final study visit was scheduled for approximately six months after birth. Antenatal visits were conducted at the John Hunter Hospital and postpartum visits were completed at the hospital or in the participants' home if they were unable to attend the hospital. Ethics approvals were provided by the Hunter New England Health Human Research Ethics Committee and the University of Newcastle Human Research Ethics Committee.

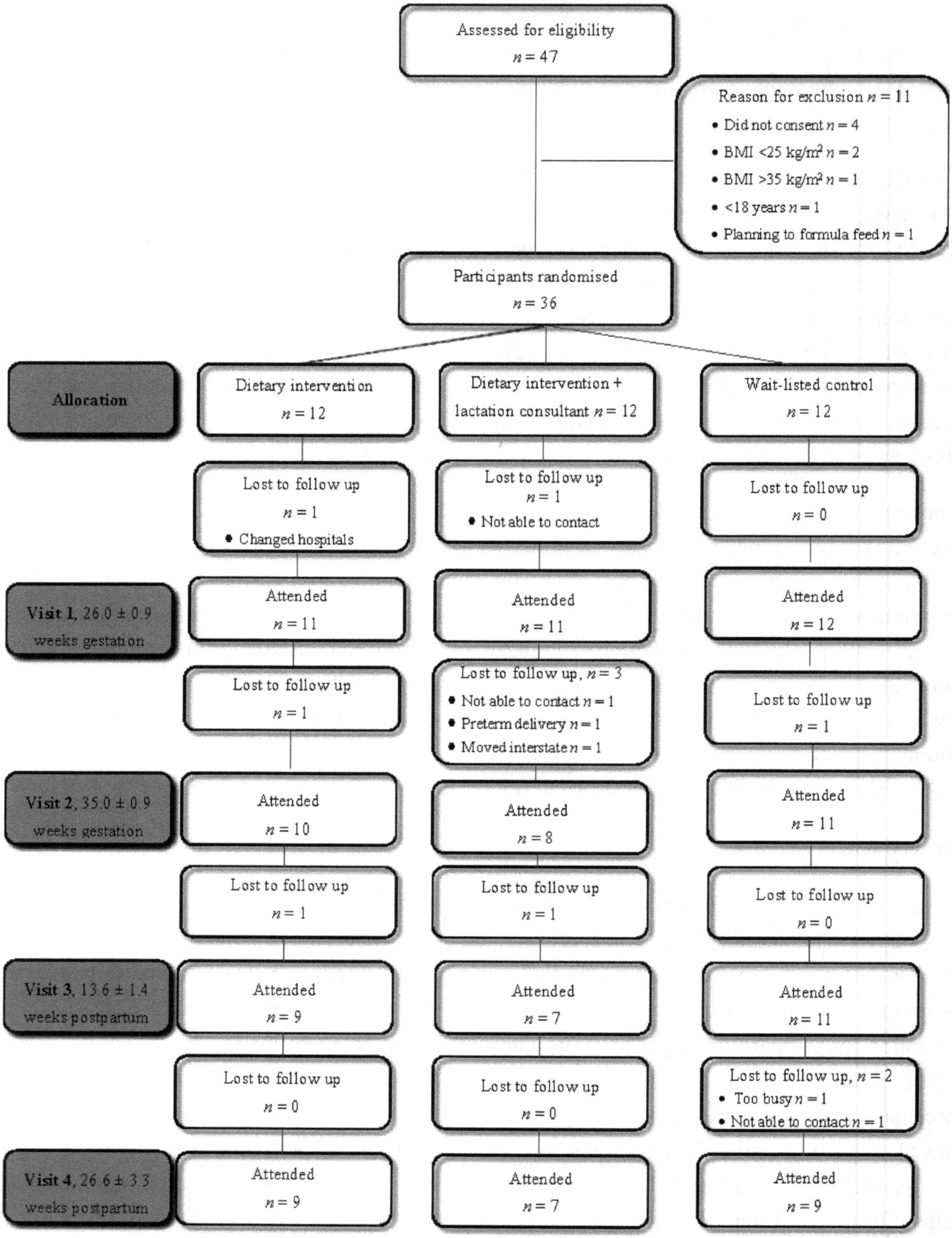

Figure 1. Flow diagram of recruitment and randomisation for a pilot randomised controlled trial.

2.1. Participants

The research dietitian circulated the study flyer in the obstetrics clinic ($n = 423$ flyers were distributed in the clinic by clinic administrators) any pregnant women who inquired were provided with written information about the study in the antenatal clinic by midwives and the study dietitian (JM), from October 2010 to September 2011. The inclusion criteria were: aged > 18 years, pre-pregnancy BMI 25–35 kg/m^2, intention to breastfeed, singleton pregnancy, English-speaking, and <26 weeks gestation at the initial screening. Women also had to agree not to participate in any other weight loss program in the postpartum period while enrolled in the study. Self-reported pre-pregnancy weight and height was recorded during the initial screening and used to calculate BMI to determine if the participants met the inclusion criteria. Previous research has demonstrated self- report compared to actual pre pregnancy weight results in the same BMI classification [28].

2.2. Study Design

2.2.1. Randomisation

Block randomisation (groups of three) using a computerised generated random number sequence was used to randomise women who were also stratified by pre-pregnancy weight status categories of overweight (BMI 25–29.99 kg/m^2) and obesity (BMI 30–35 kg/m^2). Numbered cards allocating women to an intervention group or the control group were placed in opaque, sequentially numbered envelopes. The person responsible for participant allocation (LMW) did not have direct contact with participants, therefore allocation concealment was maintained.

2.2.2. Blinding

The study dietitian (JM) was blinded to the participant's group allocation for women in the two dietary intervention groups. Blinding was maintained by ensuring the study dietitian was not aware of the group allocation until post study, and by asking the participants not to reveal their allocation. The researcher responsible for allocation concealment (LMW) contacted the study's lactation consultant directly with the participant's details for those allocated to the dietary intervention and breastfeeding support arm of the trial. The lactation consultant then contacted the participant directly to arrange follow up. By necessity the study dietitian was not blinded to the control group.

2.2.3. Dietary Intervention

Both intervention groups received the antenatal dietary intervention for postpartum weight loss, provided by an Accredited Practicing Dietitian (APD) at 35 weeks gestation (study visit 2). Specifically, women were educated to implement the self-directed weight management program "Total Eating Management System" (TEMplate System™) post-partum. The TEMplate System™ is based on social cognitive theory and includes goal setting, cognitive restructuring, and self-monitoring of food, physical activity, and weight. Energy intake was targeted at 7000 kJ/day (standard weight loss diet of 5000 kJ plus 2000 kJ per day lactation allowance), with additional 500 kJ blocks allocated based on physical activity undertaken. Participants were provided the TEMplate System™ which is based on based on healthy eating principles and the five food groups, including the lunchbox and dinner disc for maintaining meal portion control. Education was provided to ensure participants could successfully implement the following four steps to the program:

The TEMplate System™ encourages self-efficacy and uses four steps:

1. Eat a healthy breakfast;
2. Pack a daily lunch and snack box ahead of time;
3. Use TEMplate™ dinner disc to guide portion size at main meals, including four different coloured vegetables;
4. Adjust "extras" (1 extra = 500 kJ) to balance energy expenditure from physical activity and lactation, for example women exclusively breastfeeding were given advice on adding an additional 4 extras to their eating plan, partially breastfeeding were allowed an additional 2 extra servings The APD provided advice on appropriate nutrient dense "extras" that could be added to the diet.

The Wait-List Control Group Received Standard Antenatal Care and the Dietary Intervention Was Offered at Three Months Postpartum (Study Visit 3).

2.2.4. Lactation Support

One arm of the dietary intervention groups also received breastfeeding support provided by an accredited Lactation Consultant (IBCLC). "The lactation consultant gave advice on lactation issues only. There was no further dietary advice provided by the lactation consultant. During the antenatal period, participants attended two 30 min face-to-face education sessions with the IBCLC to discuss the fundamental elements of breastfeeding, previous breastfeeding experience, infant feeding expectations, goals and building rapport. A home visit was conducted up to two weeks post-delivery to ensure breastfeeding was established and for the participant to discuss any concerns. Follow up phone calls were conducted as required, to address the raised concerns of the individual participants."

2.2.5. Outcome Measures

Data collection followed many of the same procedures as had been previously employed in the Women and their children (WATCH) Study and further details are published elsewhere [29].

2.2.6. Weight and BMI

Weight was measured, to the nearest 50 grams, in indoor clothing without shoes using AND™ FV-150 K electronic weighing scales (A & D Mercury Pty Ltd., Thebarton, South Australia), which were calibrated annually according to hospital protocol. Height was measured without shoes, to the nearest millimeter, on a wall mounted Seca stadiometer (Seca Deutschland, Hamburg, Germany).

2.2.7. Biomarkers

Blood collection and analyses were outsourced to the Hunter Area Pathology Service, a National Association of Testing Authorities (NATA)-accredited laboratory. Samples were obtained at 35 weeks gestation (visit 2), three months postpartum (visit 3) and six months postpartum (visit 4). Fasting blood samples were analysed for fasting glucose (mmol/L), fasting insulin (mIU/L), glycosylated haemoglobin (HbA1c, %), lipids (total cholesterol, LDL, HDL, and triglycerides, in mmol/L), and C-reactive protein (mg/L). Homeostatic model assessment (HOMA-IR) was estimated: (glucose × insulin)/22.5.

2.2.8. Breastfeeding

Infant feeding data were obtained by the study dietitian at the three and six month follow up. The Infant Feeding Recall questionnaire was used to collect information on breastfeeding initiation, duration and exclusivity. The Current Feeding Practices questionnaire was also used to record the infant's breastfeeding and formula intake and whether the child received any of the following within the previous 24 h: vitamin or mineral supplements; medicine; plain water; sweetened or flavoured water (for example, cordials and soft drinks); fruit juice; tea or infusion; canned, powdered, or fresh milk; solid or semi-solid foods; oral rehydration salts; and other foods or fluids.

2.2.9. Further Data Collection

A 13-item questionnaire was administered in study visit 1 to determine medical history and intake of prescribed and/or non-prescribed medication including supplements. Education level, socio economic advantage and disadvantage using Socio-Economic Indexes for Areas (SEIFA) index, income and marital status were assessed by asking another six questions, modelled on the Australian Longitudinal Study of Women's Health surveys (http://alswh.org.au/). The Index of Relative Socioeconomic Advantage and Disadvantage (IRSAD) was used to provide information on social and economic status of households based on area. The IRSAD is scored one to ten with a low score indicating greater disadvantage and a higher score indicating greater advantage.

2.3. Statistical Analyses

Statistical analyses were performed using Intercooled Stata, version 11 (StataCorp LP, College Station, Texas, USA) with significance set at $\alpha = 0.05$. Normality tests were conducted to determine the distribution of data. One-way ANOVA, Kruskal-Wallis, Chi^2, and Fisher's exact tests were used to determine differences by intervention groups. Comparisons were also made between those who withdrew and those who remained in the study. Intention to treat analysis was not conducted as this was a pilot feasibility study with small numbers in each group.

3. Results

Figure 1 summarises participant recruitment, randomisation and follow-up. Thirty-six women consented (22 overweight, 14 obese), and 12 were randomised to each group, with two were lost to follow-up before the first visit. At six months postpartum, 25 of participants completed the study. Women who were lost to follow-up reported being too busy ($n = 1$), were not able to be contacted by the research team ($n = 4$), had a preterm delivery and chose to discontinue participation ($n = 1$), moved interstate ($n = 1$), or changed hospitals during antenatal care ($n = 1$).

Table 1 summarises the baseline characteristics and birth data for all participants and by group allocation. The mean age for the study population was 31 years and 85% of participants were having their first birth. Just over half the babies were female (58%) and the mean birth weight was 3.7 kg. There were no significant differences in baseline socio-demographic variables between those who withdrew and those who remained in the study, though the study was underpowered to detect any differences (data not shown).

Table 1. Baseline characteristics and birth data for pilot randomised controlled trial participants.

Participant Characteristic	All (n = 34)	Diet (n = 11)	Diet + Lactation Support (n = 11)	Control (n = 12)	p-Value
Age (years)	30.9 ± 6.0	29.5 ± 7.8	31.6 ± 5.1	31.3 ± 5.6	0.27
Height (cm)	165.4 ± 6.2	165.1 ± 6.5	166.8 ± 5.7	164.4 ± 6.5	0.44
Born in Australia, n (%)	33/34 (97)	10/11 (91)	11/11 (100)	12/12 (100)	0.65
Married or *de facto, n* (%)	25/31 (81)	7/10 (70)	8/9 (89)	10/12 (83)	0.63
Education ≥ year 12, n (%)	26/31 (84)	9/10 (90)	8/9 (89)	9/12 (75)	0.79
IRSAD ≥ 5, n (%)	23/32 (72)	7/10 (70)	9/10 (90)	7/12 (58)	0.22
Smoking, n (%)	4/34 (12)	2/11 (18)	1/11 (9)	1/12 (8)	1.00
Multiparous, n (%)	5/34 (15)	1/11 (9)	2/11 (18)	2/12 (17)	0.39
Gestational diabetes, n (%)	3/34 (9)	2/11 (18)	1/11 (9)	0/12 (0)	0.76
Infant sex, male n (%)	14/33 (42)	3/11 (27)	6/10 (60)	5/12 (42)	0.23
Birth weight (kg)	3.7 (3.3, 4.0)	3.9 (3.7, 4.1)	3.5 (3.1, 3.7)	3.5 (3.2, 4.0)	0.19

Mean ± SD for normally distributed continuous data or median (25th–75th percentile) for non-normally distributed data.

Table 2 summarises the pregnancy and postpartum weight data for the randomised controlled trial participants. Self-reported mean pre-pregnancy weight was 80.5 kg and the median BMI was 28.8 kg/m^2. By 35 weeks gestation the women had gained on average 13.6 ± 6.6 kg (mean ± SD). This is considerably higher than the Institute of Medicine's recommendations of 5–11.5 kg for women with a BMI of 25 or more [30], especially considering the final weight measurement was at 35 rather than 40 weeks gestation. Mean gestational weight gain in the dietary intervention group at 35 weeks gestation was on average 5–6 kg lower, however, this was not significant (p = 0.06) and may have occurred by chance. At three months postpartum weight retention was not significantly different between groups, however those in the dietary intervention groups (with or without lactation support) retained less weight compared to the control group. At three months postpartum, control participants commenced the dietary intervention and there was less difference in weight retention at six months postpartum. There was a trend for fewer women in the dietary intervention group to retain 5 kg or more than their pre-pregnancy weight at six months after birth, compared to the control group (p = 0.06).

Table 3 summarises the fasting biochemical data including glycaemic markers, lipids and the inflammatory biomarker CRP. There were no significant differences by group allocation.

All participants initiated breastfeeding which was to be expected on the basis of the inclusion criteria. At three months postpartum, the majority of participants had continued breastfeeding (74%). The dietary intervention with lactation support group had the highest rates of breastfeeding compared to the dietary intervention alone and the control groups though the differences were not significant.

Table 2. Weight data for pilot randomised controlled trial participants.

Time	Variable	All (n = 34)	Diet (n = 11)	Diet + Lactation Support (n = 11)	Control (n = 12)
Pre-pregnancy	Weight (kg)	80.5 ± 12.0	81.5 ± 15.1	81.6 ± 9.8	78.5 ± 11.3
	BMI (kg/m^2)	28.8 (25.4, 32.3)	27.7 (25.1, 33.7)	29.4 (25.5, 32.3)	28.9 (25.2, 32.9)
Pregnancy	Weight gain (kg) [a]	13.6 ± 6.6	9.8 ± 4.5	15.3 ± 7.2	16.0 ± 6.7
Postpartum—3 months	Weight	84.9 ± 13.7	84.2 ± 14.0	85.9 ± 14.3	84.8 ± 14.3
	BMI	30.8 ± 4.2	30.7 ± 4.1	30.6 ± 5.4	31.1 ± 3.9
	Weight retention (kg) [b]	4.6 ± 7.4	0.91 ± 7.03	4.4 ± 7.6	7.7 ± 6.8
Postpartum—6 months	Weight	85.3 ± 13.0	84.2 ± 14.7	89.9 ± 11.3	82.7 ± 13.1
	BMI	30.7 ± 3.7	30.6 ± 4.3	31.2 ± 4.4	30.3 ± 3.0
	Weight retention	3.3 ± 4.0	0.8 ± 7.2	5.6 ± 8.8	5.9 ± 4.9
	Weight ≤ pre-pregnancy, n (%)	5/25 (20)	3/9 (33)	2/7 (29)	1/9 (11)
	Weight retention ≥ 5 kg, n (%)	10/25 (40)	1/9 (11)	4/7 (57)	5/9 (56)

Mean ± SD for normally distributed continuous data or median (25th–75th percentile) for non-normally distributed data. There were no significant differences found between study groups. [a] Weight gain = Weight measured at 35 weeks gestation—self-reported pre-pregnancy weight; [b] Weight retention = Weight at visit—self-reported pre-pregnancy weight.

Table 3. Fasting biochemical data for pilot randomised controlled trial participants.

Time	Variable	All (n = 34)	Diet (n = 11)	Diet + Lactation Support (n = 11)	Control (n = 12)	p-Value
Pregnancy	Glucose (mmol/L)	4.2 ± 0.4	4.3 ± 0.5	4.2 ± 0.4	4.2 ± 0.2	0.99
	Insulin (mIU/L)	9.1 ± 3.6	8.3 ± 3.0	8.8 ± 4.4	10.1 ± 3.4	0.46
	HbA1c (%)	5.3 (5.2, 5.5)	5.3 (5.1, 5.5)	5.3 (5.1, 5.5)	5.4 (5.2, 5.6)	0.48
	HOMA-IR [a]	1.7 ± 0.8	1.6 ± 0.7	1.7 ± 0.9	1.9 ± 0.7	0.62
	Total cholesterol (mmol/L)	6.8 ± 1.2	6.7 ± 1.0	6.6 ± 1.2	7.1 ± 1.4	0.77
	Triglycerides (mmol/L)	2.3 ± 0.7	2.0 ± 0.4	2.3 ± 0.8	2.6 ± 0.7	0.11
	LDL-C (mmol/L)	3.9 ± 1.1	4.0 ± 0.7	3.6 ± 1.1	4.1 ± 1.3	0.56
	HDL-C (mmol/L)	1.9 ± 0.5	1.9 ± 0.6	1.9 ± 0.5	1.9 ± 0.4	0.95
	Total/HDL-C	3.8 ± 0.8	3.7 ± 0.8	3.7 ± 1.0	3.9 ± 0.7	0.78
	CRP (mg/L)	7.3 (4.8, 12.9)	11.1 (6.3, 13.7)	6.7 (3.0, 14.6)	7.3 (5.2, 9.5)	0.91

Table 3. *Cont.*

Time	Variable	All ($n = 34$)	Diet ($n = 11$)	Diet + Lactation Support ($n = 11$)	Control ($n = 12$)	p-Value
Postpartum—3 months	Glucose	4.6 ± 0.5	4.5 ± 0.5	4.4 ± 0.4	4.7 ± 0.5	0.58
	Insulin	5.5 (3.3, 6.8)	5.2 (4.6, 10.3)	5.5 (3.2, 6.4)	5.4 (3.2, 6.8)	0.61
	HbA1c	5.3 ± 0.2	5.3 ± 0.2	5.3 ± 0.2	5.5 ± 0.4	0.39
	HOMA-IR	1.0 (0.7, 1.4)	1.0 (0.8, 2.2)	1.2 (0.6, 1.4)	1.1 (0.6, 1.4)	0.69
	Total cholesterol	5.0 ± 1.0	5.2 ± 1.3	4.4 ± 0.6	5.2 ± 0.7	0.31
	Triglycerides	1.0 ± 0.6	1.2 ± 0.8	0.7 ± 0.2	1.0 ± 0.6	0.25
	LDL-C	3.0 ± 0.7	2.9 ± 0.7	2.6 ± 0.6	3.1 ± 0.7	0.36
	HDL-C	1.6 ± 0.5	1.7 ± 0.7	1.5 ± 0.3	1.6 ± 0.4	0.84
	Total/HDL-C	3.4 (2.5, 3.6)	3.5 (2.7, 3.8)	3.0 (2.9, 3.4)	3.4 (2.5, 4.4)	0.61
	CRP	6.2 ± 4.9	7.8 ± 6.4	5.6 ± 3.5	5.3 ± 4.1	0.56
Postpartum—6 months	Glucose	4.5 ± 0.4	4.5 ± 0.5	4.5 ± 0.4	4.6 ± 0.4	0.91
	Insulin	5.4 (3.2, 6.1)	5.8 (4.5, 10.2)	3.5 (2.7, 9.3)	5.4 (2.9, 6.0)	0.55
	HbA1c	5.3 ± 0.3	5.3 ± 0.4	5.3 ± 0.2	5.3 ± 0.3	0.88
	HOMA-IR	1.1 (0.6, 1.4)	1.1 (0.87, 1.83)	0.7 (0.5, 2.0)	1.0 (0.6, 1.3)	0.65
	Total cholesterol	4.8 ± 1.2	4.7 ± 1.6	4.8 ± 1.0	4.9 ± 1.0	0.95
	Triglycerides	0.9 (0.5, 1.2)	1.0 (0.5, 1.4)	0.8 (0.7, 1.1)	0.9 (0.5, 1.4)	0.70
	LDL-C	2.9 ± 1.0	2.7 ± 1.0	3.0 ± 1.2	3.0 ± 1.0	0.83
	HDL-C	1.3 (1.1, 1.8)	1.2 (1.1, 1.9)	1.3 (1.3, 1.3)	1.5 (1.1, 1.7)	0.94
	Total/HDL-C	3.4 (2.6, 4.3)	3.4 (2.7, 4.3)	3.7 (3.0, 4.3)	3.1 (3.0, 4.4)	0.92
	CRP	3.5 (3.0, 6.1)	3.3 (2.0, 6.1)	5.2 (2.5, 6.6)	3.1 (3.0, 4.4)	0.98

Mean ± SD for normally distributed continuous data or median (25th–75th percentile) for non-normally distributed data. [a] HOMA-IR, Homeostatic Model Assessment of Insulin Resistance: (glucose mmol/L × insulin mIU/L)/22.5.

Trial Evaluation

Fourteen of the participants who completed the study returned the evaluation questionnaire for the TEMplate™ program. Of those who returned the questionnaire, six agreed that the TEMplate™ program was easy to understand. On completion of the TEMplate™ program, the majority of participants reported that they now weigh themselves (n = 10), keep a record of what they eat (n = 5), try to be more active (n = 14), and plan (n = 9) and cook healthier meals (n = 13). Two of the participants found the TEMplate™ program too time consuming, and six found it difficult to use the program whilst also caring for a new baby. Additional barriers that were reported included time constraints (n = 7), and tiredness (n = 6). Two of the participants also suggested they would prefer face-to-face contact with a dietitian (n = 2) during the program.

4. Discussion

This pilot RCT examined the feasibility of a program that included dietary intervention and breastfeeding support for overweight and obese pregnant women, with the aim of reducing postpartum weight retention and enhancing rates of breastfeeding. As a pilot study, it was not intended to be adequately powered to show significant between group differences in outcomes of interest: weight, biomarkers, and breastfeeding. However, the results indicate that the approach is feasible and acceptable to pregnant women attending an antenatal clinic and that the methodology, including the collection of blood for biomarker assessment, and could be adapted based on qualitative feedback to a larger, adequately powered RCT.

The use of paid, dedicated research midwives to undertake the recruitment of women in an antenatal clinic setting would be an improvement on the recruitment strategy used in this pilot, given the known difficulties in recruitment in this population. Retention was at 69%, which is not ideal. However, the issues identified such as difficulty attending the primary measurement site will allow for better retention in the subsequent RCT. Women were lost to follow up for a number of reasons, in particular due to the burden of attending face to face visits. The use of a flexible delivery model, such as a web-based intervention strategy, combined with home visits for follow-up, should be considered to overcome this barrier.

Research shows the postpartum period to be associated with many adjustments for a mother, including increased time constraints, a change in priorities and child care concerns [31,32]. These adjustments can make it difficult for women to achieve a healthy lifestyle [31,32] and have been reported to contribute to the lack of success in postpartum weight loss interventions. High drop-out (up to 40%) and low attendance rates [33–35], led researchers to conduct interviews on participants from the Active Mothers Postpartum (AMP) study to further investigate lack of participation in this cohort of women [32]. Results indicate numerous barriers to achieving a healthy lifestyle at this life-stage, including: lack of time in a busy schedule; health of the family as first priority; lack of social support; lack of child care during the intervention and/or education; and location distant from the study centre [32]. This pilot study attempted to address a number of these reported issues. Women were provided with a self-management program to complete in their own time, which increased flexibility and eliminated the need for child care. Phone calls and home visits were offered for women who were unable to visit the hospital due to geographical location or who had child care issues. Additionally, in the current study the weight management education was provided during an antenatal visit towards the end of pregnancy to help prepare and organise the women for the postpartum period. Despite anticipating the known barriers in the literature to a weight loss program, there were substantial withdrawals from the program, however they predominantly occurred during the antenatal period.

Results from the evaluation suggest the majority of participants reported improved awareness of their eating and exercise behaviours as a result of the intervention. The participants indicated that they were able to record intake, monitor weight, and increase everyday exercise, plan meals and make healthier food choices using the provided program materials. Still, half of the women indicated they found it difficult to complete the program with a new baby, despite this being an intervention which they could complete in their own home. From this feedback we can deduce that any intervention in this life-stage must be goal-orientated, include self-monitoring, and be home-based, while also being quick and easy. Using web-based or mobile device technologies may be one way to enhance access within the home, to address the time and travel barriers expressed in the evaluations.

All the participants in this pilot study initiated breastfeeding, but the duration of breastfeeding was greatest in the group with additional lactation support, though small numbers meant this was not statistically significant. The provision of IBCLC support appeared to be both feasible and acceptable to overweight and obese mothers. Suboptimal breastfeeding initiation and duration rates have been frequently cited for women with a high BMI [15,25,36–39]. In a systematic review of 15 observational studies the relationship between maternal overweight and obesity and breastfeeding initiation and duration identified the rates for any breastfeeding at six months in overweight women were 17% to 52% while rates for obese women were 17% to 37% compared to normal weight women (29% to 57%) [40].

For pregnancy and postpartum metabolic markers the direction of the results was in the intended direction, indicating a potential improvement in metabolic profile due to the intervention, although not statistically significant. The pilot study was not powered to show significance. Further research in this area is warranted.

Research to manage postpartum weight retention is of increasing interest. There have been a number of lifestyle RCTs aimed at reducing postpartum weight retention or increasing weight loss [33–35,41–44]. Two of these studies had lower weight retention for both intervention and control groups compared to the current study although only one of these was significant (Control *versus* intervention: 1.0 and 1.8, $p = 0.42$; 5.1 and 2.3, $p < 0.001$) [42,43]. However, none of these studies include a breastfeeding support commencing in pregnancy; a novel component of our trial. There are a number of important methodological differences between the current study and RCTs conducted to date. The strength of the current study is the recruitment of women in the antenatal period to prepare them to achieve postpartum weight loss. Early recruitment of participants may have the added advantage of preventing gestational weight gain, although our study participants generally gained more than current recommendations [27]. Similarly, the current study uses self-reported pre-pregnancy weight, combined with weight at initial visit as objective markers of gestational weight gain and weight retention. The current study primarily focused on dietary intervention. Finally focusing on overweight and obese women targets those who may have difficulty initiating breastfeeding while supporting longer breastfeeding duration.

Our pilot study participants in the dietary intervention only group retained less weight at both three and six months postpartum compared to the two other RCTs reporting weight retention as their primary outcome [42,43]. Kinnunen *et al.* (2007) intervened during the postpartum period focusing on lifestyle change to reduce weight retention [43]. Huang, Yeh and Tsai (2011) provided weight management education during pregnancy, similar to our pilot study, however, the aim of their intervention was to limit gestational weight gain, rather than prepare the participants solely for weight loss in the postpartum period [42]. This makes it difficult to determine the postpartum impact of this intervention because gestational weight gain is a significant determinant of weight retention [45,46].

This pilot study had a number of limitations that need to be acknowledged. The primary limitation is the small sample size, making it difficult to detect significant differences in outcome variables and limiting the applicability of the study to the general population. However, as this was a feasibility study, it is more important to look at the recruitment and retention information and the evaluation data. In addition to this, the retention rate was suboptimal suggesting the need for further consideration with this population and their unique stage of life. To improve the study sample size and retention rates, regular contact with a health professional and incentives to complete the study could be considered. Additionally, providing flexible study visits to suit mothers' postpartum lifestyles may require home visits, regular phone calls, and internet support.

5. Conclusions

Overweight and obesity in women is an independent risk factor for lifestyle disease such as diabetes and heart disease [47,48]. Pregnancy can further impact this due to gestational weight gain, postpartum weight retention and lower rates of successful breastfeeding initiation and duration. Lifestyle changes, such as healthy eating and exercise, which are used in traditional weight loss programs, may be problematic for women with infants because of time constraints and changes in priorities. Despite postpartum weight retention being common and a relevant concern for women, there are currently no programs or strategies routinely offered to assist women to achieve a healthy weight after birth. The current study provides evidence to support the feasibility and preliminary efficacy of providing overweight and obese women with targeted dietary advice and breastfeeding support to improve weight, metabolic, and breastfeeding outcomes. An adequately powered RCT is now required to determine the true effect, if any, of these interventions and the costs involved in implementing those that are effective on a larger scale.

Author Contributions

JM, LM-W and CC designed the study. All authors had input into study tools and organization of RCT. RS provided access to participants and support for recruitment. JM was responsible for implementing the study and was the study dietitian who undertook the majority of the data collection. LM-W was responsible for randomization and consultation with lactation consultant. All authors contributed to the analysis and interpretation of the results. All authors contributed to writing this paper. The pilot RCT contributed to JM's Research Masters thesis.

References

1. Statistics, A.B.O. *Australian Health Survey: First Results, 2011–12*. 2012. Available online: http://www.abs.gov.au/AUSSTATS/abs@.nsf/DetailsPage/4364.0.55.0012011-12?OpenDocument (accessed on 17th December 2014).
2. Linne, Y.; Dye, L; Barkeling, B; Rossner, S. Long-Term Weight Development in Women: A 15-Year Follow-up of the Effects of Pregnancy. *Obesity* **2004**, *12*, 1166–1178.
3. Olson, C.M.; Strawderman, M.S.; Hinton, P.S.; Pearson, T.A. Gestational Weight Gain and Postpartum Behaviors Associated with Weight Change from Early Pregnancy to 1 y Postpartum. *Int. J. Obes. Relat. Metab. Disord.* **2003**, *27*, 117–127.
4. Schauberger, C.W.; Rooney, B.L.; Brimer, L.M. Factors that influence weight loss in the puerperium. *Obstet. Gynecol.* **1992**, *79*, 424–429.
5. Rothberg, B.E.G.; Magriples, U.; Kershaw, T.S.;. Rising, S.S.; Ickovics, J.R. Gestational weight gain and subsequent postpartum weight loss among young, low-income, ethnic minority women. *Am. J. Obstet. Gynecol.* **2011**, *204*, 1–11.
6. Ohlin, A.; Rossner, S. Maternal body weight development after pregnancy. *Int. J. Obes.* **1990**, *14*, 159–173.
7. Althuizen, E.; Van Poppel, M.N.M.; de Vries, J.H.; Seidell, J.C.; Mechelen, W.V. Postpartum behavior as predictor of weight change from before pregnancy to one year postpartum. *BMC Public Health* **2011**, *11*, 1–7.
8. Gunderson, E.P. Childbearing and obesity in women: Weight before, during, and after pregnancy. *Obstet. Gynecol. Clin. North Am.* **2009**, *36*, 317–332.
9. Sirimi, N.; Goulis, D.G. Obesity in pregnancy. *Hormones* **2010**, *9*, 299–306.
10. Rowlands, I.; Graves, N.; deJersey, S.; McIntyre, H.D.; Callaway, L.K. Obesity in pregnancy: Outcomes and economics. *Semin. Fetal Neonatal Med.* **2010**, *15*, 94–99.
11. Solomon, C.G.; Willett, W.C.; Carey, V.J.; Rich-Edwards, J.; Hunter, D.J.; Colditz, G.A; Stampfer, M.J.; Spelzer, F.E.; Spiegelma, D.; Manson, J.E.. A prospective study of pregravid determinants of gestational diabetes mellitus. *J. Am. Med. Assoc.* **1997**, 278, 1078–1083.
12. Sebire, N.J.; Jolly, M.; Harris, J.P.; Wadsworth, J.; Joffe, M.; Beard, R.W.; Regan, L.; Robinson, S. Maternal obesity and pregnancy outcome a study of 287213 pregnancies in London. *Int. J. Obes.* **2001**, *25*, 1175–1182.
13. Dzakpasu, S.; Fahey, J.; Kirby, R.S.; Tough, S.; Chalmers, B.; Heaman, M.; Bartholomew, S.; Biringer, A.; Darling, E.K.; Lee, L.S.; McDonald, S.D. Contribution of prepregnancy body mass index and gestational weight gain to caesarean birth in Canada. *BMC Pregnancy Childbirth* **2014**, *14*, 106.
14. Donath, S.M.; Amir, L.H. Maternal obesity and initiation and duration of breastfeeding: data from the longitudinal study of Australian children. Matern. *Child Nutr.* **2008**, *4*, 163–170.
15. Donath, S.M.; Amir, L.H. Does maternal obesity adversely affect breastfeeding initiation and duration? *J. Paediatr. Child Health* **2000**, *36*, 482–486.
16. Blumfield, M.; Hure, A.J.; MacDonald-Wicks, L.; Patterson, A.J.; Smith, R.; Collins, C.E. Disparities exist between national food group recommendations and the dietary intakes of Australian women. *BMC Women's Health* **2011**, *11*, 37.

17. Pereira, M.A.; Rifas-Shiman, S.L.; Kleinman, K.P.; Rich-Edwards, J.W.; Peterson, K.E.; Gillman, M.W. Predictors of Change in Physical Activity During and After Pregnancy: Project Viva. *Am. J. Prev. Med.* **2007**, *32*, 312–319.
18. Craigie, A.M.; Barbour, R.S.; Anderson, A.S. How can we help women lose weight after child birth? Formative findings from the WeightWell weight managment study. *Proc. Nutr. Soc.* **2010**, *69*, 1.
19. Walker, L.O.; Grobe, S.J. The Construct of Thriving in Pregnancy and Postpartum. *Nurs. Sci. Q.* **1999**, *12*, 151–157.
20. Lewallen, L.P. Healthy Behaviors and Sources of Health Information Among Low-Income Pregnant Women. *Public Health Nurs.* **2004**, *21*, 200–206.
21. Wojcicki, J.M. Maternal Prepregnancy Body Mass Index and Initiation and Duration of Breastfeeding: A Review of the Literature. *J. Women's Health* **2011**, *20*, 7.
22. Nommsen-Rivers, L.A.; Chantry, C.J.; Peerson, J.M.; Cohen, R.J.; Dewey, K.G. Delayed onset of lactogenesis among first-time mothers is related to maternal obesity and factors associated with ineffective breastfeeding. *Am. J. Clin. Nutr.* **2010**, *92*, 574–584.
23. Dewey, K.G.; Nommsen-Rivers, L.A.; Heinig, M.J.; cohen, R.J. Risk factors for suboptimal infant breastfeeding behavior, delayed onset of lactation, and excess neonatal weight loss. *Pediatrics* **2003**, *112*, 607–619.
24. Rasmussen, K.M.; Kjolhede, C.L. Prepregnant Overweight and Obesity Diminish the Prolactin Response to Suckling in the First Week Postpartum. *Pediatrics* **2004**, *113*, e465–e471.
25. Baker, J.L.; Michaelsen, K.F.; Sorensen, T.I.A.; Rasmussen, K.M. High prepregnant body mass index is associated with early termination of full and any breastfeeding in Danish women. *Am. J. Clin. Nutr.* **2007**, *86*, 404.
26. Dyson, L.; McCormick, F.; Renfrew, M. Interventions for promoting the intiation of breastfeeding. *Cochrane Database Sytematic Rev.* **2005**, *2*, CD001688.
27. Lumbiganon, P.; Martis, R.; Malinee, L.; Festin, M.R.; Ho, J.J.; Hakimi, M. Antenatal breastfeeding education for increasing breastfeeding duration. *C Collab.* **2010**, *12*, doi:10.1002/14651858. CD006425.
28. Masiero, J.V.; Tabroff, J.M.; Scannell, E. *The Accuracy of Recalled versus Measured Pre-Pregnancy Weight for the Calculation of Pre-pregnancy Body Mass Index*; University of Massachusetts Medical School: Worcester, MA, USA, 2014.
29. Hure, A.J.; Collins, C.E.; Giles, W.B.; Wright, I.M.R.; Smith, R. Protocol for the Women and their Children's Health (WATCH) study: A cohort of pregnancy and beyond. *J. Epidemiol.* **2012**, *22*, 267–275.
30. Institute of Medicine. *Weight Gain during Pregnancy: Reexamining the Guidelines*; National Academy of Sciences: Washington, DC, USA, 2009.
31. Calfas, K.J.; Marcus, B.H. Postpartum Weight Retention: A Mother's Weight to Bear? *Am. J. Prev. Med.* **2007**, *32*, 356–357.
32. Carter-Edwards, L.; Ostbye, T.; Bastian, L.; Yarnall, K.; Krause, K.; Simmons T-J.I. Barriers to adopting a healthy lifestyle: insight from postpartum women. *BMC Res. Notes* **2009**, *2*, 161.

33. Ostbye, T.; Krause, K.M.; Lovelady, C.A.; Morey, M.C.; Bastian, L.A.; Peterson, B.L.; Swamy, G.K.; Brouwer, R.J.; McBride, C.M. Active Mothers Postpartum: A Randomized Controlled Weight-Loss Intervention Trial. *Am. J. Prev. Med.* **2009**, *37*, 173–180.
34. O'Toole, M.L.; Sawicki, M.A.; Artal, R. Structured diet and physical activity prevent postpartum weight retention. *J. Womens Health (Larchmt.)* **2003**, *12*, 991–998.
35. Leermarkers, E.A.; Anglin, K.; Wing, R.R. Reducing postpartum weight retention through a correspondance intervention. *Int. J. Obes.* **1998**, *22*, 1103–1109.
36. Baker, J.L.; Michaelsen, K.F.; Rasmussen, K.M.; Sorensen, T.I.A. Maternal prepregnant body mass index, duration of breastfeeding, and timing of complementary food introduction are associated with infant weight gain. *Am. J. Clin. Nutr.* **2004**, *80*, 1579–1588.
37. Harder, T.; Bergman, R.; Kallinschnigg, G.; Plagemann, A. Duration of breastfeeding and risk of overweight: A meta-analysis. *Am. J. Epidemiol.* **2005**, *162*, 397–403.
38. Krause, K.; Lovelady, C.; Østbye, T. Predictors of Breastfeeding in Overweight and Obese Women: Data From Active Mothers Postpartum (AMP). *Matern. Child Health J.* **2011**, *15*, 367–375.
39. Li, R.; Jewell, S.; Grummer-Strawn, L. Maternal obesity and breastfeeding practices. *Am. J. Clin. Nutr.* **2003**, *77*, 931–936.
40. Amir, L.; Donath, S. A systematic review of maternal obesity and breastfeeding intention, initiation and duration. *BMC Pregnancy Childbirth* **2007**, *7*, 9.
41. Amorim Adegboye, A.; Linne, Y.; Lourenco, P. Diet or exercise, or both, for weight reduction in women after childbirth (Review). *Cochrane Collaboration* **2008**, *4*, 1–40.
42. Huang, T.; Yeh, C.; Tsai, Y. A diet and physical activity intervention for preventing weight retention among Taiwanese childbearing women: a randomised controlled trial. *Midwifery* **2011**, *27*, 257–264.
43. Kinnunen, T.; Pasanen, M.; Aittasalo, M.; Fogelholm, M.; Weiderpass, E.; Luoto, R. Reducing postpartum weight retention—A pilot trial in primary health care. *Nutr. J.* **2007**, *6*, 21.
44. Craigie, A.M.; MacLeod, M.; Barton, K.L.; Treweek, S.; anderson, A.S. Supporting postpartum weight loss in women living in deprived communities: Design implications for a randomised control trial. *Eur. J. Clin. Nutr.* **2011**, *65*, 952–958.
45. Martin, J.E.; Hure, A.J.; MacDonald-Wicks, L.; Smith, R.; Collins, C.E. Predictors of post-partum weight retention in a prospective longitudinal study. *Matern. Child Nutr.* **2014**, *10*, 496–509.
46. Gore, S.; Brown, D.; West, D. The role of postpartum weight retention in obesity among women: A review of the evidence. *Ann. Behav. Med.* **2003**, *26*, 149–159.
47. Rexrode, K.M.; Carey, V.J.; Hennekens, C.H.; Walters, E.E.; Colditz, G.A.; Stampfer, M.J.; Willett, W.C.; Manson, J.E. Abdominal Adiposity and Coronary Heart Disease in Women. *J. Am. Med. Assoc.* **1998**, *280*, 1843–1848.
48. Cameron, A.; Welborn, T.; Zimmet, P.; Dunstan, D.; Owen, N.; Salmon, J. Overweight and obesity in Australia: the 1999–2000 Australian Diabetes, Obesity and Lifestyle Study (AusDiab). *Med. J. Aust.* **2003**, *178*, 427–432.

12

The Two-Component Model for Calculating Total Body Fat from Body Density: An Evaluation in Healthy Women before, during and after Pregnancy

Elisabet Forsum [1,*], Pontus Henriksson [1] and Marie Löf [2]

1. Department of Clinical and Experimental Medicine, Linköping University, SE 581 85 Linköping, Sweden; E-Mail: pontus.henriksson@liu.se
2. Department of Biosciences and Nutrition, Karolinska Institute, NOVUM, SE 141 83 Huddinge, Sweden; E-Mail: marie.lof@ki.se

* Author to whom correspondence should be addressed; E-Mail: elisabet.forsum@liu.se

---

Abstract: A possibility to assess body composition during pregnancy is often important. Estimating body density (D_B) and use the two-component model (2CM) to calculate total body fat (TBF) represents an option. However, this approach has been insufficiently evaluated during pregnancy. We evaluated the 2CM, and estimated fat-free mass (FFM) density and variability in 17 healthy women before pregnancy, in gestational weeks 14 and 32, and 2 weeks *postpartum* based on D_B (underwater weighing), total body water (deuterium dilution) and body weight, assessed on these four occasions. TBF, calculated using the 2CM and published FFM density (TBF_{2CM}), was compared to reference estimates obtained using the three-component model (TBF_{3CM}). TBF_{2CM} minus TBF_{3CM} (mean ± 2SD) was −1.63 ± 5.67 ($p = 0.031$), −1.39 ± 7.75 ($p = 0.16$), −0.38 ± 4.44 ($p = 0.49$) and −1.39 ± 5.22 ($p = 0.043$) % before pregnancy, in gestational weeks 14 and 32 and 2 weeks *postpartum*, respectively. The effect of pregnancy on the variability of FFM density was larger in gestational week 14 than in gestational week 32. The 2CM, based on D_B and published FFM density, assessed body composition as accurately in gestational week 32 as in non-pregnant adults. Corresponding values in gestational week 14 were slightly less accurate than those obtained before pregnancy.

Keywords: before pregnancy; body composition; fat-free mass density; gestation; *postpartum*; total body fat

1. Introduction

Information regarding body composition during pregnancy is needed when estimating the requirements for dietary energy during gestation and when investigating relationships between maternal nutritional status and offspring development. Generally used body composition methods may not be appropriate during pregnancy when the body is undergoing dynamic changes to support fetal development. Based on extensive reviews of the literature Hytten [1] described how pregnancy changes the physiology of the human female including how the products of conception contribute to the composition of the pregnant body. Based on this work, van Raaij *et al.* [2] estimated average changes in fat-free mass (FFM) density and water content throughout the course of gestation. The Food and Agricultural Organization [3] and the Institute of Medicine [4] have stated that body composition methods based on these modifications [2] are satisfactory for use with pregnant women. Hopkinson *et al.* [5] evaluated these modifications in gestational week 36 and concluded that the FFM density suggested by van Raaij *et al.* [2] for women at this stage of pregnancy produce reliable mean estimates of body fat. However, except for this report [5], no validation studies have confirmed the statement quoted above [3,4].

Pregnancy is associated with retention of water, protein and mineral, *i.e.*, the components of FFM. This results in an increased water content of FFM while its concentrations of protein and mineral decrease slightly [2]. The combined effect of these changes is a decreased density of FFM [2]. This decrease is of interest when calculating total body fat (TBF) from body density (D_B) using the so-called two-component model (2CM) [6], a common procedure for assessing human body composition *in vivo*. In the past, D_B was assessed using underwater weighing whereas air-displacement plethysmography (ADP) [7] is now more common. Due to its convenience and capacity to assess D_B in subjects with varying body sizes [7,8], ADP is increasingly used and, as pointed out by Hu [9], represents an excellent alternative to underwater weighing in pregnant women. However, the use of ADP during pregnancy has been limited [10], possibly because the capacity of the 2CM to calculate TBF from D_B has been insufficiently studied during gestation. Thus studies of this capacity are needed.

As indicated above, average values for FFM hydration and FFM density are available throughout the course of pregnancy [2]. However, information regarding average FFM density is insufficient to conclude that the 2CM is satisfactory during pregnancy. It is also important to determine the variability of FFM density at each particular stage of pregnancy, since small differences in this value have a substantial impact on TBF when calculated from D_B using the 2CM [11]. Thus a high variability in FFM density is associated with a lower accuracy in estimates of TBF of individual women. In a previous study [12] conducted before, during and after pregnancy we found that the variability of FFM hydration depends on the stage of gestation. Thus the accuracy of the 2CM may well vary during the course of pregnancy. In the present paper we use data obtained in the previous study [12] to evaluate TBF results, calculated from D_B using the 2CM and based on published average FFM density values. For women in the prepregnant state we used an FFM density of 1.1 g/mL [6,13]. During pregnancy, we used the values published by van Raaij *et al.* [2] and the FFM density value published by Hopkinson *et al.* [5] was used *postpartum*. We have also calculated average FFM density and its variability.

2. Experimental Section

2.1. Subjects, Design, Body Composition Methodology and Calculations

The study was conducted on 17 healthy women before pregnancy, in gestational weeks 14 and 32, and 2 weeks *postpartum*. The ethics committee in Linköping approved the study on 19 November 1995 (95237). At the measurement before pregnancy women were 29 ± 4 years old with a body mass index (BMI) of 24.3 ± 5.3 kg/m^2. Three women (18%) were overweight (BMI = 25.0–29.9 kg/m^2) and 2 (12%) were obese (BMI ≥ 30.0 kg/m^2). This distribution of BMI values is similar to the corresponding distribution assessed for contemporary Swedish childbearing women [14]. All women delivered one healthy infant (birthweight 3770 ± 470 g) and none had generalized oedema. The subjects in this study, as well as the methods and procedures used were described previously [12]. In brief, D_B was assessed using underwater weighing where weight under water was recorded 7 times, each time with a simultaneous recording of lung volume (Volugraph 2000, Siemens-Elema, Stockholm, Sweden) [12]. Total body water (TBW) was assessed by means of deuterium dilution. After collection of background urine samples subjects received 0.05 g ^2H_2O per kg body weight *per os*. Five urine samples were collected during the following 15 days. ^{2}H-enrichments of dose and urine samples were analyzed by using an isotope ratio mass spectrometer (Deltaplus XL, Thermoquest, Bremen, Germany) as previously described [12]. ^{2}H-space was calculated using zero-time enrichment, obtained from the exponential isotope disappearance curve, providing the rate constant for ^{2}H elimination. ^{2}H-space was divided by 1.04 to obtain TBW [12]. D_B and TBW were used together with body weight to obtain reference estimates of TBF based on the three-component model (3CM) [13] where f represents the fraction of fat in the body:

$$f = (2.118/D_B) - (0.78 \times \text{TBW/body weight}) - 1.354 \quad (1)$$

TBF was also calculated from D_B based on the 2CM: [6,13]

$$1/D_B = f/0.9007 + (1 - f)/\text{FFM density} \quad (2)$$

FFM density was calculated using Equation (2) and f assessed by means of Equation (1).

2.2. Statistics

Values given are means and standard deviations (SD). Linear regression and Student's *t* test were used. The Bland and Altman [15] procedure was used to evaluate results. Thus the mean and 2SD of the difference between TBF (%), obtained using the 3CM and TBF (%) obtained using the 2CM, were calculated. This difference (y) was regressed on the average of the two estimates of TBF (%) (x). Calculation of the methodological component of the total variability in FFM density was based on propagation of error analysis [12,16]. In this calculation precision values were 1.05% [17] for TBW and 0.01 kg [18] for body weight. Precision for D_B was assessed on 4 occasions in one weight-stable, non-pregnant woman with a weight and volume of 56.6 kg and 53.9 L, respectively, and was 0.0016 g/mL corresponding to 0.371 L (0.7%) for body volume [12]. As described previously [12], the methodological error was based on measurement errors expressed in two different ways, *i.e.*, in % of an appropriate mean value or in kg and L [12]. Biological variability was calculated from total observed variability and the propagated methodological error [12]. Significance was accepted when $p < 0.05$. Statistical calculations were conducted using SPSS Statistics 21 (IBM, Armonk, NY, USA).

3. Results

3.1. Total Body Fat Calculated by Means of the 2CM versus the 3CM

Table 1 shows body weight (kg), TBW (kg), D_B (g/mL) and TBF (%), assessed by means of the 2CM and the 3CM, of the women before pregnancy, in gestational weeks 14 and 32, and 2 weeks *postpartum*. As shown in the table, the FFM density suggested for the particular stage of reproduction was used in the 2CM. The 2CM provides lower estimates of TBF (%) than those obtained by means of the 3CM and this difference was significant before pregnancy and 2 weeks *postpartum*.

Table 1. Body weight, total body water, body density and total body fat assessed by means of two- and three-component models in healthy women [12] before pregnancy, at gestational weeks 14 and 32 and 2 weeks *postpartum* [1].

	Before Pregnancy	**Gestational Week 14**	**Gestational Week 32**	**2 Weeks *Postpartum***
Body weight (kg)	66.6 ± 12.8	68.4 ± 13.2	77.3 ± 13.0	71.5 ± 12.8
Total body water (kg)	31.5 ± 4.0	32.5 ± 4.3	38.1 ± 4.4	33.6 ± 4.2
Body density (g/mL)	1.029 ± 0.019	1.027 ± 0.021	1.021 ± 0.018	1.020 ± 0.017
Total body fat (%)				
Two-component model	31.4 ± 9.0 [2]	31.8 ± 10.1 [3]	32.7 ± 8.8 [4]	33.8 ± 8.5 [5,6]
Three-component model [7]	33.0 ± 7.9	33.2 ± 7.7	33.1 ± 7.9	35.2 ± 6.8
p for difference [8]	0.031	0.16	0.49	0.043

[1] Mean ± SD, $n = 17$; [2] Calculated using Equation (2) and fat-free mass density 1.1 g/mL [6,13]; [3] Calculated using Equation (2) and fat-free mass density 1.099 g/mL [2]; [4] Calculated using Equation (2) and fat-free mass density 1.092 g/mL [2]; [5] Calculated using Equation (2) and fat-free mass density 1.094 g/mL [5]; [6] The corresponding result calculated using Equation (2) and fat-free mass density 1.1 g/mL [6,13] is 35.4% ± 8.3% total body fat, which does not differ significantly from the corresponding value, assessed by means of the three-component model; [7] Calculated using Equation (1); [8] Student's t test for paired observations.

Figure 1 shows TBF (%) of the women in the study, obtained by means of the 2CM (x) and the 3CM (y), and plotted around the line of identity. The regression equations were $y = 0.84x + 6.8$, $r = 0.95$, $p < 0.001$ (before pregnancy), $y = 0.72x + 10.3$, $r = 0.94$, $p < 0.001$ (gestational week 14), $y = 0.87x + 4.5$, $r = 0.97$, $p < 0.001$ (gestational week 32) and $y = 0.78x + 8.9$, $r = 0.96$, $p < 0.001$ (2 weeks *postpartum*). Figure 1 demonstrates that the 2CM and the 3CM agree fairly well on all measurement occasions.

Figure 1. Total body fat, assessed using a three-component model (y) *versus* total body fat, assessed using a two-component model (x) in 17 healthy women [12] plotted around the line of identity. The fat-free mass density used in the two-component model is also given. (**A**) Before pregnancy, FFM density = 1.1 g/mL [6,13]; (**B**) Gestational week 14, FFM density = 1.099 g/mL [2]; (**C**) Gestational week 32, FFM density = 1.092 g/mL [2]; (**D**) 2 weeks *postpartum*, FFM density = 1.094 g/mL [5]. FFM, fat-free mass; TBF_{3CM}, total body fat assessed using a three-component model; TBF_{2CM}, total body fat, assessed using a two-component model.

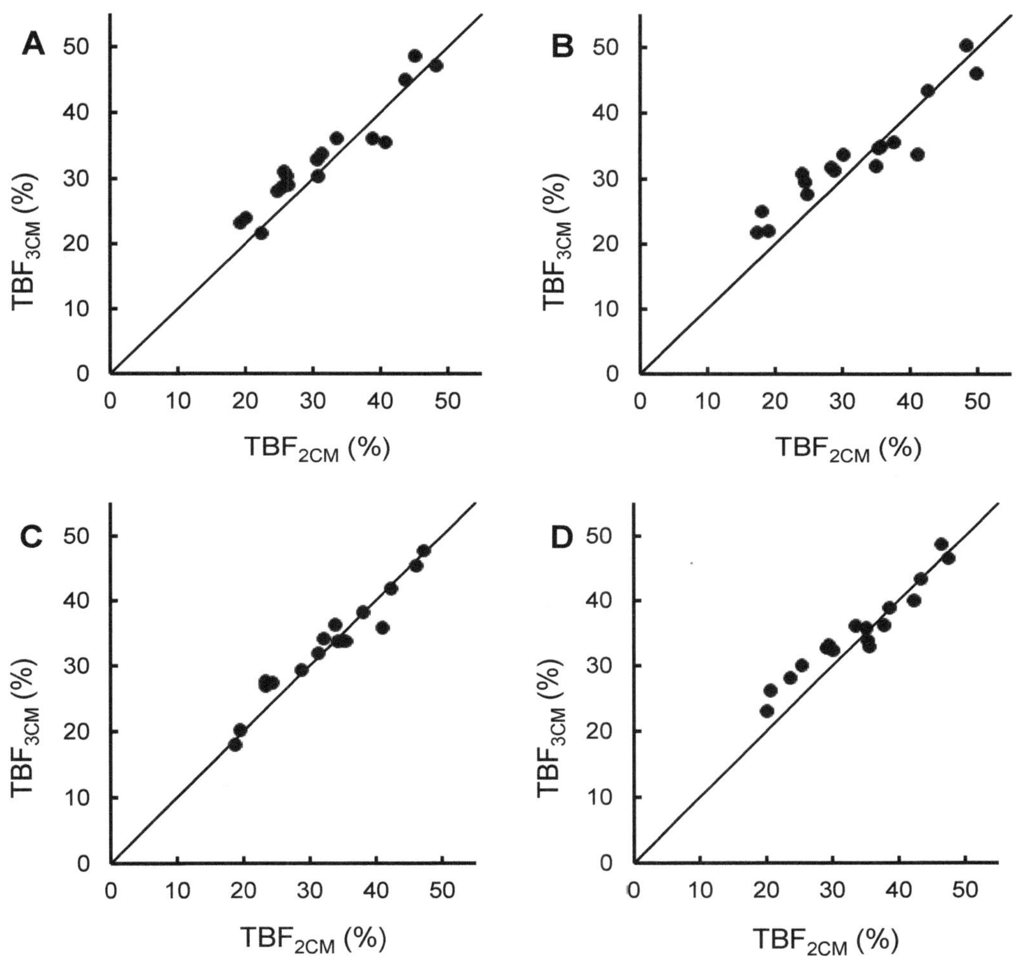

Figure 2 shows a Bland and Altman evaluation of our data. 2SD corresponds to 7.75% and 4.44% TBF at gestational weeks 14 and 32, respectively. The corresponding values before pregnancy and 2 weeks *postpartum* were 5.67% and 5.22% TBF, respectively. At gestational week 14 and 2 weeks *postpartum*, significant relationships were found between TBF (%), assessed by means of the 2CM minus TBF (%) assessed by means of the 3CM, on the one hand, and the average of these two estimates, on the other hand. The corresponding relationships before pregnancy and in gestational week 32 were not significant.

Figure 2. A Bland and Altman evaluation of a two-component model [1], based on body density, for assessing TBF (%) in women before pregnancy, at gestational weeks 14 and 32 and 2 weeks *postpartum* when compared to reference estimates of TBF (%) obtained by means of a three-component model [2]. The figure shows the average and 2SD of the difference between the two estimates and the correlation coefficient (r) and p-value for the relationship obtained when ($TBF_{2CM} - TBF_{3CM}$) (%) (y) is regressed on ($TBF_{2CM} + TBF_{3CM}$)/2 (%) (x). When r is significant ($p < 0.05$), the regression equation for this relationship is given. (**A**) Before pregnancy, ($TBF_{2CM} - TBF_{3CM}$) = −1.63%, 2SD = 5.67%, $r = 0.39$ ($p = 0.12$); (**B**) Gestational week 14, ($TBF_{2CM} - TBF_{3CM}$) = −1.39%, 2SD = 7.75%, $r = 0.61$ ($p = 0.009$), $y = 0.27x - 10.2$; (**C**) Gestational week 32, ($TBF_{2CM} - TBF_{3CM}$) = −0.38%, 2SD = 4.44%, $r = 0.40$ ($p = 0.12$); (**D**) 2 weeks *postpartum*: ($TBF_{2CM} - TBF_{3CM}$) = −1.39%, 2SD = 5.22%, $r = 0.63$ ($p = 0.006$), $y = 0.22x - 8.9$. Using Equation (2) and the fat-free mass density 1.1 g/mL [6,13]: ($TBF_{2CM} - TBF_{3CM}$) = −0.25%, 2SD = 5.93%, $r = 0.59$ ($p = 0.014$), $y = 0.19x - 6.6$. TBF, total body fat; TBF_{2CM}, total body fat assessed using the two-component model; TBF_{3CM}, total body fat assessed using the three-component model.

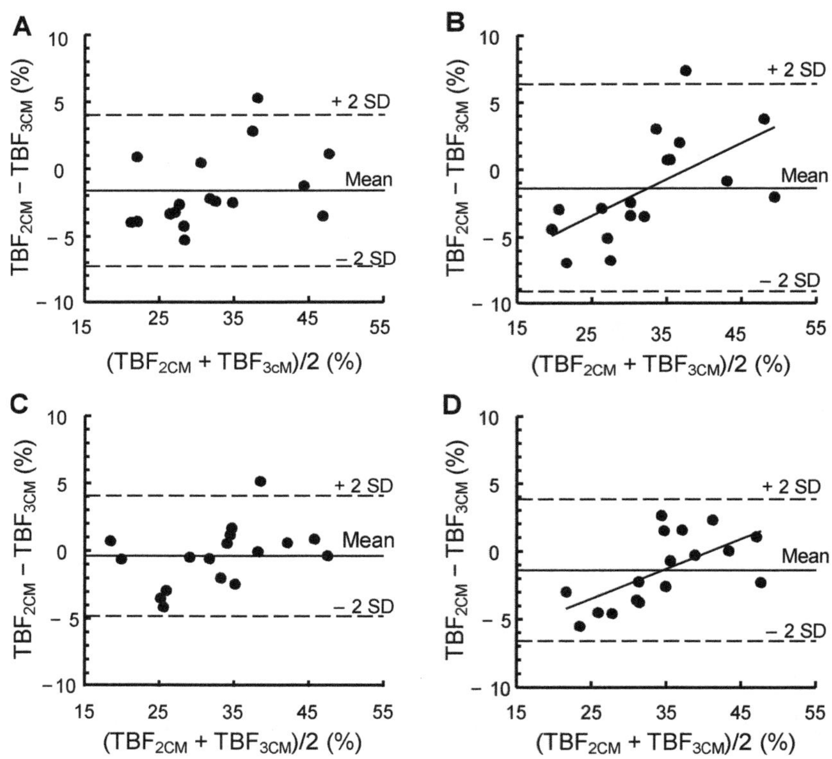

[1] The two-component model is based on Equation (2) and the fat-free mass density 1.1 g/mL (before pregnancy) [6,13], 1.099 g/mL (gestational week 14) [2], 1.092 g/mL (gestational week 32) [2] and 1.094 g/mL (2 weeks *postpartum*) [5]; [2] $n = 17$.

3.2. FFM Density and Its Variability

Table 2 shows estimated average FFM density and its variability before pregnancy, at gestational weeks 14 and 32, and 2 weeks *postpartum*. FFM density was 1.106, 1.104, 1.093 and 1.099 g/mL, before pregnancy, at gestational weeks 14 and 32, and 2 weeks postpartum, respectively. No significant differences between these values and the corresponding values published by van Raaij *et al.* [2] were observed at gestational weeks 14 or 32. Table 2 also shows the biological variability of FFM density, estimated on the same occasions and based on the two sets of methodological errors. These two sets are described in footnotes 3 and 4 of Table 2. Before pregnancy, biological variability was 0.007 and 0.009 g/mL when using the first and second sets of assumptions, respectively. The impact of pregnancy on the biological variability of FFM density was smaller in gestational week 32 than in gestational week 14, and this was the case for both sets of assumptions.

4. Discussion

The 2CM is considered to be capable of generating useful body composition results in healthy adult subjects in the general population if a valid figure for FFM density is used [7]. The data in Figure 1 show that there is considerable agreement between the 2CM and the 3CM regarding their capacity to assess TBF (%) before, during and after pregnancy, although the results of the two models may differ for individual women. Thus our data support previous statements [3,4] that the 2CM, based on appropriate FFM density values, can provide useful body composition results also during pregnancy. However, as discussed below, the accuracy of such results may vary during pregnancy.

In this paper, we use a 3CM to obtain reference estimates of TBF before, during and after pregnancy, although a four-component model (4CM) is generally regarded as the best option when evaluating simpler body composition methods [5,6]. A commonly used 4CM calculates TBF from body weight, TBW, D_B and body mineral and has the advantage over a 3CM of avoiding assumptions about the mineral content of the body [6]. However, the theoretical errors in estimates of TBF (%), associated with variations in FFM composition, are not very different between the 4CM and the 3CM [11]. This can be reconciled with results in women showing that the water content of FFM was significantly related to the difference in TBF (%) assessed by means of a 2CM *versus* a 4CM, while the corresponding relationship for the mineral content of FFM was weaker and not significant [19]. Thus a 3CM, based on TBW, D_B and body weight can provide useful reference estimates of body composition in healthy women.

Application of a 4CM in pregnant women is not regarded as appropriate since an assessment of body mineral requires the use of dual-energy X-ray absorptiometry, a technique that is unacceptable for such subjects due to radiation exposure. The body mineral content increases during gestation due to the contribution of the fetus. In gestational week 32, the fetus increases the contents of osseous and non-osseous minerals in the pregnant body, by about 1% each [6,20,21]. Such changes have only a minor impact on TBF (%), calculated by means of the 3CM, since Elia estimated that increases in the body mineral content as high as 20%–25% affect such estimates by less than one unit TBF (%) [11]. Furthermore, for women in gestational week 36, Hopkinson *et al.* [5] compared the 3CM to the 4CM and found the results to be in close agreement. In this comparison, the body mineral content required by the 4CM was measured 2 weeks postpartum and the authors [5] reckoned that the magnitude of changes in this variable between week 36 of gestation and 2 weeks postpartum was too small to have any appreciable effect on the results. Based on this evidence, we conclude that the 3CM provides useful reference estimates of body composition also in pregnant women.

Table 2. Average and total variability of FFM density in women before, during and after pregnancy. The contributions to total variability of methodological error and biological variability using two sets of assumptions are also shown.

	Average FFM density [1]	Total variability of FFM density	Propagation of error analysis 1 [2]				Propagation of error analysis 2 [3]			
			Methodological error		Biological variability		Methodological error		Biological variability	
	g/mL	SD	SD	% [4]	SD	% [4]	SD	% [4]	SD	% [4]
Before pregnancy	1.106	0.010	0.007	49	0.007	51	0.006	33	0.009	67
Gestational week 14	1.104	0.014	0.007	28	0.012	72	0.006	18	0.013	82
Gestational week 32	1.093	0.008	0.007	96	0.002	4	0.005	47	0.006	53
2 weeks *postpartum*	1.099	0.009	0.007	70	0.005	30	0.006	41	0.007	59

[1] Calculated using Equation (2) and a fraction of fat in the body (f) calculated using Equation (1). [2] Errors for total body water and body volume are expressed in % of an appropriate mean value. The calculations are based on the following precision values [12]: body weight 0.01 kg; total body water 1.05% corresponding to 0.331 kg in women before pregnancy, 0.341 kg in gestational week 14, 0.400 kg in gestational week 32, and 0.352 kg 2 weeks *postpartum*; body volume 0.7% corresponding to 0.455 L in women before pregnancy, 0.467 L in gestational week 14, 0.531 L in gestational week 32, and 0.492 L 2 weeks *postpartum*. [3] Errors for total body water and body volume are expressed in kg and L, respectively. The calculations are based on the following precision values [12]: 0.01 kg for body weight; 0.331 L for total body water and 0.371 L for body volume. [4] Percentage of total variability. $n = 17$; FFM, fat-free mass.

Our estimated FFM density of women prior to pregnancy is in agreement with the figure, 1.1 g/mL, which is the value generally regarded as an appropriate average for the general population [7]. However, it may be relevant to note that the 2CM underestimated TBF of our women before pregnancy when this FFM density was used and Fields *et al.* [19] reported a similar underestimate by the 2CM in their study on healthy women also using this FFM density. This suggests that women may have a slightly higher FFM density than 1.100 g/mL, which is the value for the reference body [6]. However, confirming this suggestion is difficult, since available techniques for assessing FFM density *in vivo* may not be accurate enough. Small variations in this variable between different populations of women may also be present.

We estimated average FFM density 2 weeks *postpartum* at 1.099 g/mL, which is slightly higher than 1.094 g/mL as reported by Hopkinson *et al.* [5]. A consequence of using this lower value is that the 2CM underestimates TBF (%) *postpartum*. Furthermore, as shown by the Bland and Altman evaluation, the magnitude of the difference between the two models is associated with TBF (%) of the women. Using an FFM density of 1.1 g/mL 2 weeks *postpartum* produces more satisfactory average estimates of TBF (%), but, as indicated in Figure 2, the difference between the models regarding TBF (%) is still associated with TBF (%) of the women.

Our results regarding the biological variability of FFM density were obtained using two sets of methodological errors. As previously discussed [12] we found both sets to be reasonable and justified and we were not able to determine whether one was superior to the other. Prior to pregnancy, we found the biological variability of FFM density to be 0.007 and 0.009 g/mL, respectively, using the two sets of methodological errors. This is comparable to the published values of 0.0084 g/mL [6] and 0.0073 g/mL [22]. This rather large biological variability of FFM density has a negative impact on the accuracy of the 2CM in non-pregnant women. The finding that the biological variability in FFM density is lower at gestational week 32 but higher at gestational week 14 when compared to the value before pregnancy is a corollary of our previous findings [12] regarding the biological variability of FFM hydration at gestational weeks 14 and 32 *versus* before pregnancy. These observations are consistent with data in Figure 2 showing that the 2SD value at gestational week 32 is only 4.44% TBF as opposed to 5.67% and 7.75% TBF before pregnancy and at gestational week 14, respectively. These observations indicate that the accuracy of the 2CM, when based on published FFM density values [2], is better at gestational week 32 than at gestational week 14.

Published values for FFM density in pregnant women [2] are based on data by Hytten [1], collected in British women several decades ago. Nevertheless, the differences between these values [2] and our estimates of FFM density during pregnancy were small and not significant. This supports the conclusion that the FFM density values by van Raaij *et al.* [2] produce valid average estimates of TBF of women when used in a 2CM at gestational weeks 14 and 32. Furthermore, we suggest that these observations can be reconciled with the statement that the influence of pregnancy on FFM density and composition is predictable and part of the regulatory processes needed to meet the physiological changes inherent in this physiological state.

A limitation of this study is that the number of women is small, while a strength is that the same women were studied before, during and after pregnancy. This made it possible to demonstrate how pregnancy influences FFM density and its variability which is important information for assessing body composition during pregnancy. It is also relevant to emphasize that our results were obtained in healthy women being pregnant with one fetus and may not be valid for women not meeting these criteria. Furthermore, our results were obtained in women with a BMI distribution typical for Swedish women [14] and may not be appropriate in populations with a different pattern of body weight.

5. Conclusions

This study confirmed that FFM density values at gestational weeks 14 and 32 are in close agreement with those published by van Raaij *et al.* [2]. We found the corresponding value 2 weeks *postpartum* to be close to 1.1 g/mL which is the figure commonly regarded as an appropriate average for healthy non-pregnant adults. Furthermore, our results showed that a 2CM, based on estimates of D_B and the FFM density values reported by van Raaij *et al.* [2], is able to generate body composition results in gestational week 32 that are at least as accurate as those obtained in the pre-pregnant state with the same methodology when using a FFM density of 1.1 g/mL. Corresponding values obtained in gestational week 14 were found to be slightly less accurate than those obtained before pregnancy.

Acknowledgments

Supported by grants from the Swedish Research Council (project No. 15402), the Swedish Research Council Formas (222-2006-614, 222-2008-1332), the Medical Faculty, Linköping University, and the County Council of Östergötland.

Author Contributions

All authors contributed to data analysis and manuscript preparation. Elisabet Forsum had the prime responsibility for the final content. All authors read and approved the final manuscript.

References

1. Hytten, F.E. Nutrition. In *Clinical Physiology in Obstetrics*; Hytten, F.E., Chamberlain, G., Eds.; Blackwell Scientific Publications: Oxford, UK, 1980; pp. 163–192.
2. Van Raaij, J.M.A.; Peek, M.E.M.; Vermaat-Miedema, S.H.; Schonk, C.M.; Hautvast, J.G.A.J. New equations for estimating body fat mass in pregnancy from body density or total body water. *Am. J. Clin. Nutr.* **1988**, *48*, 24–29.
3. Food and Agricultural Organization of the United Nations. Energy requirements of pregnancy. In *Human Energy Requirements*; Report of a Joint FAO/WHO/UNU Expert Consultation, Food and Nutrition Technical Report Series 1; Food and Agricultural Organization of the United Nations: Rome, Italy, 2004; pp. 53–62.
4. Institute of Medicine and National Research Council. *Weight Gain during Pregnancy—Reexaming the Guidelines*; Rasmussen, K.M., Yaktine, A.L., Eds.; The National Academies Press: Washington, DC, USA, 2009; p. 80.
5. Hopkinson, J.M.; Butte, N.F.; Ellis, K.J.; Wong, W.W.; Puyan, M.R.; O'Brian Smith, E. Body fat estimation in late pregnancy and early postpartum: Comparison of two-, three-, and four-component models. *Am. J. Clin. Nutr.* **1997**, *65*, 432–438.

6. Going, S.B. Densitometry. *Human Body Composition*; Roche, A.F., Heymsfield, S.B., Lohman, T.G., Eds.; Human Kinetics: Champaign, IL, USA, 1996; pp. 3–23.
7. Fields, D.A.; Goran, M.I.; McCrory, M.A. Body-composition assessment via air-displacement plethysmography in adults and children: A review. *Am. J. Clin. Nutr.* **2002**, *75*, 453–467.
8. Ginde, S.R.; Geliebter, A.; Rubiano, F.; Silva, A.M.; Wang, J.; Heshka, S.; Heymsfield, S.B. Air displacement plethysmography: Validation in overweight and obese subjects. *Obes. Res.* **2005**, *13*, 1232–1237.
9. Hu, F.B. Measurements of adiposity and body composition. In *Obesity Epidemiology*; Oxford University Press: New York, NY, USA, 2008; pp. 53–83.
10. Widen, E.M.; Gallagher, D. Body composition changes in pregnancy: Measurements, predictors and outcomes. *Eur. J. Clin. Nutr.* **2014**, *68*, 643–652.
11. Elia, M. Body composition analysis: An evaluation of 2 component models, multicomponent models and bedside techniques. *Clin. Nutr.* **1992**, *11*, 114–127.
12. Lof, M.; Forsum, E. Hydration of fat-free mass in healthy women with special reference to the effect of pregnancy. *Am. J. Clin. Nutr.* **2004**, *80*, 960–965.
13. Siri, W.E. Body composition from fluid spaces and density: Analysis of methods. In *Techniques for Measuring Body Composition*; Brozek, J., Henschel, A., Eds.; National Academy of Sciences/National Research Council: Washington, DC, USA, 1961; pp. 223–244.
14. Swedish Maternity Care Registry—2012 Annual Report. Available online: http://www.ucr.uu.se/mhv/index.php/arsrapporter (accessed on 13 September 2014).
15. Bland, J.M.; Altman, D.G. Statistical methods for assessing agreement between two methods of clinical measurement. *Lancet* **1986**, *1*, 307–310.
16. Kendall, M.; Stewart, A. *The Advanced Theory of Statistics*, 4th ed.; Griffin & Co Ltd.: London, UK, 1977; pp. 246–247.
17. Wells, J.; Fuller, N.; Dewit, O.; Fewtrell, M.; Elia, M.; Cole, T. Four-component model of body composition in children: Density and hydration of fat-free mass and comparison with simpler models. *Am. J. Clin. Nutr.* **1999**, *69*, 904–912.
18. Murgatroyd, P.; Coward, W. An improved method for estimating changes in whole-body fat and protein mass in man. *Br. J. Nutr.* **1989**, *62*, 311–314.
19. Fields, D.A.; Wilson, G.D.; Gladden, L.B.; Hunter, G.R.; Pascoe, D.D.; Goran, M.I. Comparison of the BOD POD with the four-compartment model in adult females. *Med. Sci. Sports. Exerc.* **2001**, *33*, 1605–1610.
20. Widdowson, E.M. Changes in body proportions and composition during growth. In *Scientific Foundations of Pediatrics*, 2nd ed.; Davis, J.A., Dobbing, J., Eds.; Heinemann Medical Books Ltd.: London, UK, 1981; pp. 330–342.
21. Fomon, S.J.; Haschke, F.; Ziegler, E.E.; Nelson, S.E. Body composition of reference children from birth to age 10 years. *Am. J. Clin. Nutr.* **1982**, *35*, 1169–1175.
22. Fuller, N.J.; Jebb, S.A.; Laskey, M.A.; Coward, W.A.; Elia, M. Four-component model for the assessment of body composition in humans: Comparison with alternative methods, and evaluation of the density and hydration of fat-free mass. *Clin. Sci.* **1992**, *82*, 687–693.

Permissions

All chapters in this book were first published by MDPI; hereby published with permission under the Creative Commons Attribution License or equivalent. Every chapter published in this book has been scrutinized by our experts. Their significance has been extensively debated. The topics covered herein carry significant findings which will fuel the growth of the discipline. They may even be implemented as practical applications or may be referred to as a beginning point for another development.

The contributors of this book come from diverse backgrounds, making this book a truly international effort. This book will bring forth new frontiers with its revolutionizing research information and detailed analysis of the nascent developments around the world.

We would like to thank all the contributing authors for lending their expertise to make the book truly unique. They have played a crucial role in the development of this book. Without their invaluable contributions this book wouldn't have been possible. They have made vital efforts to compile up to date information on the varied aspects of this subject to make this book a valuable addition to the collection of many professionals and students.

This book was conceptualized with the vision of imparting up-to-date information and advanced data in this field. To ensure the same, a matchless editorial board was set up. Every individual on the board went through rigorous rounds of assessment to prove their worth. After which they invested a large part of their time researching and compiling the most relevant data for our readers.

The editorial board has been involved in producing this book since its inception. They have spent rigorous hours researching and exploring the diverse topics which have resulted in the successful publishing of this book. They have passed on their knowledge of decades through this book. To expedite this challenging task, the publisher supported the team at every step. A small team of assistant editors was also appointed to further simplify the editing procedure and attain best results for the readers.

Apart from the editorial board, the designing team has also invested a significant amount of their time in understanding the subject and creating the most relevant covers. They scrutinized every image to scout for the most suitable representation of the subject and create an appropriate cover for the book.

The publishing team has been an ardent support to the editorial, designing and production team. Their endless efforts to recruit the best for this project, has resulted in the accomplishment of this book. They are a veteran in the field of academics and their pool of knowledge is as vast as their experience in printing. Their expertise and guidance has proved useful at every step. Their uncompromising quality standards have made this book an exceptional effort. Their encouragement from time to time has been an inspiration for everyone.

The publisher and the editorial board hope that this book will prove to be a valuable piece of knowledge for researchers, students, practitioners and scholars across the globe.

List of Contributors

Wonsuk Yoo
Department of Preventive Medicine, University of Tennessee Health Science Center, 66 N. Pauline, Memphis, TN 38163, USA

Frances A. Tylavsky
Department of Preventive Medicine, University of Tennessee Health Science Center, 600 Jefferson St. Room 337 Memphis, TN 38105, USA
Department of Preventive Medicine, University of Tennessee Health Science Center, 66 N. Pauline, Memphis, TN 38163, USA

Eszter Völgyi
Department of Pediatrics (primary), Department of Preventive Medicine, University of Tennessee Health Science Center, Le Bonheur Children's Hospital, Research Building, 50 North Dunlap Street, Room 477R, Memphis, TN 38103, USA
Department of Preventive Medicine, University of Tennessee Health Science Center, 66 N. Pauline, Memphis, TN 38163, USA

Kecia N. Carroll
Department of Pediatrics, Vanderbilt University Medical Center, 2200 Children's Way, Nashville, TN 37232, USA
Division of General Pediatrics, Department of Pediatrics, Vanderbilt University School of Medicine, 313 Oxford House, Nashville, TN 37232-4313, USA

Marion E. Hare
Department of Preventive Medicine, University of Tennessee Health Science Center, 66 N. Pauline, Memphis, TN 38163, USA
Department of Pediatrics, University of Tennessee Health Science Center, 50 N. Dunlap, Memphis, TN 38103, USA

Karen Ringwald-Smith
St. Jude Children's Research Hospital, 262 Danny Thomas Place, Memphis, TN 38105, USA

Chandrika Piyathilake
Department of Nutrition Sciences, University of Alabama at Birmingham, 326 Webb Nutrition Sciences Building, 1675 University Blvd., AL 35294, USA

Michelle Blumfield and Clare Collins
School of Health Sciences, University of Newcastle, Callaghan, New South Wales 2308, Australia
Mothers and Babies Research Centre, Hunter Medical Research Institute, John Hunter Hospital, Level 3, Endocrinology, Locked Bag 1, Hunter Region Mail Centre, New South Wales 2310, Australia

Alexis Hure
School of Medicine and Public Health, Faculty of Health, University of Newcastle, Callaghan, New South Wales 2308, Australia

Roger Smith
School of Medicine and Public Health, Faculty of Health, University of Newcastle, Callaghan, New South Wales 2308, Australia
Mothers and Babies Research Centre, Hunter Medical Research Institute, John Hunter Hospital, Level 3, Endocrinology, Locked Bag 1, Hunter Region Mail Centre, Newcastle 2310, New South Wales, Australia

Stephen Simpson
School of Biological Sciences, University of Sydney, Sydney, New South Wales 2006, Australia

David Raubenheimer
Institute of Natural Sciences, Massey University, Albany 0632, New Zealand
Charles Perkins Centre, School of Biological Sciences, University of Sydney, Sydney, New South Wales 2006, Australia

Kristyn Dunlop
Department of Physiology and Pharmacology, Western University, London, ON N6A-5C1, Canada

Megan Cedrone and James F. Staples
Department of Biology, Western University, London, ON N6A 5B7, Canada

Timothy R.H. Regnault
Department of Physiology and Pharmacology, Western University, London, ON N6A-5C1, Canada
Department of Obstetrics and Gynecology, Western University, London, ON N6H-5W9, Canada
Lawson Health Research Institute, London, ON N6C-2R5, Canada
Children's Health Research Institute, London, ON N6C-2V5, Canada

Kimberly A. Vonnahme and Joel S. Caton
Department of Animal Sciences, North Dakota State University, Fargo, ND 58102, USA

Caleb O. Lemley
Department of Animal and Dairy Sciences, Mississippi State University, Mississippi State, MS 39762, USA

Allison M. Meyer
Division of Animal Sciences, University of Missouri, Columbus, MO 65210, USA

Roshan T. Ramlal, Charles van der Horst, Margaret Bentley and Linda Adair
University of North Carolina, Chapel Hill, NC 27599, USA

Martin Tembo, Alice Soko and Maggie Chigwenembe
UNC Project Malawi, Tidziwe Center, Mzimba Road, Lilongwe, Malawi

Caroline C. King, Sascha Ellington and Denise J. Jamieson
U.S. Centers for Disease Control and Prevention, 4770 Buford Highway, Atlanta, GA 30341, USA

Charles Chasel,
UNC Project Malawi, Tidziwe Center, Mzimba Road, Lilongwe, Malawi
Division of Epidemiology and Biostatistics, Faculty of Health Sciences, University of Witwatersrand, Johannesburg, 2193, South Africa

Michelle L. Blumfield and Clare E. Collins
School of Health Sciences, Faculty of Health and Medicine, University of Newcastle, Callaghan, New South Wales 2308, Australia
Priority Research Centre in Physical Activity and Nutrition, Faculty of Health and Medicine, University of Newcastle, Callaghan, New South Wales 2308, Australia

Caryl Nowson
School of Exercise and Nutrition Science, Deakin University, Geelong, Victoria 3216, Australia

Alexis J. Hure
School of Medicine and Public Health, Faculty of Health and Medicine, University of Newcastle, Callaghan, New South Wales 2308, Australia

Stephen J. Simpson
Charles Perkins Centre, School of Biological Sciences, University of Sydney, Sydney, New South Wales 2006, Australia

Song Zhang, Paige L. Barker, Kimberley J. Botting, Isabella C. McMillen, Christine M. McMillan and Janna L. Morrison
Early Origins of Adult Health Research Group, Sansom Institute for Health Research, University of South Australia, Adelaide, SA 5001, Australia

Claire T. Roberts
The Robinson Research Institute, University of Adelaide, Adelaide, SA 5005, Australia

Vladislava Zohdi and M. Jane Black
Department of Anatomy and Developmental Biology, Monash University, Melbourne, VIC 3800, Australia

Kyungjoon Lim
Neuropharmacology Laboratory, Baker IDI Heart and Diabetes Institute, St Kilda Rd Central, Melbourne 8008, Australia

James T. Pearson
Department of Physiology, Monash University, Melbourne, VIC 3800, Australia
Monash Biomedical Imaging, Monash University, Melbourne, VIC 3800, Australia

Ryan James Wood-Bradley and Sanna Barrand
School of Medicine, Deakin University, Waurn Ponds, Victoria 3216, Australia

Anais Giot
Insitut Politechnique LaSalle Beauvais, 60026 Beauvais Cedex, Picardie, France

James Andrew Armitage
School of Medicine, Deakin University, Waurn Ponds, Victoria 3216, Australia
Department of Anatomy and Developmental Biology, Monash University, Clayton, Victoria 3800, Australia

Uriyoán Colón-Ramos
Department of Global Health, Milken Institute School of Public Health, George Washington University, 950 New Hampshire Avenue, Washington, DC 20037, USA

Susan B. Racette
Program in Physical Therapy, Department of Medicine, and Institute for Public Health, Washington University School of Medicine, 4444 Forest Park Avenue, St. Louis, MO 63108, USA

Jody Ganiban
Clinical and Developmental Psychology, Department of Psychology, Columbian College of Arts and Sciences, George Washington University, Room 304 Building GG 2125 St. NW, Washington, DC 20052, USA

Thuy G. Nguyen
Department of Preventive Medicine, University of Tennessee Health Science Center, 600 Jefferson St. Room 337 Memphis, TN 38105, USA

Mehmet Kocak
Division of Biostatistics and Epidemiology, Department of Preventive Medicine, College of Medicine, University of Tennessee Health Science Center, 66 N. Pauline Street, Suite-633, Office 619, Memphis, TN 38105, USA

Julia Martin
School of Health Sciences, Faculty of Health and Medicine, University of Newcastle, Callaghan, Newcastle 2308, New South Wales, Australia

Lesley MacDonald-Wicks
School of Health Sciences, Faculty of Health and Medicine, University of Newcastle, Callaghan, New South Wales 2308, Australia
Priority Research Centre in Physical Activity and Nutrition, Faculty of Health and Medicine, University of Newcastle, Callaghan, New South Wales 2308, Australia

Clare E Collins
School of Health Sciences, Faculty of Health and Medicine, University of Newcastle, Callaghan, Newcastle 2308, New South Wales, Australia
Priority Research Centre in Physical Activity and Nutrition, Faculty of Health and Medicine, University of Newcastle, Callaghan, Newcastle 2308, New South Wales, Australia

Elisabet Forsum and Pontus Henriksson
Department of Clinical and Experimental Medicine, Linköping University, SE 581 85 Linköping, Sweden

Marie Löf
Department of Biosciences and Nutrition, Karolinska Institute, NOVUM, SE 141 83 Huddinge, Sweden

Index

Printed in the USA
CPSIA information can be obtained
at www.ICGtesting.com
LVHW082259151223
766290LV00007B/210

9 781639 277636